Endocrine and Metabolic Disorders

SOURCEBOOK

Third Edition

Health Reference Series

Third Edition

Endocrine and Metabolic Disorders

SOURCEBOOK

Basic Consumer Health Information about Hormonal and Metabolic Disorders That Affect the Body's Growth, Development, and Functioning, Including Disorders of the Pancreas, Ovaries and Testes, and Pituitary, Thyroid, Parathyroid, and Adrenal Glands, with Facts about Growth Disorders, Addison Disease, Cushing Syndrome, Conn Syndrome, Diabetic Disorders, Multiple Endocrine Neoplasia, Inborn Error of Metabolism, and More

Along with Information about Endocrine Functioning, Diagnostic and Screening Tests, a Glossary of Related Terms, and Directories of Additional Resources

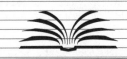

OMNIGRAPHICS

615 Griswold, Ste. 901, Detroit, MI 48226

Bibliographic Note
Because this page cannot legibly accommodate all the copyright notices, the Bibliographic
Note portion of the Preface constitutes an extension of the copyright notice.

* * *

Health Reference Series
Keith Jones, *Managing Editor*
***

OMNIGRAPHICS
A PART OF RELEVANT INFORMATION
***

Copyright © 2017 Omnigraphics
ISBN 978-0-7808-1543-8
E-ISBN 978-0-7808-1544-5

Library of Congress Cataloging-in-Publication Data

Names: Omnigraphics, Inc.

Title: Endocrine and metabolic disorders sourcebook: basic consumer health
information about hormonal and metabolic disorders that affect the body's growth,
development, and functioning, including disorders of the pancreas, ovaries and
testes, and pituitary, thyroid, parathyroid, and adrenal glands, with facts about
growth disorders, addison disease, cushing syndrome, conn syndrome, diabetic
disorders, multiple endocrine neoplasia, inborn errors of metabolism, and more
along with information about endocrine functioning, diagnostic and screening
tests, a glossary of related terms, and directories of additional resources.

Description: Third edition. | Detroit, MI: Omnigraphics, [2017] | Includes
bibliographical references and index.

Identifiers: LCCN 2016047068 (print) | LCCN 2016047751 (ebook) |
ISBN 9780780815438 (hardcover: alk. paper) | ISBN 9780780815445 (ebook)
| ISBN 9780780815445 (eBook)

Subjects: LCSH: Endocrine glands--Diseases--Popular works. | Metabolism--
Disorders--Popular works.

Classification: LCC RC648 .E418 2017 (print) | LCC RC648 (ebook) | DDC
616.4/8--dc23

LC record available at https://lccn.loc.gov/2016047068

Table of Contents

Part V: Pancreatic and Diabetic Disorders

Part VI: Disorders of the Ovaries and Testes

Part VII: Other Disorders of Endocrine and Metabolic Functioning

Part VIII: Additional Help and Information

Preface

About This Book

The endocrine system includes the pituitary, adrenal, and thyroid glands, the pancreas, and the ovaries and testes. These glands secrete hormones that regulate metabolism, the process that supplies the body's cells with energy. Abnormal levels of hormones, whether too high or too low, disrupt normal functioning and compromise health. Sometimes the symptoms of dysfunction appear so gradually they are hardly noticed. Hypothyroidism, for example, can remain undetected for years. Diabetes, the most common endocrine disorder in the United States, afflicts more than 29 million Americans, yet one-third are unaware they have it.

Endocrine and Metabolic Disorders Sourcebook, Third Edition, provides updated information about the endocrine system and its role in the regulation of human growth, organ function, and metabolic control. Readers will learn about growth disorders, hypothyroidism, diabetic disorders, Addison disease, Cushing syndrome, pheochromocytoma, multiple endocrine neoplasia type 1, inborn errors of metabolism, and other disorders, including facts about symptoms, diagnosis, and treatment. A glossary and directories of resources provide additional help and information.

How to Use This Book

This book is divided into parts and chapters. Parts focus on broad areas of interest. Chapters are devoted to single topics within a part.

Part I: Endocrine Functioning and Metabolism describes the endocrine system, the various endocrine glands and their hormones, and the processes of metabolism and energy balance. Chemicals that disrupt the endocrine process are discussed. Individual chapters explain prenatal tests, newborn screening, genetic counseling and genetic testing.

Part II: The Pituitary Gland and Growth Disorders discusses growth disorders and explains the growth hormone evaluation process. It also describes pituitary tumors, prolactinomas, and other diseases related to the pituitary gland, including acromegaly, and diabetes insipidus.

Part III: Thyroid and Parathyroid Gland Disorders offers facts about proper thyroid functioning and common dysfunctions, including Hashimoto thyroiditis, hypothyroidism, hyperthyroidism, and Graves disease. It also describes disorders of the parathyroid glands and discusses related cancers.

Part IV: Adrenal Gland Disorders provides facts about diseases of adrenal insufficiency, including Addison disease, Conn syndrome, Cushing syndrome, and pheochromocytoma, along with information about adrenal gland cancer and congenital adrenal conditions. The management of adrenal insufficiency and the use of laparoscopic techniques for adrenal gland removal are also described.

Part V: Pancreatic and Diabetic Disorders provides information about pancreas function tests and the management of pancreatitis, insulin resistance, diabetes mellitus, and hypoglycemia. Facts about pancreatic and islet cell cancer and Zollinger-Ellison syndrome are also included.

Part VI: Disorders of the Ovaries and Testes describes disorders that result when sex gland hormone production is not balanced. These include hypogonadism, gynecomastia, menstrual problems, polycystic ovarian syndrome, premature ovarian failure, precocious puberty and turner syndrome.

Part VII: Other Disorders of Endocrine and Metabolic Functioning presents information about inherited enzyme deficiencies and other syndromes and diseases that result from, or impact, hormonal and metabolic processes.

Part VIII: Additional Help and Information includes a glossary of related terms, a guide to resources for children with special needs, and a directory of organizations able to provide more information about endocrine and metabolic disorders.

Bibliographic Note

This volume contains documents and excerpts from publications issued by the following U.S. government agencies: Centers for Disease Control and Prevention (CDC); *Eunice Kennedy Shriver* National Institute of Child Health and Human Development (NICHD); Genetic and Rare Diseases Information Center (GARD); Genetics Home Reference (GHR); National Cancer Institute (NCI); National Center for Biotechnology Information (NCBI); National Heart Lung and Blood Institute (NHLBI); National Human Genome Research Institute (NHGRI); National Institute of Diabetes and Digestive and Kidney Diseases (NIDDK); National Institute of Neurological Disorders and Stroke (NINDS); National Institute on Aging (NIA); National Institutes of Health (NIH); Office on Women's Health (OWH); and U.S. Environmental Protection Agency (EPA).

In addition, this volume contains copyrighted documents from the following organization: The Nemours Foundation

It may also contain original material produced by Omnigraphics and reviewed by medical consultants.

About the Health Reference Series

The *Health Reference Series* is designed to provide basic medical information for patients, families, caregivers, and the general public. Each volume takes a particular topic and provides comprehensive coverage. This is especially important for people who may be dealing with a newly diagnosed disease or a chronic disorder in themselves or in a family member. People looking for preventive guidance, information about disease warning signs, medical statistics, and risk factors for health problems will also find answers to their questions in the *Health Reference Series*. The *Series*, however, is not intended to serve as a tool for diagnosing illness, in prescribing treatments, or as a substitute for the physician/patient relationship. All people concerned about medical symptoms or the possibility of disease are encouraged to seek professional care from an appropriate healthcare provider.

A Note about Spelling and Style

Health Reference Series editors use *Stedman's Medical Dictionary* as an authority for questions related to the spelling of medical terms and the *Chicago Manual of Style* for questions related to grammatical structures, punctuation, and other editorial concerns. Consistent adherence is not always possible, however, because the individual volumes within the *Series* include many documents from a wide variety of different producers, and the editor's primary goal is to present material from each source as accurately as is possible. This sometimes means that information in different chapters or sections may follow other guidelines and alternate spelling authorities.

Medical Review

Omnigraphics contracts with a team of qualified, senior medical professionals who serve as medical consultants for the *Health Reference Series*. As necessary, medical consultants review reprinted and originally written material for currency and accuracy. Citations including the phrase, "Reviewed (month, year)" indicate material reviewed by this team. Medical consultation services are provided to the *Health Reference Series* editors by:

Dr. Vijayalakshmi, MBBS, DGO, MD
Dr. K. Sivanandham, MBBS, DCH, MS (Research), PhD

Our Advisory Board

We would like to thank the following board members for providing initial guidance on the development of this series:

- Dr. Lynda Baker, Associate Professor of Library and Information Science, Wayne State University, Detroit, MI

- Nancy Bulgarelli, William Beaumont Hospital Library, Royal Oak, MI

- Karen Imarisio, Bloomfield Township Public Library, Bloomfield Township, MI

- Karen Morgan, Mardigian Library, University of Michigan-Dearborn, Dearborn, MI

- Rosemary Orlando, St. Clair Shores Public Library, St. Clair Shores, MI

Health Reference Series *Update Policy*

The inaugural book in the *Health Reference Series* was the first edition of *Cancer Sourcebook* published in 1989. Since then, the *Series* has been enthusiastically received by librarians and in the medical community. In order to maintain the standard of providing high-quality health information for the layperson the editorial staff at Omnigraphics felt it was necessary to implement a policy of updating volumes when warranted.

Medical researchers have been making tremendous strides, and it is the purpose of the *Health Reference Series* to stay current with the most recent advances. Each decision to update a volume is made on an individual basis. Some of the considerations include how much new information is available and the feedback we receive from people who use the books. If there is a topic you would like to see added to the update list, or an area of medical concern you feel has not been adequately addressed, please write to:

Managing Editor
Health Reference Series
Omnigraphics
615 Griswold, Ste. 901
Detroit, MI 48226

Part One

Endocrine Functioning and Metabolism

Chapter 1

Introduction to the Endocrine System

Although we rarely think about them, the glands of the endocrine system and the hormones they release influence almost every cell, organ, and function of our bodies. The endocrine system is instrumental in regulating mood, growth and development, tissue function, and metabolism, as well as sexual function and reproductive processes.

In general, the endocrine system is in charge of body processes that happen slowly, such as cell growth. Faster processes like breathing and body movement are controlled by the nervous system. But even though the nervous system and endocrine system are separate systems, they often work together to help the body function properly.

About the Endocrine System

The foundations of the endocrine system are the hormones and glands. As the body's chemical messengers, hormones transfer information and instructions from one set of cells to another. Although many different hormones circulate throughout the bloodstream, each one affects only the cells that are genetically programmed to receive and respond to its message. Hormone levels can be influenced by factors such as stress, infection, and changes in the balance of fluid and minerals in blood.

Text in this chapter is excerpted from "Endocrine System," © 1995–2016. The Nemours Foundation/KidsHealth®. Reprinted with permission.

A gland is a group of cells that produces and secretes, or gives off, chemicals. A gland selects and removes materials from the blood, processes them, and secretes the finished chemical product for use somewhere in the body.

Some types of glands release their secretions in specific areas. For instance, exocrine glands, such as the sweat and salivary glands, release secretions in the skin or inside of the mouth. Endocrine glands, on the other hand, release more than 20 major hormones directly into the bloodstream, where they can move to cells in other parts of the body.

What the Endocrine System Does

Once a hormone is secreted, it travels from the endocrine gland through the bloodstream to target cells designed to receive its message. Along the way to the target cells, special proteins bind to some of the hormones. The special proteins act as carriers that control the amount of hormone that is available to interact with and affect the target cells.

Also, the target cells have receptors that latch onto only specific hormones, and each hormone has its own receptor, so that each hormone will communicate only with specific target cells that possess receptors for that hormone. When the hormone reaches its target cell, it locks onto the cell's specific receptors and these hormone-receptor combinations transmit chemical instructions to the inner workings of the cell.

When hormone levels reach a certain normal or necessary amount, further secretion is controlled by important body mechanisms to maintain that level of hormone in the blood. This regulation of hormone secretion may involve the hormone itself or another substance in the blood related to the hormone.

For example, if the thyroid gland has secreted adequate amounts of thyroid hormones into the blood, the pituitary gland senses the normal levels of thyroid hormone in the bloodstream and adjusts its release of thyrotropin, the pituitary hormone that stimulates the thyroid gland to produce thyroid hormones.

Another example is parathyroid hormone, which increases the level of calcium in the blood. When the blood calcium level rises, the parathyroid glands sense the change and decrease their secretion of parathyroid hormone. This turnoff process is called a negative feedback system.

Problems with the Endocrine System

Too much or too little of any hormone can be harmful to the body. For example, if the pituitary gland produces too much growth hormone,

4

a child may grow excessively tall. If it produces too little, a child may be abnormally short.

Controlling the production of or replacing specific hormones can treat many endocrine disorders in children and adolescents, some of which include:

Adrenal insufficiency. This condition is characterized by decreased function of the adrenal cortex and the consequent underproduction of adrenal corticosteroid hormones. The symptoms of adrenal insufficiency may include weakness, fatigue, abdominal pain, nausea, dehydration, and skin changes. Doctors treat adrenal insufficiency by giving replacement corticosteroid hormones.

Cushing syndrome. Excessive amounts of glucocorticoid hormones in the body can lead to Cushing syndrome. In children, it most often results when a child takes large doses of synthetic corticosteroid drugs (such as prednisone) to treat autoimmune diseases such as lupus. If the condition is due to a tumor in the pituitary gland that produces excessive amounts of corticotropin and stimulates the adrenals to overproduce corticosteroids, it's known as Cushing disease.

Symptoms may take years to develop and include obesity, growth failure, muscle weakness, easy bruising of the skin, acne, high blood pressure, and psychological changes. Depending on the specific cause, doctors may treat this condition with surgery, radiation therapy, chemotherapy, or drugs that block the production of hormones.

Type 1 diabetes. Previously known as juvenile diabetes, this condition happens when the pancreas doesn't produce enough insulin. In children and teens, it's usually the result of an autoimmune disorder in which specific immune system cells and antibodies produced by the immune system attack and destroy the cells of the pancreas that produce insulin. Symptoms include excessive thirst, hunger, urination (peeing), and weight loss.

Type 1 diabetes can cause long-term complications, including kidney problems, nerve damage, blindness, and early coronary heart disease and stroke. To control their blood sugar levels and reduce the risk of developing diabetes complications, kids need regular injections of insulin.

Type 2 diabetes. Unlike type 1 diabetes, in which the body can't produce normal amounts of insulin, in type 2 diabetes the body can't respond to insulin normally. Children and teens who have it tend to be overweight, and it is believed that excess body fat plays a role in this insulin resistance. In fact, the rate of type 2 diabetes in kids has risen along with the dramatically increasing rates of obesity among kids.

The symptoms and possible complications of type 2 diabetes are basically the same as those of type 1. Some kids and teens can control their blood sugar level with dietary changes, exercise, and oral medications, but many will need to take insulin injections like those with type 1 diabetes.

Growth hormone problems. Too much growth hormone in children who are still growing will make their bones and other body parts grow excessively, resulting in gigantism. This rare condition is usually caused by a pituitary tumor and can be treated by removing the tumor.

In contrast, when the pituitary gland fails to produce adequate amounts of growth hormone, a child's growth in height is impaired. Hypoglycemia (low blood sugar) may also occur in kids with growth hormone deficiency, particularly in infants and young children with the condition.

Hyperthyroidism. Hyperthyroidism is a condition in which the levels of thyroid hormones in the blood are excessively high. Symptoms may include weight loss, nervousness, tremors, excessive sweating, increased heart rate and blood pressure, protruding eyes, and a swelling in the neck from an enlarged thyroid gland (goiter).

In kids this is usually caused by Graves disease, an autoimmune disorder in which specific antibodies produced by the immune system stimulate the thyroid gland to become overactive. The disease may be controlled with medications or by removal or destruction of the thyroid gland through surgery or radiation treatments.

Hypothyroidism. Hypothyroidism is when the levels of thyroid hormones in the blood are abnormally low. Thyroid hormone deficiency slows body processes and may lead to fatigue, a slow heart rate, dry skin, weight gain, constipation, and, in kids, slowing of growth and delayed puberty.

Hashimoto thyroiditis, which results from an autoimmune process that damages the thyroid and blocks thyroid hormone production, is the most common cause of hypothyroidism in kids. Infants can also be born with an absent or underdeveloped thyroid gland, resulting in hypothyroidism. It can be treated with oral thyroid hormone replacement.

Precocious puberty. Body changes associated with puberty may occur at an abnormally young age in some kids if the pituitary hormones that stimulate the gonads to produce sex hormones rise prematurely. An injectable medication is available that can suppress the secretion of these pituitary hormones (known as gonadotropins) and arrest the progression of sexual development in most of these children.

Chapter 2

Endocrine Gland Hormones

Chapter Contents

Section 2.1

Endocrine Glands and Their Hormones

This section contains text excerpted from the following sources: Text
under the heading "Why Are Hormones Important?" is excerpted
from "Endocrine Disruption," U.S. Environmental Protection Agency
(EPA), August 30, 2016; Text beginning with the heading "Endocrine
Glands in the Body" is excerpted from "Endocrine System," National
Cancer Institute (NCI), July 1, 2002. Reviewed October 2016.

Why Are Hormones Important?

Hormones act as chemical messengers that are released into the
blood stream to act on an organ in another part of the body. Although
hormones reach all parts of the body, only target cells with compat-
ible receptors are equipted to respond. Over 50 hormones have been
identified in humans and other vertebrates.

Hormones control or regulate many biological processes and are
often produced in exceptionally low amounts within the body. Examples of such processes include:

- Blood sugar control (insulin);

- Differentiation, growth, and function of reproductive organs (testosterone (T) and estradiol); and

- Body growth and energy production (growth hormone and thyroid hormone)

Much like a lock and key, many hormones act by binding to receptors that are produced within cells. When a hormone binds to a receptor, the receptor carries out the hormone's instructions, either by alter-
ing the cell's existing proteins or turning on genes that will builld a
new protein. The hormone-receptor complex switches on or switches
off specific biological processes in cells, tissues, and organs.

Some examples of hormones include:

- Estrogens are the group of hormones responsible for female sexual development. They are produced primarily by the ovaries
  and in small amounts by the adrenal glands.

- Androgens are responsible for male sex characteristics. Testosterone, the sex hormone produced by the testicles, is an androgen.

- The thyroid gland secretes two main hormones, thyroxine and triiodothyronine, into the bloodstream. These thyroid hormones stimulate all the cells in the body and control biological processes such as growth, reproduction, development, and metabolism.

The endocrine system, made up of all the body's different hormones, regulates all biological processes in the body from conception through adulthood and into old age, including the development of the brain and nervous system, the growth and function of the reproductive system, as well as the metabolism and blood sugar levels. The female ovaries, male testes, and pituitary, thyroid, and adrenal glands are major constituents of the endocrine system.

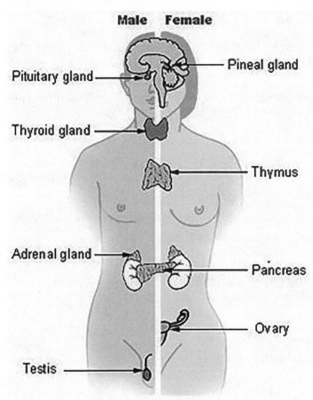

Figure 2.1. *Major Endocrine Glands*

Endocrine Glands in the Body

The endocrine system is made up of the endocrine glands that secrete hormones. Although there are eight major endocrine glands scattered throughout the body, they are still considered to be one system because they have similar functions, similar mechanisms of influence, and many important interrelationships.

Some glands also have non-endocrine regions that have functions other than hormone secretion. For example, the pancreas has a major exocrine portion that secretes digestive enzymes and an endocrine portion that secretes hormones. The ovaries and testes secrete hormones and also produce the ova and sperm. Some organs, such as the stomach, intestines, and heart, produce hormones, but their primary function is not hormone secretion.

Pituitary and Pineal Glands

Pituitary Gland

The pituitary gland or hypophysis is a small gland about 1 centimeter in diameter or the size of a pea. It is nearly surrounded by bone as it rests in the sella turcica, a depression in the sphenoid bone. The gland is connected to the hypothalamus of the brain by a slender stalk called the infundibulum.

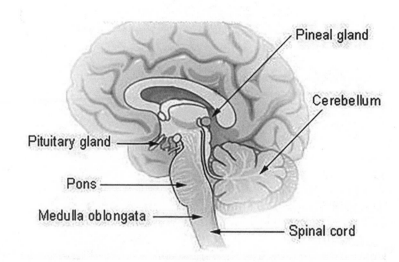

Figure 2.2. *Pituitary and Pineal Glands*

There are two distinct regions in the gland: the anterior lobe (adenohypophysis) and the posterior lobe (neurohypophysis). The activity of the adenohypophysis is controlled by releasing hormones from the hypothalamus. The neurohypophysis is controlled by nerve stimulation.

Hormones of the Anterior Lobe (Adenohypophysis)

Growth hormone is a protein that stimulates the growth of bones, muscles, and other organs by promoting protein synthesis. This hormone drastically affects the appearance of an individual because it influences height. If there is too little growth hormone in a child, that person may become a pituitary dwarf of normal proportions but small stature. An excess of the hormone in a child results in an exaggerated bone growth, and the individual becomes exceptionally tall or a giant.

Thyroid-stimulating hormone, or thyrotropin, causes the glandular cells of the thyroid to secrete thyroid hormone. When there is a hypersecretion of thyroid-stimulating hormone, the thyroid gland enlarges and secretes too much thyroid hormone.

Adrenocorticotropic hormone reacts with receptor sites in the cortex of the adrenal gland to stimulate the secretion of cortical hormones, particularly cortisol.

Gonadotropic hormones react with receptor sites in the gonads, or ovaries and testes, to regulate the development, growth, and function of these organs.

Prolactin hormone promotes the development of glandular tissue in the female breast during pregnancy and stimulates milk production after the birth of the infant.

Hormones of the Posterior Lobe (Neurohypophysis)

Antidiuretic hormone promotes the reabsorption of water by the kidney tubules, with the result that less water is lost as urine. This mechanism conserves water for the body. Insufficient amounts of antidiuretic hormone cause excessive water loss in the urine.

Oxytocin causes contraction of the smooth muscle in the wall of the uterus. It also stimulates the ejection of milk from the lactating breast.

Pineal Gland

The pineal gland, also called pineal body or epiphysis cerebri, is a small cone-shaped structure that extends posteriorly from the third ventricle of the brain. The pineal gland consists of portions of neurons, neuroglial cells, and specialized secretory cells called pinealocytes. The pinealocytes synthesize the hormone melatonin and secrete it directly into the cerebrospinal fluid, which takes it into the blood. Melatonin affects reproductive development and daily physiologic cycles.

Thyroid and Parathyroid Glands

Thyroid Gland

The thyroid gland is a very vascular organ that is located in the neck. It consists of two lobes, one on each side of the trachea, just below the larynx or voice box. The two lobes are connected by a narrow band of tissue called the isthmus. Internally, the gland consists of follicles, which produce thyroxine and triiodothyronine hormones. These hormones contain iodine.

About 95 percent of the active thyroid hormone is thyroxine, and most of the remaining 5 percent is triiodothyronine. Both of these require iodine for their synthesis. Thyroid hormone secretion is regulated by a negative feedback mechanism that involves the amount of circulating hormone, hypothalamus, and adenohypophysis.

If there is an iodine deficiency, the thyroid cannot make sufficient hormone. This stimulates the anterior pituitary to secrete thyroid-stimulating hormone, which causes the thyroid gland to increase in size in a vain attempt to produce more hormones. But it cannot produce more hormones because it does not have the necessary raw material, iodine. This type of thyroid enlargement is called simple goiter or iodine deficiency goiter.

Calcitonin is secreted by the parafollicular cells of the thyroid gland. This hormone opposes the action of the parathyroid glands by reducing the calcium level in the blood. If blood calcium becomes too high, calcitonin is secreted until calcium ion levels decrease to normal.

Parathyroid Gland

Four small masses of epithelial tissue are embedded in the connective tissue capsule on the posterior surface of the thyroid glands. These are parathyroid glands, and they secrete parathyroid hormone or parathormone. Parathyroid hormone is the most important regulator of blood calcium levels. The hormone is secreted in response to low blood calcium levels, and its effect is to increase those levels.

Hypoparathyroidism, or insufficient secretion of parathyroid hormone, leads to increased nerve excitability. The low blood calcium levels trigger spontaneous and continuous nerve impulses, which then stimulate muscle contraction.

Adrenal Gland

The adrenal, or suprarenal, gland is paired with one gland located near the upper portion of each kidney. Each gland is divided into an outer cortex and an inner medulla. The cortex and medulla of the adrenal gland, like the anterior and posterior lobes of the pituitary, develop from different embryonic tissues and secrete different hormones. The adrenal cortex is essential to life, but the medulla may be removed with no life-threatening effects.

The hypothalamus of the brain influences both portions of the adrenal gland but by different mechanisms. The adrenal cortex is regulated by negative feedback involving the hypothalamus and adrenocorticotropic hormone; the medulla is regulated by nerve impulses from the hypothalamus.

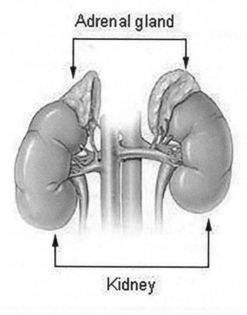

Figure 2.3. *Adrenal Gland*

Hormones of the Adrenal Cortex

The adrenal cortex consists of three different regions, with each region producing a different group or type of hormones. Chemically, all the cortical hormones are steroid.

Mineralocorticoids are secreted by the outermost region of the adrenal cortex. The principal mineralocorticoid is aldosterone, which acts to conserve sodium ions and water in the body.

Glucocorticoids are secreted by the middle region of the adrenal cortex. The principal glucocorticoid is cortisol, which increases blood glucose levels.

The third group of steroids secreted by the adrenal cortex is the gonadocorticoids, or sex hormones. These are secreted by the innermost region. Male hormones, androgens, and female hormones, estrogens, are secreted in minimal amounts in both sexes by the adrenal cortex, but their effect is usually masked by the hormones from the testes and ovaries. In females, the masculinization effect of androgen secretion may become evident after menopause, when estrogen levels from the ovaries decrease.

Hormones of the Adrenal Medulla

The adrenal medulla develops from neural tissue and secretes two hormones, epinephrine and norepinephrine. These two hormones are secreted in response to stimulation by sympathetic nerve, particularly during stressful situations. A lack of hormones from the adrenal medulla produces no significant effects. Hypersecretion, usually from a tumor, causes prolonged or continual sympathetic responses.

Pancreas—Islets of Langerhans

The pancreas is a long, soft organ that lies transversely along the posterior abdominal wall, posterior to the stomach, and extends from the region of the duodenum to the spleen. This gland has an exocrine portion that secretes digestive enzymes that are carried through a duct to the duodenum. The endocrine portion consists of the pancreatic islets, which secrete glucagons and insulin.

Alpha cells in the pancreatic islets secrete the hormone glucagons in response to a low concentration of glucose in the blood. Beta cells in the pancreatic islets secrete the hormone insulin in response to a high concentration of glucose in the blood.

Gonads

The gonads, the primary reproductive organs, are the testes in the male and the ovaries in the female. These organs are responsible for producing the sperm and ova, but they also secrete hormones and are considered to be endocrine glands.

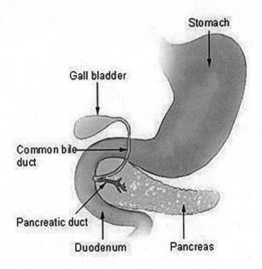

Figure 2.4. *Pancreas*

Testes

Male sex hormones, as a group, are called androgens. The principal androgen is testosterone, which is secreted by the testes. A small amount is also produced by the adrenal cortex. Production of testosterone begins during fetal development, continues for a short time after birth, nearly ceases during childhood, and then resumes at puberty. This steroid hormone is responsible for:

- The growth and development of the male reproductive structures.

- Increased skeletal and muscular growth.

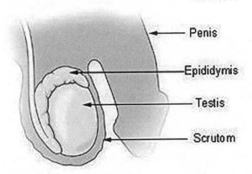

Figure 2.5. *Testis*

17

- Enlargement of the larynx accompanied by voice changes.

- Growth and distribution of body hair.

- Increased male sexual drive.

Testosterone secretion is regulated by a negative feedback system that involves releasing hormones from the hypothalamus and gonadotropins from the anterior pituitary.

Ovaries

Two groups of female sex hormones are produced in the ovaries, the estrogens and progesterone. These steroid hormones contribute to the development and function of the female reproductive organs and sex characteristics. At the onset of puberty, estrogens promotes:

- The development of the breasts.

- Distribution of fat evidenced in the hips, legs, and breast.

- Maturation of reproductive organs such as the uterus and vagina.

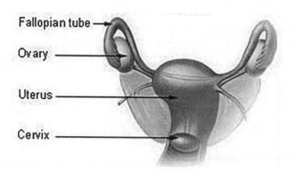

Figure 2.6. *Ovary*

Progesterone causes the uterine lining to thicken in preparation for pregnancy. Together, progesterone and estrogens are responsible for the changes that occur in the uterus during the female menstrual cycle.

Other Endocrine Glands

In addition to the major endocrine glands, other organs have some hormonal activity as part of their function. These include the thymus, stomach, small intestines, heart, and placenta.

Thymosin, produced by the thymus gland, plays an important role in the development of the body's immune system.

The lining of the stomach, the gastric mucosa, produces a hormone, called gastrin, in response to the presence of food in the stomach. This hormone stimulates the production of hydrochloric acid and the enzyme pepsin, which are used in the digestion of food.

The mucosa of the small intestine secretes the hormones secretin and cholecystokinin. Secretin stimulates the pancreas to produce a bicarbonate-rich fluid that neutralizes the stomach acid. Cholecysto-kinin stimulates contraction of the gallbladder, which releases bile. It also stimulates the pancreas to secrete digestive enzyme.

The heart also acts as an endocrine organ in addition to its major role of pumping blood. Special cells in the wall of the upper chambers of the heart, called atria, produce a hormone called atrial natriuretic hormone, or atriopeptin.

The placenta develops in the pregnant female as a source of nourishment and gas exchange for the developing fetus. It also serves as a temporary endocrine gland. One of the hormones it secretes is human chorionic gonadotropin, which signals the mother's ovaries to secrete hormones to maintain the uterine lining so that it does not degenerate and slough off in menstruation.

Section 2.2

Hormones Regulate the Digestive Process

This section includes text excerpted from "Your Digestive System and How It Works," National Institute of Diabetes and Digestive and Kidney Diseases (NIDDK), September 2013.

What Is the Digestive System?

The digestive system is made up of the gastrointestinal (GI) tract—also called the digestive tract—and the liver, pancreas, and gallbladder. The GI tract is a series of hollow organs joined in a long, twisting tube from the mouth to the anus. The hollow organs that make up the GI tract are the mouth, esophagus, stomach, small intestine, large intestine—which includes the rectum—and anus. Food enters the mouth and passes to the anus through the hollow organs of the GI tract. The liver, pancreas, and gallbladder are the solid organs of the digestive system. The digestive system helps the body digest food.

Bacteria in the GI tract, also called gut flora or microbiome, help with digestion. Parts of the nervous and circulatory systems also play roles in the digestive process. Together, a combination of nerves, hormones, bacteria, blood, and the organs of the digestive system completes the complex task of digesting the foods and liquids a person consumes each day.

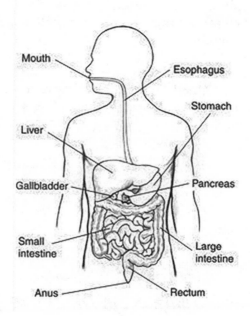

Figure 2.7. *Digestive System*

Why Is Digestion Important?

Digestion is important for breaking down food into nutrients, which the body uses for energy, growth, and cell repair. Food and drink must be changed into smaller molecules of nutrients before the blood absorbs them and carries them to cells throughout the body. The body breaks down nutrients from food and drink into carbohydrates, protein, fats, and vitamins.

How Does Digestion Work?

Digestion works by moving food through the GI tract. Digestion begins in the mouth with chewing and ends in the small intestine. As food passes through the GI tract, it mixes with digestive juices, causing large molecules of food to break down into smaller molecules. The body then absorbs these smaller molecules through the walls of the small intestine into the bloodstream, which delivers them to the rest of the body. Waste products of digestion pass through the large intestine and out of the body as a solid matter called stool.

How Do Digestive Juices in Each Organ of the GI Tract Break down Food?

Digestive juices contain enzymes—substances that speed up chemical reactions in the body—that break food down into different nutrients.

Salivary glands. Saliva produced by the salivary glands moistens food so it moves more easily through the esophagus into the stomach. Saliva also contains an enzyme that begins to break down the starches from food.

Glands in the stomach lining. The glands in the stomach lining produce stomach acid and an enzyme that digests protein.

Pancreas. The pancreas produces a juice containing several enzymes that break down carbohydrates, fats, and proteins in food. The pancreas delivers digestive juice to the small intestine through small tubes called ducts.

Liver. The liver produces a digestive juice called bile. The gallbladder stores bile between meals. When a person eats, the gallbladder squeezes bile through the bile ducts, which connect the gallbladder and liver to the small intestine. The bile mixes with the fat in food. The bile acids dissolve fat into the watery contents of the intestine, much like how detergents dissolve grease from a frying pan, so the intestinal and pancreatic enzymes can digest the fat molecules.

Small intestine. Digestive juice produced by the small intestine combines with pancreatic juice and bile to complete digestion. The body completes the breakdown of proteins, and the final breakdown of starches produces glucose molecules that absorb into the blood.

Bacteria in the small intestine produce some of the enzymes needed to digest carbohydrates.

How Is the Digestive Process Controlled?

Hormone and nerve regulators control the digestive process.

Hormone Regulators

The cells in the lining of the stomach and small intestine produce and release hormones that control the functions of the digestive system. These hormones stimulate production of digestive juices and regulate appetite.

Nerve Regulators

Two types of nerves help control the action of the digestive system: extrinsic and intrinsic nerves.

Extrinsic, or outside, nerves connect the digestive organs to the brain and spinal cord. These nerves release chemicals that cause the muscle layer of the GI tract to either contract or relax, depending on whether food needs digesting. The intrinsic, or inside, nerves within the GI tract are triggered when food stretches the walls of the hollow organs. The nerves release many different substances that speed up or delay the movement of food and the production of digestive juices.

Section 2.3

Can Hormones Prevent Aging?

This section includes text excerpted from "Can We Prevent Aging?" National Institute on Aging (NIA), National Institutes of Health (NIH), February 2012. Reviewed October 2016.

What Are Hormones

Hormones are chemical messengers that set in motion different processes to keep our bodies working properly. For example, they are involved in regulating our metabolism, immune function, sexual reproduction, and growth. Hormones are made by specialized groups of cells within the body's glands. The glands—such as the pituitary, thyroid, adrenals, ovaries, and testes—release hormones into the body as needed to stimulate, regulate, and control the function of other tissues and organs involved in biological processes. Most hormones are typically found in very low concentrations in the bloodstream. But a hormone's concentration will fluctuate depending on the body's activity or time of day.

We cannot survive without hormones. As children, hormones help us grow up. In our teenage years, they drive puberty. As we get older, some hormone levels naturally decline.

There are hormones that naturally decline with age, including:

- Human growth hormone

- Testosterone

- Estrogen and progesterone (as part of menopausal hormone therapy)

- Dehydroepiandrosterone (DHEA)

How Hormones Work

A hormone acts upon a cell much like a key unlocking a door. After being released by a gland, a hormone molecule travels through the blood until it finds a cell with the right fit. The hormone latches onto a cell via the cell's receptor. When this happens a signal is sent into the cell. These signals may instruct the cell to multiply, make proteins or enzymes, or perform other vital tasks. Some hormones can even cause a cell to release other hormones.

A hormone may fit with many types of cells but may not affect all cells in the same way. For example, one hormone may stimulate one cell to perform a task, but it might also turn off a different cell. Additionally, how a cell responds to a hormone may change throughout life.

Hormone Therapy

Levels of some hormones change naturally over the lifespan. Some hormones increase with age, like parathyroid hormone that helps regulate the amount of calcium in the blood and bone. Some tend to decrease over time, such as testosterone in men and estrogen in women. When the body fails to make enough of a hormone because of a disease or disorder, a doctor may prescribe hormone supplements.

These come in many forms such as pills, shots, topicals (gels, creams, and sprays applied to the skin), and medicated skin patches.

Truth is that, to date, no research has shown that hormone therapies add years to life or prevent age-related frailty. And, while some drugs have real health benefits for people with clinical hormone deficiencies due to a disease or disorder, they also can cause harmful side effects. That's why people who have a diagnosed hormone deficiency should still only take hormones prescribed by a doctor and under a doctor's supervision.

In some cases, the U.S. Food and Drug Administration (FDA) may have approved a hormone (or hormone therapy) for one purpose, but it is prescribed by physicians for another. This off-label use may occur when physicians believe that research, such as clinical studies, demonstrates a drug's usefulness for another condition. However, consumers should be aware that off-label use of any drug may not have been tested and verified to the same degree as the original use of the drug.

Some Dangers of Hormone Therapy and "Anti-Aging" Supplements

Higher concentrations of hormones in your body are not necessarily better. And, a decrease in hormone concentration with age is not necessarily a bad thing. The body maintains a delicate balance between how much hormone it produces and how much it needs to function properly. Natural hormone production fluctuates throughout the day. That means that the amount of hormone in your blood when you wake up may be different 2, 12, or 20 hours later.

If you take hormone supplements, especially without medical supervision, you can adversely affect this tightly controlled, regulated system. Replacement or supplemental hormones cannot replicate your body's natural variation. Because hormonal balance is so intricate, too much of a hormone in your system may actually cause the opposite of the intended effect. For example, taking a hormone supplement can cause your own hormone regulation to stop working. Or, your body may process the supplements differently than the naturally produced hormone, causing an alternate, undesired effect. It is also possible that a supplement could amplify negative side effects of the hormone naturally produced by the body. At this point, scientists do not know all the consequences.

Some hormone-like products are sold over the counter without a prescription. Using them can be dangerous. Products that are marketed as dietary supplements are not approved or regulated by the FDA. That is, companies making dietary supplements do not need to provide any proof that their products are safe and effective before selling them. There is no guarantee that the "recommended" dosage is safe, that the same amount of active ingredients is in every bottle, or that the substance is what the company claims. What you bought over the counter may not have been thoroughly studied, and potential negative side effects may not be understood or defined. In addition, these over-the-counter products may interfere with your other medications. National Institute on Aging (NIA) does not recommend taking any supplement touted as an "anti-aging" remedy because there is no proof of effectiveness and the health risks of short- and long-term use are largely unknown.

Effect of Hormones on Aging

Human Growth Hormone

Growth hormone is important for normal growth and development, as well as for maintaining tissues and organs. It is made by the pituitary gland, a pea-sized structure located at the base of the brain.

Research supports supplemental use of human growth hormone (hGH) injections in certain circumstances. For instance, hGH injections can help children who do not produce enough growth hormone. Sometimes hGH injections may be prescribed for young adults whose obesity is the result of having had their pituitary gland surgically removed. These uses are different from taking hGH as an "anti-aging" strategy. As with other hormones, growth hormone levels often decline with age, but this decrease is not necessarily bad. At least one epidemiological study suggests that people who have high levels of naturally produced growth hormone are more apt to die at younger ages than those with lower levels of the hormone.

Although there is no conclusive evidence that hGH can prevent aging or halt age-related physical decline, some clinics market hGH for that purpose, and some people spend a great deal of money on such supplements. Shots can cost more than $15,000 a year. These shots are only available by prescription and should be administered by a doctor. But, because of the unknown risks—and the evidence suggests that side effects strongly overcome any possible benefits—it is hard to find a doctor who will prescribe hGH shots. Over-the-counter dietary supplements, known as human growth hormone releasers, are currently being marketed as low-cost alternatives to hGH shots. But claims of their anti-aging effects, like all those regarding hGH, are unsubstantiated.

Research is starting to paint a fuller picture of the effects of hGH, but there is still much to learn. For instance, study findings indicate that injections of hGH can increase muscle mass; however, it seems to have little impact on muscle strength or function. Questions about potential side effects, such as diabetes, joint pain, and fluid buildup leading to high blood pressure or heart failure, remain unanswered, too. A report that children who were treated with pituitary growth hormone have an increased risk of cancer created a heightened concern about the dangers of hGH injections. Whether or not older people treated with hGH for extended periods have an increased risk of cancer is unknown. To date, only small, short-term studies have looked specifically at hGH as an "anti-aging" therapy for older people. Additional research is necessary to assess the potential risks and benefits of hGH.

Testosterone

Testosterone is a vital sex hormone that plays an important role in puberty. In men, testosterone not only regulates sex drive (libido), it also helps regulate bone mass, fat distribution, muscle mass and strength, and the production of red blood cells and sperm. Testosterone isn't exclusively a male hormone—women produce small amounts as well.

As men age, they often produce somewhat less testosterone, especially compared to years of peak testosterone production during adolescence and early adulthood. Normal testosterone production ranges widely, and it is unclear what amount of decline or how low a level of testosterone will cause adverse effects.

"Male menopause," a condition supposedly caused by diminishing testosterone levels in aging men, has been increasingly reported about in recent years. There is very little scientific evidence that this condition, also known as andropause or viropause, exists. The likelihood that an aging man will experience a major shutdown of testosterone production similar to a woman's menopause is very remote. In fact, many of the changes that take place in older men often are incorrectly attributed to decreasing testosterone levels. For instance, some men experiencing erectile difficulty (impotence) may be tempted to blame it on lowered testosterone, but many cases of erectile problems are due to circulatory problems.

For men whose bodies make very little or no testosterone, testosterone replacement may offer benefits. FDA-approved testosterone drugs come in different forms, including patches, injections, and topical gels. Men whose testes (the reproductive glands that make testosterone and sperm) have been damaged or whose pituitary glands have been harmed or destroyed by trauma, infections, or tumors may also be prescribed testosterone. Treatment with testosterone drugs can help men with exceptionally low testosterone levels maintain strong muscles and bones and increase their sex drive. It is unclear if men who are at the lower end of the normal range for testosterone production would benefit from treatment.

More research is needed to learn what effects testosterone drug therapy may have in healthy older men without these extreme deficiencies. NIA is investigating the role of testosterone therapy in delaying or preventing frailty and helping with other age-related health issues. Results from preliminary studies involving small groups of men are inconclusive. Specifically, it remains unclear to what degree testosterone supplements can help men maintain strong muscles and sturdy bones, sustain robust sexual activity, or sharpen memory.

There are also concerns about the long-term, harmful effects that testosterone drugs might have on the aging body. Most epidemiological studies suggest that higher natural levels of testosterone are not associated with a higher incidence of prostate cancer—the second leading cause of cancer death among men. However, scientists do not know if taking testosterone drugs increases men's risk for developing prostate cancer or promoting the growth of an existing tumor. There is also uncertainty about effects of testosterone treatment on the cardiovascular system in older men, especially men with mobility limitations and other diseases. Future studies will address this issue to ensure that older men receiving testosterone treatment are not exposed to unnecessary risks.

The bottom line: there is no scientific proof that testosterone treatment in healthy men will help them age better. Until more scientifically rigorous studies are conducted, it is not known if the possible benefits of testosterone therapy outweigh any of its potential risks. NIA continues to conduct research to gather more evidence about the effects of testosterone treatment in aging men.

Hormones in Women

Estrogen and progesterone are two hormones that play an important part in women's menstrual cycle and pregnancy. Estrogen also helps maintain bone strength and may reduce the risk of heart disease and memory problems before menopause. Both estrogen and progesterone are produced naturally by the ovaries. However, after menopause, the ovaries make much less of these hormones. For more than 60 years, millions of women have used estrogen to relieve their menopausal symptoms, especially hot flashes and vaginal dryness. Some women may also be prescribed estrogen to prevent or treat osteoporosis—loss of bone strength—that often happens after menopause. The use of estrogen (by a woman whose uterus has been removed) or estrogen with progesterone or a progestin, a synthetic form of progesterone (by a woman with a uterus), to treat the symptoms of menopause is called menopausal hormone therapy (MHT), formerly known as hormone replacement therapy (HRT).

There is a rich research base investigating estrogen. Many large, reliable long-term studies of estrogen and its effects on the body have been conducted. Yet, much remains unknown. In fact, the history of estrogen research demonstrates why it is important to examine both the benefits and risks of any hormone therapy before it becomes widely used. Here's what scientists know:

- **Endometrial problems**—While estrogen helps some women with symptom management during and after menopause, it can raise the risk of certain problems. Estrogen may cause a thickening of the lining of the uterus (endometrium) and increase the risk of endometrial cancer. To lessen these risks, doctors now prescribe progesterone or a progestin, in combination with estrogen, to women with a uterus to protect the lining.

- **Heart disease**—The role of estrogen in heart disease is complex. Early studies suggested MHT could lower postmenopausal women's risk for heart disease—the number one killer of women in the United States. But results from the NIH Women's Health Initiative (WHI) suggest that using estrogen with or without a progestin after menopause does not protect women from heart disease and may even increase their risk.

WHI scientists reported that using estrogen plus progestin actually elevates some postmenopausal women's chance of developing heart disease, stroke, blood clots, and breast cancer, but women also experienced fewer hip fractures and cases of colorectal cancer. The scientists published another report, this time on postmenopausal women who used estrogen alone, which had some similar findings: women had an increased risk of stroke and blood clots, but fewer hip fractures. Then, a closer analysis of the WHI results indicated that younger women, ages 50 to 59 at the start of the trial, who used estrogen alone, had significantly less calcified plaque in their coronary arteries than women not using estrogen. Increased plaque in coronary arteries is a risk factor for heart attacks. Scientists also noted that the risk of heart attack increased in women who started MHT more than 10 years after menopause (especially if these women had menopausal symptoms). There was no evidence of increased risk of heart attack in women who began MHT within 10 years of going through menopause.

- **Dementia**—Some observational studies have suggested that estrogen may protect against Alzheimer disease. However, testing in clinical trials in older, postmenopausal women has challenged that view. Researchers leading the WHI Memory Study (WHIMS), a substudy of the WHI, reported that women age 65 and older who took one kind of estrogen combined with progestin were at twice the risk for developing dementia compared to women who did not take any hormones. The scientists reported that using the same kind of estrogen alone also increased the risk of developing dementia in women age 65 and older compared to women not taking any hormones. What possibly accounts for the different findings between the observational and clinical studies? One central issue may be timing. The women in the WHIMS trial started treatment a decade or more after menopause. In observational studies that reported estrogen's positive effects on cognition, the majority of women began treatment soon after menopause. This has led researchers to wonder if it may be advantageous to begin treatment earlier, at a time closer to menopause. Additionally, it appears that progesterone and progestins (progesterone-like compounds) differ in their impact on brain health.

Despite research thus far, there are still many unknowns about the risks and benefits of MHT. For instance, because women in their early 50's were only a small part of the WHI, scientists do not yet know if certain risks are applicable to younger women who use estrogen to relieve their symptoms during the menopausal transition.

You may also have heard about another approach to hormone therapy for women—"bioidentical hormones." These are hormones derived from plants, such as soy or yams, that have identical chemical structures to hormones produced by the human body. The term "bioidentical hormones" is now also being applied to the use of compounded hormones. Large clinical trials of these compounded hormones have not been done, and many bioidentical hormones that are available without a prescription are not regulated or approved for safety and efficacy by the FDA. FDA-regulated bioidentical hormones, such as estradiol and progesterone, are available by prescription for women considering MHT.

For middle-age and older women, the decision to take hormones is far more complex and difficult than ever before. Questions about MHT remain. Would using a different estrogen and/or progestin or different dose change the risks? Would the results be different if the hormones were given as a patch or cream, rather than a pill? Would taking progestin less often be as effective and safe? Does starting MHT around the time of menopause, compared to years later, change the risks? Can we predict which women will benefit or be harmed by using MHT? As these and other questions are addressed by research, women should continue to review the pros and cons of MHT with their doctors. They should assess the benefits as well as personal risks to make an informed decision about whether or not this therapy is right for them.

DHEA

Dehydroepiandrosterone, or DHEA, is made from cholesterol by the adrenal glands, which sit on top of each kidney. It is converted by the body into two other important hormones: testosterone and estrogen.

For most people, DHEA production peaks in the mid-20's and then gradually declines with age. The effects of this decline, including its role in the aging process, are unclear. Even so, some proponents claim that over-the-counter DHEA supplements can improve energy and strength and boost immunity. Claims are also made that supplements increase muscle and decrease fat. To date, there is no conclusive scientific evidence that DHEA supplements have any of these benefits.

The conversion of naturally produced DHEA into estrogen and testosterone is highly individualized. There is no way to predict who will make more or less of these hormones. Having an excess of testosterone or estrogen in your body could be risky.

Scientists do not yet know the effects of long-term (defined as over 1 year) use of DHEA supplements. Early indications are that these supplements, even when taken briefly, may have detrimental effects on the body, including liver damage. But the picture is not clear. Two short-term studies showed that taking DHEA supplements has no harmful effects on blood, prostate, or liver function. However, these studies were too small to lead to broader conclusions about the safety or efficacy of DHEA supplementation.

Researchers are working to find more definite answers about DHEA's effects on aging, muscles, and the immune system. In the meantime, if you are thinking about taking DHEA supplements, be aware that the effects are not fully known and might turn out to cause more harm than good.

Chapter 3

Metabolism Basics

Our bodies get the energy they need from food through metabolism, the chemical reactions in the body's cells that convert the fuel from food into the energy needed to do everything from moving to thinking to growing.

Specific proteins in the body control the chemical reactions of metabolism, and each chemical reaction is coordinated with other body functions. In fact, thousands of metabolic reactions happen at the same time—all regulated by the body—to keep our cells healthy and working.

Metabolism is a constant process that begins when we're conceived and ends when we die. It is a vital process for all life forms—not just humans. If metabolism stops, a living thing dies.

Here's an example of how the process of metabolism works in humans—and it begins with plants. First, a green plant takes in energy from sunlight. The plant uses this energy and the molecule chlorophyll (which gives plants their green color) to build sugars from water and carbon dioxide in a process known as photosynthesis.

When people and animals eat the plants (or, if they're carnivores, when they eat animals that have eaten the plants), they take in this energy (in the form of sugar), along with other vital cell-building chemicals.

The body's next step is to break the sugar down so that the energy released can be distributed to, and used as fuel by, the body's cells.

Text in this chapter is excerpted from "Metabolism," © 1995–2016. The Nemours Foundation/KidsHealth®. Reprinted with permission.

Enzymes

After food is eaten, molecules in the digestive system called enzymes break proteins down into amino acids, fats into fatty acids, and carbohydrates into simple sugars (for example, glucose). In addition to sugar, both amino acids and fatty acids can be used as energy sources by the body when needed. These compounds are absorbed into the blood, which transports them to the cells.

After they enter the cells, other enzymes act to speed up or regulate the chemical reactions involved with "metabolizing" these compounds. During these processes, the energy from these compounds can be released for use by the body or stored in body tissues, especially the liver, muscles, and body fat.

In this way, the process of metabolism is really a balancing act involving two kinds of activities that go on at the same time—the *building up* of body tissues and energy stores and the *breaking down* of body tissues and energy stores to generate more fuel for body functions:

- **Anabolism**, or constructive metabolism, is all about building and storing. It supports the growth of new cells, the maintenance of body tissues, and the storage of energy for use in the future. During anabolism, small molecules are changed into larger, more complex molecules of carbohydrates, protein, and fat.

- **Catabolism**, or destructive metabolism, is the process that produces the energy required for all activity in the cells. In this process, cells break down large molecules (mostly carbohydrates and fats) to release energy. This energy release provides fuel for anabolism, heats the body, and enables the muscles to contract and the body to move. As complex chemical units are broken down into more simple substances, the waste products released in the process of catabolism are removed from the body through the skin, kidneys, lungs, and intestines.

The Endocrine System

Several of the hormones of the endocrine system are involved in controlling the rate and direction of metabolism. Thyroxine, a hormone produced and released by the thyroid gland, plays a key role in determining how fast or slow the chemical reactions of metabolism proceed in a person's body.

Another gland, the pancreas secretes hormones that help determine whether the body's main metabolic activity at a particular time will be anabolic or catabolic. For example, after eating a meal, usually more anabolic activity happens because eating increases the level of glucose—the body's most important fuel—in the blood. The pancreas senses this increased level of glucose and releases the hormone insulin, which signals cells to increase their anabolic activities.

Metabolism is a complicated chemical process, so it's not surprising that many people think of it in its simplest sense: as something that influences how easily our bodies gain or lose weight. That's where calories come in. A calorie is a unit that measures how much energy a particular food provides to the body. A chocolate bar has more calories than an apple, so it provides the body with more energy—and sometimes that can be too much of a good thing. Just as a car stores gas in the gas tank until it is needed to fuel the engine, the body stores calories—primarily as fat. If you overfill a car's gas tank, it spills over onto the pavement. Likewise, if a person eats too many calories, they "spill over" in the form of excess body fat.

The number of calories someone burns in a day is affected by how much that person exercises, the amount of fat and muscle in his or her body, and the person's **basal metabolic rate (BMR)**. BMR is a measure of the rate at which a person's body "burns" energy, in the form of calories, while at rest.

The BMR can play a role in a person's tendency to gain weight. For example, someone with a low BMR (who therefore burns fewer calories while at rest or sleeping) will tend to gain more pounds of body fat over time than a similar-sized person with an average BMR who eats the same amount of food and gets the same amount of exercise.

What Factors Influence BMR?

To a certain extent, BMR is inherited. Sometimes health problems can affect BMR, but people can change their BMR in certain ways. For example, exercising more not only will cause someone to burn more calories directly from the extra activity itself, but becoming more physically fit will increase BMR as well.

BMR is also influenced by body composition—people with more muscle and less fat generally have higher BMRs.

Metabolic Disorders

In a broad sense, a metabolic disorder is any disease that is caused by an abnormal chemical reaction in the body's cells. Most disorders involve either abnormal levels of enzymes or hormones, or problems with how those enzymes or hormones work.

When the metabolism of body chemicals is blocked or defective, it can cause a buildup of toxic substances in the body or a lack of substances needed for normal body function, either of which can lead to serious symptoms.

Some metabolic diseases are inherited. These are called inborn errors of metabolism. When babies are born, they're tested for many of these in a newborn screening test. Many inborn errors of metabolism can lead to serious complications or even death if they're not controlled with diet or medicine from an early age.

G6PD deficiency: Glucose-6-phosphate dehydrogenase (G6PD) is just one of the many enzymes that play a role in cell metabolism. G6PD is produced by red blood cells (RBCs) and helps the body metabolize carbohydrates. Without enough normal G6PD to help RBCs handle certain harmful substances, the cells can be damaged or destroyed, leading to hemolytic anemia. In a process called hemolysis, RBCs are destroyed prematurely, and the bone marrow (the soft, spongy part of the bone that produces new blood cells) may not be able to produce enough new red blood cells.

Kids with G6PD deficiency may be pale and tired and have a rapid heartbeat and breathing. They may also have an enlarged spleen or jaundice (yellowing of the skin and eyes). G6PD deficiency is usually treated by stopping medicines or treating the illness or infection causing the stress on the RBCs.

Galactosemia: Babies born with this inborn error of metabolism lack the enzyme that converts galactose (one of two sugars found in lactose) into glucose, a sugar the body is able to use. As a result, milk (including breast milk) and other dairy products must be eliminated from the diet. Otherwise, galactose can build up in the system and damage the body's cells and organs, leading to blindness, severe intellectual disability, growth deficiency, and even death.

Hyperthyroidism: This is when an overactive thyroid gland releases too much of the hormone thyroxine, which increases BMR. It causes symptoms such as weight loss, increased heart rate and blood pressure, protruding eyes, and a swelling in the neck from an enlarged thyroid (goiter). The disease may be controlled with medicines or through surgery or radiation treatments.

Hypothyroidism: This is when an absent or underactive thyroid (due to a developmental problem or thyroid disease) causes the release of too little of the hormone thyroxine, which lowers BMR.

If not treated, this condition can result in stunted growth and intellectual disability in infants and young children. Hypothyroidism slows body processes and causes fatigue (tiredness), slow heart rate, excessive weight gain, and constipation. Kids and teens with this condition can be treated with oral thyroid hormone.

Phenylketonuria: Also known as PKU, this is caused by a defect in the enzyme that breaks down the amino acid phenylalanine. This amino acid is necessary for normal growth in infants and children and for normal protein production. However, if too much of it builds up in the body, brain tissue is affected and intellectual disability happens.

Early diagnosis and dietary restriction of the amino acid can prevent or lessen the severity of these complications.

Type 1 diabetes: This is when the pancreas doesn't produce and secrete enough insulin. Symptoms of this disease include excessive thirst and urination, hunger, and weight loss. Over the long term, it can cause kidney problems, pain due to nerve damage, blindness, and heart and blood vessel disease. Kids and teens with type 1 diabetes need to get regular insulin injections and to control their blood sugar levels to reduce the risk of developing complications.

Type 2 diabetes: This is when the body can't respond normally to insulin. Symptoms are similar to those of type 1 diabetes. Many kids who develop type 2 diabetes are overweight, which is thought to play a role in their decreased responsiveness to insulin. Some can be treated successfully with dietary changes, exercise, and oral medicine, but insulin injections are necessary in other cases. Controlling blood sugar levels reduces the risk of developing the same kinds of long-term health problems that happen with type 1 diabetes.

Chapter 4

Energy Balance

What Is Energy Balance?

Energy is another word for "calories." Your energy balance is the balance of calories consumed through eating and drinking compared to calories burned through physical activity. What you eat and drink is ENERGY IN. What you burn through physical activity is ENERGY OUT.

You burn a certain number of calories just by breathing air and digesting food. You also burn a certain number of calories (ENERGY OUT) through your daily routine. For example, children burn calories just being students—walking to their lockers, carrying books, and so on—and adults burn calories walking to the bus stop, going shopping, etc.

An important part of maintaining energy balance is the amount of ENERGY OUT (physical activity) that you do. People who are more **physically active** burn **more** calories than those who are not as physically active.

The same amount of ENERGY IN (calories consumed) and ENERGY OUT (calories burned) over time = weight stays the same

---

This chapter contains text excerpted from the following sources: Text beginning with the heading "What Is Energy Balance?" is excerpted from "Healthy Weight Basics," National Heart, Lung, and Blood Institute (NHLBI), February 13, 2013; Text beginning with the heading "Body Mass Index" is excerpted from "Healthy Weight," Centers for Disease Control and Prevention (CDC), May 15, 2015.

More IN than OUT over time = weight gain
More OUT than IN over time = weight loss

Your ENERGY IN and OUT don't have to balance every day. It's having a balance **over time** that will help you stay at a healthy weight for the long term. Children need to balance their energy, too, but they're also growing and that should be considered as well. Energy balance in children happens when the amount of ENERGY IN and ENERGY OUT supports natural growth without promoting excess weight gain.

That's why you should take a look at the Estimated Calorie Requirement chart (Table 4.1), to get a sense of how many calories (ENERGY IN) you and your family need on a daily basis.

Estimated Calorie Requirements

This calorie requirement chart presents estimated amounts of calories needed to maintain energy balance (and a healthy body weight) for various gender and age groups at three different levels of physical activity. The estimates are rounded to the nearest 200 calories and were determined using an equation from the Institute of Medicine (IOM).

Table 4.1. Estimated Calorie Requirements (in kilocalories) for Each Gender and Age Group at Three Levels of Physical Activity

Gender	Age (years)	Activity Level		
		Sedentary	Moderately Active	Active
Child	2–3	1,000	1,000–1,400	1,000–1,400
Female	4–8	1,200	1,400–1,600	1,400–1,800
Female	9–13	1,600	1,600–2,000	1,800–2,000
Female	14–18	1,800	2,000	2,400
Female	19–30	2,000	2,000–2,200	2,400
Female	31–50	1,800	2,000	2,200
Female	51+	1,600	1,800	2,000–2,200
Male	4–8	1,400	1,400–1,600	1,600–2,000
Male	9–13	1,800	1,800–2,200	2,000–2,600
Male	14–18	2,200	2,400–2,800	2,800–3,200
Male	19–30	2,400	2,600–2,800	3,000

Table 4.1. Continued

Gender	Age (years)	Activity Level		
		Sedentary	Moderately Active	Active
Male	31–50	2,200	2,400–2,600	2,800–3,000
Male	51+	2,000	2,200–2,400	2,400–2,800

• These levels are based on Estimated Energy Requirements (EER) from the *IOM Dietary Reference Intakes* macronutrients report, calculated by gender, age, and activity level for reference-sized individuals. "Reference size," as determined by IOM, is based on median height and weight for ages up to age 18 years of age and median height and weight for that height to give a BMI of 21.5 for adult females and 22.5 for adult males.

• Sedentary means a lifestyle that includes only the light physical activity associated with typical day-to-day life.

• Moderately active means a lifestyle that includes physical activity equivalent to walking about 1.5 to 3 miles per day at 3 to 4 miles per hour, in addition to the light physical activity associated with typical day-to-day life.

• Active means a lifestyle that includes physical activity equivalent to walking more than 3 miles per day at 3 to 4 miles per hour, in addition to the light physical activity associated with typical day-to-day life.

• The calorie ranges shown are to accommodate needs of different ages within the group. For children and adolescents, more calories are needed at older ages. For adults, fewer calories are needed at older ages.

Body Mass Index

What Is Body Mass Index?

Body Mass Index (BMI) is a person's weight in kilograms divided by the square of height in meters. BMI does not measure body fat directly, but research has shown that BMI is moderately correlated with more direct measures of body fat obtained from skinfold thickness measurements, bioelectrical impedance, densitometry (underwater weighing), dual energy X-ray absorptiometry (DXA) and other methods.

Furthermore, BMI appears to be as strongly correlated with various metabolic and disease outcome as are these more direct measures of body fatness. In general, BMI is an inexpensive and easy-to-perform method of screening for weight category, for example underweight, normal or healthy weight, overweight, and obesity.

How Is BMI Used?

A high BMI can be an indicator of high body fatness. BMI can be used as a screening tool but is not diagnostic of the body fatness or health of an individual.

To determine if a high BMI is a health risk, a healthcare provider would need to perform further assessments. These assessments might include skinfold thickness measurements, evaluations of diet, physical activity, family history, and other appropriate health screenings.

How Is BMI Interpreted for Adults?

For adults 20 years old and older, BMI is interpreted using standard weight status categories. These categories are the same for men and women of all body types and ages.

The standard weight status categories associated with BMI ranges for adults are shown in the following table.

Table 4.2. Weight Status and BMI

BMI	Weight Status
Below 18.5	Underweight
18.5–24.9	Normal or Healthy Weight
25.0–29.9	Overweight
30.0 and Above	Obese

Physical Activity for a Healthy Weight

Why Is Physical Activity Important?

Regular physical activity is important for good health, and it's especially important if you're trying to lose weight or to maintain a healthy weight.

- When losing weight, more physical activity increases the number of calories your body uses for energy or "burns off." The burning of calories through physical activity, combined with reducing the number of calories you eat, creates a "calorie deficit" that results in weight loss.

- Most weight loss occurs because of decreased caloric intake. However, evidence shows the only way to *maintain* weight loss is to be engaged in regular physical activity.

- Most importantly, physical activity reduces risks of cardiovascular disease and diabetes beyond that produced by weight reduction alone.

Physical activity also helps to—

- maintain weight

- reduce high blood pressure

- reduce risk for type 2 diabetes, heart attack, stroke, and several forms of cancer

- reduce arthritis pain and associated disability

- reduce risk for osteoporosis and falls

- reduce symptoms of depression and anxiety

How Much Physical Activity Do I Need?

When it comes to weight management, people vary greatly in how much physical activity they need. Here are some guidelines to follow:

To maintain your weight: Work your way up to 150 minutes of moderate-intensity aerobic activity, 75 minutes of vigorous-intensity aerobic activity, or an equivalent mix of the two each week. Strong scientific evidence shows that physical activity can help you maintain your weight over time. However, the exact amount of physical activity needed to do this is not clear since it varies greatly from person to person. It's possible that you may need to do more than the equivalent of 150 minutes of moderate-intensity activity a week to maintain your weight.

To lose weight and keep it off: You will need a high amount of physical activity unless you also adjust your diet and reduce the amount of calories you're eating and drinking. Getting to and staying at a healthy weight requires both regular physical activity and a healthy eating plan.

Chapter 5

Endocrine Disruptors

What Are Endocrine Disruptors?

Endocrine disruptors are chemicals that may interfere with the production or activity of hormones in the human endocrine system. These chemicals may occur naturally or be manufactured. The term "endocrine disruptors" describes a diverse group of chemicals that are suspected or known to affect human hormones. Effects on human hormones can range from minor to serious depending on the specific endocrine receptor and the amount of exposure. Because these chemicals are found in products you use every day and you are exposed to many endocrine receptors at the same time, it is difficult to determine the public health effects of these chemicals.

The human endocrine system is responsible for controlling and coordinating many body functions, including the production of hormones. The human endocrine system includes the pancreas, pituitary, thyroid, adrenal, and male and female reproductive glands.

Endocrine disruptors interfere with the production, release, transport, metabolism, or elimination of the body's natural hormones. They can mimic naturally occurring hormones, potentially causing overproduction or underproduction of hormones. They may also interfere or block the way natural hormones and their receptors are made or controlled.

This chapter includes text excerpted from "Endocrine Disruptors," National Institutes of Health (NIH), March 31, 2016.

Endocrine disruptors include dioxins, polychlorinated biphenyls (PCBs), dichloro diphenyl trichloroethane (DDT), and some other pesticides. Suspected endocrine disruptors include phytoestrogens and fungal estrogens, the herbicide atrazine, phenols such as BPA (bisphenol A), and plasticizers such as phthalates. Many products and industrial processes use and release several naturally–occurring heavy metals that affect hormone actions and reproduction, including arsenic, cadmium, lead, and mercury.

Some endocrine disruptors known to cause harmful human health effects have been banned in the United States. Even some prescription drugs like DES (diethylstilbestrol) have had unexpected effects on the endocrine system. The general use of DDT has been banned by the U.S. Environmental Protection Agency (EPA) because it posed unacceptable risks to the environment and potential harm to human health.

How Might I Be Exposed to Endocrine Disruptors?

Chemicals that might be endocrine disruptors are commonplace in daily life. You can be exposed to endocrine disruptors by breathing, eating, drinking, or touching them. Exposure can occur through air, water, soil, food, and consumer products. You may be exposed through contaminated food, contaminated groundwater or drinking water, combustion sources, and contaminants in consumer products.

At home, you can be exposed to minute amounts of possible endocrine disruptors through food, beverages, and medicines. You can be exposed if you use products that contain endocrine disruptors, such as plastics, cleaning products, bottles, and cans. You can be exposed if you eat contaminated species, including contaminated fish. You can be exposed to the herbicide atrazine if you live or work on a farm.

You may be exposed if you use pesticides and other garden chemicals. You can be exposed by leakage from landfill areas. Sewage discharge and runoff may carry pollution that includes endocrine disruptors from factories, fields, and yards into waterways.

At work, you may be exposed to endocrine disruptors if you work at a facility that manufactures products or uses processes containing these chemicals or burns medical waste. You may be exposed if you work on a farm or facility that uses pesticides and herbicides.

How Can Endocrine Disruptors Affect My Health?

Different types of endocrine disruptors can affect your health in different ways. It is important to remember that the amount of exposure to an endocrine disruptor may be as important as how toxic the endocrine disruptor is. According to the World Health Organization's (WHO's) International Programme on Chemical Safety, there is still uncertainty about some links between human health effects and exposure to endocrine disruptors. Some endocrine disruptors are listed as human carcinogens or as "reasonably anticipated to be human carcinogens" in the *Thirteenth Report on Carcinogens* published by the National Toxicology Program (NTP). Arsenic, cadmium, and 2,3,7,8-Tetrachlorodibenzo-p-dioxin (TCDD dioxin) are human carcinogens. DDT, lead, PCBs, and di(2-ethylhexyl) phthalates are anticipated to be human carcinogens.

Endocrine disruptors may interfere with the production or activity of hormones in the endocrine system. They may cause reduced fertility and an increase in some diseases, including endometriosis and some cancers. Human health concerns about endocrine disruptors include reproductive effects, such as sperm levels, reproductive abnormalities, and early puberty. Exposure of infants and fetuses to endocrine disruptors can affect the developing reproductive and nervous systems and organs. Other human health concerns include nervous system and immune functions.

If you think your health has been affected by exposure to endocrine disruptors, contact your healthcare professional.

For poisoning emergencies or questions about possible poisons, contact your local poison control center at 1-800-222-1222.

Chapter 6

Diagnostic Tests and Procedures for Endocrine and Metabolic Disorders

Diagnostic tests and procedures are vital tools that help physicians confirm or rule out the presence of a neurological disorder or other medical condition. A century ago, the only way to make a positive diagnosis for many neurological disorders was by performing an autopsy after a patient had died. But decades of basic research into the characteristics of disease, and the development of techniques that allow scientists to see inside the living brain and monitor nervous system activity as it occurs, have given doctors powerful and accurate tools to diagnose disease and to test how well a particular therapy may be working.

Perhaps the most significant changes in diagnostic imaging over the past 20 years are improvements in spatial resolution (size, intensity, and clarity) of anatomical images and reductions in the time needed to send signals to and receive data from the area being imaged. These advances allow physicians to simultaneously see the structure of the brain and the changes in brain activity as they occur. Scientists

This chapter includes text excerpted from "Neurological Diagnostic Tests and Procedures," National Institute of Neurological Disorders and Stroke (NINDS), November 19, 2015.

continue to improve methods that will provide sharper anatomical images and more detailed functional information.

Researchers and physicians use a variety of diagnostic imaging techniques and chemical and metabolic analyses to detect, manage, and treat neurological disease. Some procedures are performed in specialized settings, conducted to determine the presence of a particular disorder or abnormality. Many tests that were previously conducted in a hospital are now performed in a physician's office or at an outpatient testing facility, with little if any risk to the patient. Depending on the type of procedure, results are either immediate or may take several hours to process.

What Are Some of the More Common Screening Tests?

Laboratory screening tests of blood, urine, or other substances are used to help diagnose disease, better understand the disease process, and monitor levels of therapeutic drugs. Certain tests, ordered by the physician as part of a regular check-up, provide general information, while others are used to identify specific health concerns. For example, blood and blood product tests can detect brain and/or spinal cord infection, bone marrow disease, hemorrhage, blood vessel damage, toxins that affect the nervous system, and the presence of antibodies that signal the presence of an autoimmune disease. Blood tests are also used to monitor levels of therapeutic drugs used to treat epilepsy and other neurological disorders. Genetic testing of DNA extracted from white cells in the blood can help diagnose Huntington disease and other congenital diseases. Analysis of the fluid that surrounds the brain and spinal cord can detect meningitis, acute and chronic inflammation, rare infections, and some cases of multiple sclerosis. Chemical and metabolic testing of the blood can indicate protein disorders, some forms of muscular dystrophy and other muscle disorders, and diabetes. Urinalysis can reveal abnormal substances in the urine or the presence or absence of certain proteins that cause diseases including the mucopolysaccharidoses.

Genetic testing or counseling can help parents who have a family history of a neurological disease determine if they are carrying one of the known genes that cause the disorder or find out if their child is affected. Genetic testing can identify many neurological disorders, including spina bifida, in utero (while the child is inside the mother's womb). Genetic tests include the following:

- Amniocentesis, usually done at 14–16 weeks of pregnancy, tests a sample of the amniotic fluid in the womb for genetic defects

(the fluid and the fetus have the same DNA). Under local anesthesia, a thin needle is inserted through the woman's abdomen
and into the womb. About 20 milliliters of fluid (roughly 4
teaspoons) is withdrawn and sent to a lab for evaluation. Test
results often take 1–2 weeks.

- Chorionic villus sampling (CVS), is performed by removing and
  testing a very small sample of the placenta during early pregnancy. The sample, which contains the same DNA as the fetus,
  is removed by catheter or fine needle inserted through the cervix
  or by a fine needle inserted through the abdomen. It is tested for
  genetic abnormalities and results are usually available within
  2 weeks. CVS should not be performed after the tenth week of
  pregnancy.

- Uterine ultrasound is performed using a surface probe with gel.
  This noninvasive test can suggest the diagnosis of conditions
  such as chromosomal disorders.

What Is a Neurological Examination?

A neurological examination assesses motor and sensory skills, the
functioning of one or more cranial nerves, hearing and speech, vision,
coordination and balance, mental status, and changes in mood or
behavior, among other abilities. Items including a tuning fork, flash-
light, reflex hammer, ophthalmoscope, and needles are used to help
diagnose brain tumors, infections such as encephalitis and meningitis,
and diseases such as Parkinson disease, Huntington disease, amyo-
trophic lateral sclerosis (ALS), and epilepsy. Some tests require the
services of a specialist to perform and analyze results.

X-rays of the patient's chest and skull are often taken as part of a
neurological work-up. X-rays can be used to view any part of the body,
such as a joint or major organ system. Fluoroscopy is a type of X-ray
that uses a continuous or pulsed beam of low-dose radiation to produce
continuous images of a body part in motion. Fluoroscopy can be used
to evaluate the flow of blood through arteries.

What Are Some Diagnostic Tests Used to Diagnose Neurological Disorders?

Based on the result of a neurological exam, physical exam, patient
history, X-rays of the patient's chest and skull, and any previous
screening or testing, physicians may order one or more of the following

diagnostic tests to determine the specific nature of a suspected neurological disorder or injury. These diagnostics generally involve either nuclear medicine imaging, in which very small amounts of radioactive materials are used to study organ function and structure, or diagnostic imaging, which uses magnets and electrical charges to study human anatomy.

The following list of available procedures—in alphabetical rather than sequential order—includes some of the more common tests used to help diagnose a neurological condition.

- Angiography is a test used to detect blockages of the arteries or veins. A cerebral angiogram can detect the degree of narrowing or obstruction of an artery or blood vessel in the brain, head, or neck. It is used to diagnose stroke and to determine the location and size of a brain tumor, aneurysm, or vascular malformation.

- Biopsy involves the removal and examination of a small piece of tissue from the body. Muscle or nerve biopsies are used to diagnose neuromuscular disorders and may also reveal if a person is a carrier of a defective gene that could be passed on to children.

- Brain scans are imaging techniques used to diagnose tumors, blood vessel malformations, or hemorrhage in the brain. These scans are used to study organ function or injury or disease to tissue or muscle. Types of brain scans include computed tomography, magnetic resonance imaging, and positron emission tomography.

- Cerebrospinal fluid analysis involves the removal of a small amount of the fluid that protects the brain and spinal cord. The fluid is tested to detect any bleeding or brain hemorrhage, diagnose infection to the brain and/or spinal cord, identify some cases of multiple sclerosis and other neurological conditions, and measure intracranial pressure.

- Computed tomography (CT) scan, is a noninvasive, painless process used to produce rapid, clear two-dimensional images of organs, bones, and tissues. Neurological CT scans are used to view the brain and spine. They can detect bone and vascular irregularities, certain brain tumors and cysts, herniated discs, epilepsy, encephalitis, spinal stenosis (narrowing of the spinal canal), a blood clot or intracranial bleeding in patients with stroke, brain damage from head injury, and other disorders.

- Discography is often suggested for patients who are considering lumbar surgery or whose lower back pain has not responded to conventional treatments. This outpatient procedure is usually performed at a testing facility or a hospital.

- An intrathecal contrast-enhanced CT scan (also called cisternography) is used to detect problems with the spine and spinal nerve roots. This test is most often performed at an imaging center.

- Electroencephalography (EEG), monitors brain activity through the skull. EEG is used to help diagnose certain seizure disorders, brain tumors, brain damage from head injuries, inflammation of the brain and/or spinal cord, alcoholism, certain psychiatric disorders, and metabolic and degenerative disorders that affect the brain. EEGs are also used to evaluate sleep disorders, monitor brain activity when a patient has been fully anesthetized or loses consciousness, and confirm brain death.

- Electromyography, or EMG, is used to diagnose nerve and muscle dysfunction and spinal cord disease. It records the electrical activity from the brain and/or spinal cord to a peripheral nerve root (found in the arms and legs) that controls muscles during contraction and at rest. An EMG is usually done in conjunction with a nerve conduction velocity (NCV) test, which measures electrical energy by assessing the nerve's ability to send a signal. This two-part test is conducted most often in a hospital.

- Electronystagmography (ENG) describes a group of tests used to diagnose involuntary eye movement, dizziness, and balance disorders, and to evaluate some brain functions. The test is performed at an imaging center.

- Evoked potentials (also called evoked response) measure the electrical signals to the brain generated by hearing, touch, or sight. These tests are used to assess sensory nerve problems and confirm neurological conditions including multiple sclerosis, brain tumor, acoustic neuroma (small tumors of the inner ear), and spinal cord injury.

- Magnetic resonance imaging (MRI) uses computer-generated radio waves and a powerful magnetic field to produce detailed images of body structures including tissues, organs, bones, and nerves. Neurological uses include the diagnosis of brain and spinal cord tumors, eye disease, inflammation, infection, and vascular irregularities that may lead to stroke. MRI can also detect and monitor degenerative disorders such as multiple sclerosis and can document brain injury from trauma.

- Myelography involves the injection of a water- or oil-based contrast dye into the spinal canal to enhance X-ray imaging of the spine. Myelograms are used to diagnose spinal nerve injury, herniated discs, fractures, back or leg pain, and spinal tumors.

- Positron emission tomography (PET) scans provide two- and three-dimensional pictures of brain activity by measuring radioactive isotopes that are injected into the bloodstream. PET scans of the brain are used to detect or highlight tumors and diseased tissue, measure cellular and/or tissue metabolism, show blood flow, evaluate patients who have seizure disorders that do not respond to medical therapy and patients with certain memory disorders, and determine brain changes following injury or drug abuse, among other uses.

- A polysomnogram measures brain and body activity during sleep. It is performed over one or more nights at a sleep center.

- Single photon emission computed tomography (SPECT), a nuclear imaging test involving blood flow to tissue, is used to evaluate certain brain functions. The test may be ordered as a follow-up to an MRI to diagnose tumors, infections, degenerative spinal disease, and stress fractures.

- Thermography uses infrared sensing devices to measure small temperature changes between the two sides of the body or within a specific organ. Also known as digital infrared thermal imaging, thermography may be used to detect vascular disease of the head and neck, soft tissue injury, various neuromusculoskeletal disorders, and the presence or absence of nerve root compression.

- Ultrasound imaging, also called ultrasound scanning or sonography, uses high-frequency sound waves to obtain images inside the body. Neurosonography (ultrasound of the brain and spinal column) analyzes blood flow in the brain and can diagnose stroke, brain tumors, hydrocephalus (build-up of cerebrospinal fluid in the brain), and vascular problems. It can also identify or rule out inflammatory processes causing pain.

Chapter 7

Comprehensive Metabolic Panel

A comprehensive metabolic panel (CMP) is a blood test that provides information about:

- how the kidney and liver are functioning
- sugar (glucose) and protein levels in the blood
- the body's electrolyte and fluid balance

Why It's Done

A CMP may be ordered as part of routine medical exam or physical, or to help diagnose conditions such as diabetes, or liver or kidney disease. The CMP may also be used to monitor chronic conditions, or when a patient is taking medications that can cause certain side effects. The CMP helps evaluate:

- Glucose, a type of sugar used by the body for energy. Abnormal levels can indicate diabetes or hypoglycemia (low blood sugar).

- Calcium, which plays an important role in muscle contraction, transmitting messages through the nerves, and the release of hormones. Elevated or decreased calcium levels may indicate

---

a hormone imbalance or problems with the kidneys, bones, or pancreas.

• Albumin and total blood protein, which are needed to build and maintain muscles, bones, blood, and organ tissue. The CMP measures albumin specifically (the major blood protein produced by the liver), as well as the amount of all proteins in the blood. Low levels may indicate liver or kidney disease or nutritional problems.

• Sodium, potassium, carbon dioxide, and chloride (electrolytes), which help regulate the body's fluid levels and its acid-base balance. They also play a role in regulating heart rhythm, muscle contraction, and brain function. Abnormal levels also may occur with heart disease, kidney disease, or dehydration.

• Blood urea nitrogen (BUN) and creatinine, which are waste products filtered out of the blood by the kidneys. Increased concentrations in the blood may signal a decrease in kidney function.

• Alkaline phosphatase (ALP), alanine amino transferase (ALT), aspartate amino transferase (AST), and bilirubin; ALP, ALT, and AST are liver enzymes; bilirubin is produced by the liver. Elevated concentrations may indicate liver dysfunction.

Preparation

It may help to have your child wear a short-sleeved shirt to allow easier access for the technician to draw the blood. Usually no special preparation is needed, but sometimes your doctor may ask for the test to be performed after fasting. That means your child may be asked not to eat for 8 to 12 hours before the test.

The Procedure

A health professional will usually draw the blood from a vein. For an infant, the blood may be obtained by puncturing the heel with a small needle (lancet). If the blood is being drawn from a vein, the skin surface is cleaned with antiseptic, and an elastic band (tourniquet) is placed around the upper arm to apply pressure and cause the veins to swell with blood. A needle is inserted into a vein (usually in the arm inside of the elbow or on the back of the hand) and blood is withdrawn and collected in a vial or syringe.

After the procedure, the elastic band is removed. Once the blood has been collected, the needle is removed and the area is covered with cotton or a bandage to stop the bleeding. Collecting blood for this test will only take a few minutes.

What to Expect

Either method (heel or vein withdrawal) of collecting a sample of blood is only temporarily uncomfortable and can feel like a quick pinprick. Afterward, there may be some mild bruising, which should go away in a few days.

Getting the Results

The blood sample will be processed by a machine. Parts of a CMP may be available in minutes in an emergency, but more commonly the full test results come after a few hours or the next day.

If any of the CMP results are abnormal, further testing may be necessary to determine what's causing the problem and how to treat it.

Risks

The CMP test is considered a safe procedure. However, as with many medical tests, some problems can occur with having blood drawn, such as:

- fainting or feeling lightheaded

- hematoma (blood accumulating under the skin causing a lump or bruise)

- pain associated with multiple punctures to locate a vein

Chapter 8

Prenatal Tests

What Do Prenatal Tests Find?

Prenatal tests can help identify health problems that could endanger both a woman and her unborn child, some of which are treatable. However, these tests do have limitations. As an expectant parent, it's important to educate yourself about them and to think about what you would do if a health problem was detected in either you or your baby.

Prenatal tests are given in the first, second, and third trimesters. In a mother, they can determine key things about her health that can affect her baby's health, such as:

- her blood type
- whether she has gestational diabetes, anemia, or other health conditions
- her immunity to certain diseases
- whether she has a sexually transmitted disease (STD) or cervical cancer

In a developing child, prenatal tests can identify:

- treatable health problems that can affect the baby's health
- characteristics of the baby, including size, sex, age, and placement in the uterus

---

Text in this chapter is excerpted from "Prenatal Tests: FAQs," © 1995–2016. The Nemours Foundation/KidsHealth®. Reprinted with permission.

- the chance that a baby has certain birth defects or genetic problems

- certain types of fetal abnormalities, like heart problems

The last two items on this list may seem the same, but there's a key difference. Some prenatal tests are screening tests and only reveal the possibility of a problem. Other prenatal tests are diagnostic, which means that they can determine—with a fair degree of certainty—whether a fetus has a specific problem. In the interest of making the more specific determination, the screening test may be followed by a diagnostic test.

Who Gets Prenatal Tests?

Certain prenatal tests are considered routine—that is, almost all pregnant women receiving prenatal care get them. They include things like checking urine levels for protein, sugar, or signs of infection.

Other non-routine tests are recommended only for certain women, especially those with high-risk pregnancies. These may include women who:

- are age 35 or older

- are adolescents

- have had a premature baby

- have had a baby with a birth defect—especially heart or genetic problems

- are carrying more than one baby

- have high blood pressure, diabetes, lupus, heart disease, kidney problems, cancer, a sexually transmitted disease, asthma, or a seizure disorder

- have an ethnic background in which genetic disorders are common (or a partner who does)

- have a family history of mental retardation (or a partner who does)

Although your healthcare provider (who may be your OB-GYN, family doctor, or a certified nurse-midwife) may recommend these tests, it's ultimately up to you to decide whether to have them.

Also, if you or your partner have a family history of genetic problems, you may want to consult with a genetic counselor to help you look at the history of problems in your family and to determine the risk to your children.

To decide which tests are right for you, it's important to carefully discuss with your healthcare provider:

- what these tests are supposed to measure

- how reliable they are

- the potential risks

- your options and plans if the results indicate a disorder or defect

Where Can I Get More Information?

Some prenatal tests can be stressful, and because many aren't definitive, even a negative result may not completely relieve any anxiety you might be experiencing. Because many women who have abnormal tests end up having healthy babies and because some of the problems that are detected can't be treated, some women decide not to have some of the tests.

One important thing to consider is what you'll do in the event that a birth defect or chromosomal abnormality is discovered. Your healthcare provider or a genetic counselor can help you establish priorities, give you the facts, and discuss your options.

It's also important to remember that tests are offered to women— they are not mandatory. You should feel free to ask your healthcare provider why he or she is ordering a certain test, what the risks and benefits are, and, most important, what the results will—and won't— tell you.

If you think that your healthcare provider isn't answering your questions adequately, you should say so. Things you might want to ask include:

- How accurate is this test?

- What are you looking to get from these test results? What do you hope to learn?

- How long before I get the results?

- Is the procedure painful?

- Is the procedure dangerous to me or the fetus?

- Do the potential benefits outweigh the risks?

- What could happen if I don't undergo this test?

- How much will the test cost?

- Will the test be covered by insurance?

- What do I need to do to prepare?

You also can ask your healthcare provider for literature about each type of test.

How Can I Give My Baby a Good Start?

The best way for mothers-to-be to avoid birth defects and problems with the pregnancy is to take precautions, such as:

- not smoking (and avoiding secondhand smoke)

- avoiding alcohol and other drugs

- checking with the doctor about the safety of prescription and over-the-counter medications

- avoiding fumes, chemicals, radiation, and excessive heat

- eating a healthy diet

- taking prenatal vitamins—if possible, even before becoming pregnant

- getting exercise (after discussing it with the doctor)

- getting plenty of rest

- getting prenatal care—if possible, beginning with a preconception visit to the doctor to see if anything needs to change before you get pregnant

Chapter 9

Newborn Screening for Metabolic Disorders

About Newborn Screening

Newborn screening is the practice of testing every newborn for certain harmful or potentially fatal disorders that aren't otherwise apparent at birth.

Many of these are metabolic disorders (often called "inborn errors of metabolism") that interfere with the body's use of nutrients to maintain healthy tissues and produce energy. Other disorders that screening can detect include problems with hormones or the blood.

In general, metabolic and other inherited disorders can hinder an infant's normal physical and mental development in a variety of ways. And parents can pass along the gene for a certain disorder without even knowing that they're carriers.

With a simple blood test, doctors often can tell whether newborns have certain conditions that eventually could cause problems. Although these conditions are considered rare and most babies are given a clean bill of health, early diagnosis and proper treatment can make the difference between lifelong impairment and healthy development.

Text in this chapter is excerpted from "Newborn Screening Tests," © 1995–2016. The Nemours Foundation/KidsHealth®. Reprinted with permission.

Screening: Past, Present, and Future

In the early 1960s, scientist Robert Guthrie, PhD, developed a blood test that could determine whether newborns had the metabolic disorder phenylketonuria (PKU). People with PKU lack an enzyme needed to process the amino acid phenylalanine, which is necessary for normal growth in kids and for normal protein use throughout life. However, if too much phenylalanine builds up, it damages brain tissue and eventually can cause substantial developmental delay.

If kids born with PKU are put on a special diet right away, they can avoid the developmental delay the condition caused in past generations and lead normal lives.

Since the development of the PKU test, researchers have developed additional blood tests that can screen newborns for other disorders that, unless detected and treated early, can cause physical problems, developmental delay, and in some cases, death.

The federal government has set no national standards, so screening requirements vary from state to state and are determined by individual state public health departments. Many states have mandatory newborn screening programs, but parents can refuse the testing for their infant if they choose.

Almost all states now screen for more than 30 disorders. One screening technique, the tandem mass spectrometry (or MS/MS), can screen for more than 20 inherited metabolic disorders with a single drop of blood.

Which Tests Are Offered?

Traditionally, state decisions about what to screen for have been based on weighing the costs against the benefits. "Cost" considerations include:

- the risk of false positive results (and the worry they cause)

- the availability of treatments known to help the condition

- financial costs

So what can you do? Your best strategy is to stay informed. Discuss this issue with both your obstetrician or healthcare provider and your future baby's doctor before you give birth. Know what tests are routinely done in your state and in the hospital where you'll deliver (some hospitals go beyond what's required by state law).

If your state isn't offering screening for the expanded panel of disorders, you may want to ask your doctors about supplemental screening, though you'll probably have to pay for additional tests yourself.

If you're concerned about whether your infant was screened for certain conditions, ask your child's doctor for information about which tests were done and whether further tests are recommended.

Newborn screening varies by state and is subject to change, especially given advancements in technology. However, the disorders listed here are the ones typically included in newborn screening programs.

PKU

When this disorder is detected early, feeding an infant a special formula low in phenylalanine can prevent mental retardation. A low-phenylalanine diet will need to be followed throughout childhood and adolescence and perhaps into adult life. This diet cuts out all high-protein foods, so people with PKU often need to take a special artificial formula as a nutritional substitute.

Incidence: 1 in 10,000 to 25,000.

Congenital Hypothyroidism

This is the disorder most commonly identified by routine screening. Affected babies don't have enough thyroid hormone and so develop retarded growth and brain development. (The thyroid, a gland at the front of the neck, releases chemical substances that control metabolism and growth.)

If the disorder is detected early, a baby can be treated with oral doses of thyroid hormone to permit normal development.

Incidence: 1 in 4,000.

Galactosemia

Babies with galactosemia lack the enzyme that converts galactose (one of two sugars found in lactose) into glucose, a sugar the body is able to use. As a result, milk (including breast milk) and other dairy products must be eliminated from the diet. Otherwise, galactose can build up in the system and damage the body's cells and organs, leading to blindness, severe mental retardation, growth deficiency, and even death.

Incidence: 1 in 60,000 to 80,000. Several less severe forms of galactosemia that may be detected by newborn screening may not require any intervention.

Sickle Cell Disease

Sickle cell disease is an inherited blood disease in which red blood cells mutate into abnormal "sickle" shapes and can cause episodes of pain, damage to vital organs such as the lungs and kidneys, and even death. Young children with sickle cell disease are especially prone to certain dangerous bacterial infections, such as pneumonia (inflammation of the lungs) and meningitis (inflammation of the brain and spinal cord).

Studies suggest that newborn screening can alert doctors to begin antibiotic treatment before infections occur and to monitor symptoms of possible worsening more closely. The screening test can also detect other disorders affecting hemoglobin (the oxygen-carrying substance in the blood).

Incidence: about 1 in every 500 African-American births and 1 in every 1,000 to 1,400 Hispanic-American births; also occurs with some frequency among people of Mediterranean, Middle Eastern, and South Asian descent.

Biotinidase Deficiency

Babies with this condition don't have enough biotinidase, an enzyme that recycles biotin (a B vitamin) in the body. The deficiency may cause seizures, poor muscle control, immune system impairment, hearing loss, mental retardation, coma, and even death. If the deficiency is detected in time, however, problems can be prevented by giving the baby extra biotin.

Incidence: 1 in 72,000 to 126,000.

Congenital Adrenal Hyperplasia

This is actually a group of disorders involving a deficiency of certain hormones produced by the adrenal gland. It can affect the development of the genitals and may cause death due to loss of salt from the kidneys. Lifelong treatment through supplementation of the missing hormones manages the condition.

Incidence: 1 in 12,000.

Maple Syrup Urine Disease (MSUD)

Babies with MSUD are missing an enzyme needed to process three amino acids that are essential for the body's normal growth. When not processed properly, these can build up in the body, causing urine to smell like maple syrup or sweet, burnt sugar. These babies usually have little appetite and are extremely irritable.

If not detected and treated early, MSUD can cause mental retardation, physical disability, and even death. A carefully controlled diet that cuts out certain high-protein foods containing those amino acids can prevent this. Like people with PKU, those with MSUD are often given a formula that supplies the necessary nutrients missed in the special diet they must follow.

Incidence: 1 in 250,000.

Tyrosinemia

Babies with this amino acid metabolism disorder have trouble processing the amino acid tyrosine. If it accumulates in the body, it can cause mild retardation, language skill difficulties, liver problems, and even death from liver failure. Treatment requires a special diet and sometimes a liver transplant. Early diagnosis and treatment seem to offset long-term problems, although more information is needed.

Incidence: not yet determined. Some babies have a mild self-limited form of tyrosinemia.

Cystic Fibrosis

Cystic fibrosis (CF) is a genetic disorder that particularly affects the lungs and digestive system and makes kids who have it more vulnerable to repeated lung infections. There is no known cure—treatment involves trying to prevent serious lung infections (sometimes with antibiotics) and providing adequate nutrition. Early detection may help doctors reduce the problems associated with CF, but the real impact of newborn screening has yet to be determined.

Incidence: 1 in 2,000 Caucasian babies; less common in African-Americans, Hispanics, and Asians.

MCAD Deficiency

MCAD (medium chain acyl CoA dehydrogenase) deficiency is a fatty acid metabolism disorder. Kids who have it are prone to repeated episodes of low blood sugar (hypoglycemia), which can cause seizures and interfere with normal growth and development. Treatment involves making sure kids don't fast (skip meals) and supplies extra nutrition (usually by intravenous nutrients) when they're ill. Early detection and treatment can help affected children live normal lives.

Toxoplasmosis

Toxoplasmosis is a parasitic infection that can be transmitted through the mother's placenta to an unborn child. The disease-causing organism can invade the brain, eye, and muscles, possibly resulting in blindness and mental retardation. The benefit of early detection and treatment is uncertain.

Incidence: 1 in 1,000. But only one or two states screen for toxoplasmosis.

Hearing Screening

Most but not all states require newborns hearing to be screened before they're discharged from the hospital. If your baby isn't examined then, be sure that he or she does get screened within the first 3 weeks of life.

Kids develop critical speaking and language skills in their first few years. A hearing loss that's caught early can be treated to help prevent interference with that development.

Should I Request Additional Tests?

If you answer "yes" to any of these questions, talk to your doctor and perhaps a genetic counselor about additional tests:

• Do you have a family history of an inherited disorder?

• Have you previously given birth to a child who's affected by a disorder?

• Did an infant in your family die because of a suspected metabolic disorder?

• Do you have another reason to believe that your child may be at risk for a certain condition?

How Screening Is Done

In the first 2 or 3 days of life, your baby's heel will be pricked to obtain a small blood sample for testing. Most states have a state or regional laboratory perform the analyses, although some use a private lab.

It's generally recommended that the sample be taken after the first 24 hours of life. Some tests, such as the one for PKU, may not be as sensitive if they're done too soon after birth. However, because mothers and newborns are often discharged within a day, some babies may be tested within the first 24 hours. If this happens, experts recommend that a repeat sample be taken no more than 1 to 2 weeks later. It's especially important that the PKU screening test be run again for accurate results. Some states routinely do two tests on all infants.

Getting the Results

Different labs have different procedures for notifying families and pediatricians of the results. Some may send the results to the hospital where your child was born and not directly to your child's doctor, which may mean a delay in getting the results to you.

And although some states have a system that allows doctors to access the results via phone or computer, others may not. Ask your doctor how you'll get the results and when you should expect them.

If a test result comes back abnormal, try not to panic. This does not necessarily mean that your child has the disorder in question. A screening test is not the same as diagnostic test. The initial screening provides only preliminary information that must be followed up with more specific diagnostic testing.

If testing confirms that your child does have a disorder, your doctor may refer you to a specialist for further evaluation and treatment. Keep in mind that dietary restrictions and supplements, along with proper medical supervision, often can prevent most of the serious physical and mental problems that were associated with metabolic disorders in the past.

You also may wonder whether the disorder can be passed on to any future children. You'll want to discuss this with your doctor and perhaps a genetic counselor. Also, if you have other children who weren't screened for the disorder, consider having testing done. Again, speak with your doctor.

Chapter 10

Genetics and Chromosome Abnormalities

Genetics research studies how individual genes or groups of genes are involved in health and disease. Understanding genetic factors and genetic disorders is important in learning more about preventing birth defects, developmental disabilities, and other unique conditions among children.

Some genetic changes have been associated with an increased risk of having a child with a birth defect or developmental disability. Genetics also can help us understand how birth defects and developmental disabilities happen.

How We Get Our Genes

People get (inherit) their chromosomes, which contain their genes, from their parents. Chromosomes come in pairs and humans have 46 chromosomes, in 23 pairs. Children randomly get one of each pair of chromosomes from their mother and one of each pair from their father. The chromosomes that form the 23rd pair are called the sex chromosomes. They decide if a person is male or female. A female has two X chromosomes, and a male has one X and one Y chromosome. Each

This chapter contains text excerpted from the following sources: Text in this chapter begins with excerpts from "Family Health History and Genetics," Centers for Disease Control and Prevention (CDC), March 3, 2015; Text beginning with the heading "What Are Chromosomes?" is excerpted from "Chromosome Abnormalities," National Human Genome Research Institute (NHGRI), January 6, 2016.

daughter gets an X from her mother and an X from her father. Each son gets an X from his mother and a Y from his father.

Genetic Disorders

Genetic disorders can happen for many reasons. Genetic disorders often are described in terms of the chromosome that contains the gene. If the gene is on one of the first 22 pairs of chromosomes, called the autosomes, the genetic disorder is called an autosomal condition. If the gene is on the X chromosome, the disorder is called X-linked.

Genetic disorders also are grouped by how they run in families. Disorders can be dominant or recessive, depending on how they cause conditions and how they run in families.

Dominant

Dominant diseases can be caused by only one copy of a gene with a DNA mutation. If one parent has the disease, each child has a 50 percent chance of inheriting the mutated gene.

Recessive

For recessive diseases, both copies of a gene must have a DNA mutation in order to get one of these diseases. If both parents have one copy of the mutated gene, each child has a 25 percent chance of having the disease, even though neither parent has it. In such cases, each parent is called a carrier of the disease. They can pass the disease on to their children, but do not have the disease themselves.

Single Gene Disorders

Some genetic diseases are caused by a DNA mutation in one of a person's genes. For example, suppose part of a gene usually has the sequence TAC. A mutation can change the sequence to TTC in some people. This change in sequence can change the way that the gene works, for example by changing the protein that is made. Mutations can be passed down to a child from his or her parents. Or, it can happen for the first time in the sperm or egg, so that the child will have the mutation but the parents will not. Single gene disorders can be autosomal or X-linked.

For example, sickle cell disease is an autosomal single gene disorder. It is caused by a mutation in a gene found on chromosome 11. Sickle cell disease causes anemia and other complications. Fragile X syndrome, on the other hand, is an X-linked single gene disorder. It is caused by a change in a gene on the X chromosome. It is the most common known cause of intellectual disability and developmental disability that can be inherited (passed from one generation to the next).

Complex Conditions

A complex disease is caused by both genes and environmental factors. Complex diseases are also called multifactorial. Many birth defects and developmental disabilities are complex conditions. For example, while some orofacial clefts are associated with single gene disorders, the majority most likely are caused by changes in several genes acting together with environmental exposures.

What Are Chromosomes?

Chromosomes are the structures that hold genes. Genes are the individual instructions that tell our bodies how to develop and function; they govern physical and medical characteristics, such as hair color, blood type and susceptibility to disease.

Many chromosomes have two segments, called "arms," separated by a pinched region known as the centromere. The shorter arm is called the "p" arm. The longer arm is called the "q" arm.

How Many Chromosomes Do Humans Have?

The typical number of chromosomes in a human cell is 46: 23 pairs, holding an estimated total of 20,000 to 25,000 genes. One set of 23 chromosomes is inherited from the biological mother (from the egg), and the other set is inherited from the biological father (from the sperm).

Of the 23 pairs of chromosomes, the first 22 pairs are called "autosomes." The final pair is called the "sex chromosomes." Sex chromosomes determine an individual's sex: females have two X chromosomes (XX), and males have an X and a Y chromosome (XY). The mother and father each contribute one set of 22 autosomes and one sex chromosome.

What Are Chromosome Abnormalities?

There are many types of chromosome abnormalities. However, they can be organized into two basic groups: numerical abnormalities and structural abnormalities.

- **Numerical Abnormalities:** When an individual is missing one of the chromosomes from a pair, the condition is called monosomy. When an individual has more than two chromosomes instead of a pair, the condition is called trisomy.

An example of a condition caused by numerical abnormalities is Down syndrome, which is marked by mental retardation, learning difficulties, a characteristic facial appearance and poor muscle tone (hypotonia) in infancy. An individual with Down syndrome has three copies of chromosome 21 rather than two; for that reason, the condition is also known as Trisomy 21. An example of monosomy, in which an individual lacks a chromosome, is Turner syndrome. In Turner syndrome, a female is born with only one sex chromosome, an X, and is usually shorter than average and unable to have children, among other difficulties.

- **Structural Abnormalities:** A chromosome's structure can be altered in several ways.

- **Deletions:** A portion of the chromosome is missing or deleted.

- **Duplications:** A portion of the chromosome is duplicated, resulting in extra genetic material.

- **Translocations:** A portion of one chromosome is transferred to another chromosome. There are two main types of translocation. In a reciprocal translocation, segments from two different chromosomes have been exchanged. In a Robertsonian translocation, an entire chromosome has attached to another at the centromere.

- **Inversions:** A portion of the chromosome has broken off, turned upside down, and reattached. As a result, the genetic material is inverted.

- **Rings:** A portion of a chromosome has broken off and formed a circle or ring. This can happen with or without loss of genetic material.

Most chromosome abnormalities occur as an accident in the egg or sperm. In these cases, the abnormality is present in every cell of the body. Some abnormalities, however, happen after conception; then some cells have the abnormality and some do not.

Chromosome abnormalities can be inherited from a parent (such as a translocation) or be "*de novo*" (new to the individual). This is why, when a child is found to have an abnormality, chromosome studies are often performed on the parents.

How Do Chromosome Abnormalities Happen?

Chromosome abnormalities usually occur when there is an error in cell division. There are two kinds of cell division, mitosis and meiosis.

- **Mitosis** results in two cells that are duplicates of the original cell. One cell with 46 chromosomes divides and becomes two cells with 46 chromosomes each. This kind of cell division occurs throughout the body, except in the reproductive organs. This is the way most of the cells that make up our body are made and replaced.

- **Meiosis** results in cells with half the number of chromosomes, 23, instead of the normal 46. This is the type of cell division that occurs in the reproductive organs, resulting in the eggs and sperm.

In both processes, the correct number of chromosomes is supposed to end up in the resulting cells. However, errors in cell division can result in cells with too few or too many copies of a chromosome. Errors can also occur when the chromosomes are being duplicated.

Other factors that can increase the risk of chromosome abnormalities are:

- **Maternal Age:** Women are born with all the eggs they will ever have. Some researchers believe that errors can crop up in the eggs' genetic material as they age. Older women are at higher risk of giving birth to babies with chromosome abnormalities than younger women. Because men produce new sperm throughout their lives, paternal age does not increase risk of chromosome abnormalities.

- **Environment:** Although there is no conclusive evidence that specific environmental factors cause chromosome abnormalities, it is still possible that the environment may play a role in the occurrence of genetic errors.

Chapter 11

Genetic Counseling

If you and your partner are newly pregnant, you may be amazed at the number and variety of prenatal tests available to you. Blood tests, urine tests, monthly medical exams, screening tests, and family history tracking—each helps to assess the health of you and your baby, and to predict any potential health risks.

You may also have the option of genetic testing. These tests identify the likelihood of passing certain genetic diseases or disorders (those caused by a defect in the genes—the tiny, DNA-containing units of heredity that determine the characteristics and functioning of the entire body) to your children.

Some of the more familiar genetic disorders are:

- Down syndrome

- Cystic fibrosis

- Sickle cell disease

- Tay-sachs disease (a fatal disease affecting the central nervous system)

If your history suggests that genetic testing would be helpful, you may be referred to a genetic counselor. Or, you might decide to seek out genetic counseling yourself.

But what do genetic counselors do, and how can they help your family?

What Is Genetic Counseling?

Genetic counseling is the process of:

- evaluating family history and medical records

- ordering genetic tests

- evaluating the results of this investigation

- helping parents understand and reach decisions about what to do next

Genetic tests are done by analyzing small samples of blood or body tissues. They determine whether you, your partner, or your baby carry genes for certain inherited disorders.

Genes are made up of DNA molecules, which are the building blocks of heredity. They're grouped together in specific patterns within a person's chromosomes, forming the unique "blueprint" for every physical and biological characteristic of that person.

Humans have 46 chromosomes, arranged in pairs in every living cell of our bodies. When the egg and sperm join at conception, half of each chromosomal pair is inherited from each parent. This newly formed combination of chromosomes then copies itself again and again during fetal growth and development, passing identical genetic information to each new cell in the growing fetus.

Current science suggests that every human has about 25,000 genes per cell. An error in just one gene (and in some instances, even the alteration of a single piece of DNA) can sometimes be the cause for a serious medical condition.

Some diseases, such as Huntington disease (a degenerative nerve disease) and Marfan syndrome (a connective tissue disorder), can be inherited from just one parent. But most disorders, including cystic fibrosis, sickle cell anemia, and Tay-Sachs disease, cannot occur unless both the mother and father pass along the gene.

Other genetic conditions, such as Down syndrome, are usually not inherited. In general, they result from an error (mutation) in the cell division process during conception or fetal development. Still others, such as achondroplasia (the most common form of dwarfism), may either be inherited or the result of a genetic mutation.

Genetic tests don't yield easy-to-understand results. They can reveal the presence, absence, or malformation of genes or chromosomes. Deciphering what these complex tests mean is where a genetic counselor comes in.

About Genetic Counselors

Genetic counselors are professionals who have completed a master's program in medical genetics and counseling skills. They then pass a certification exam administered by the American Board of Genetic Counseling.

Genetic counselors can help identify and interpret the risks of an inherited disorder, explain inheritance patterns, suggest testing, and lay out possible scenarios. (They refer you to a doctor or a laboratory for the actual tests.) They will explain the meaning of the medical science involved, provide support, and address any emotional issues raised by the results of the genetic testing.

Who Should See One?

Most couples planning a pregnancy or who are expecting don't need genetic counseling. About 3 percent of babies are born with birth defects each year, according to the Centers for Disease Control and Prevention (CDC)—and of the malformations that do occur, the most common are also among the most treatable. Cleft palate and clubfoot, two of the more common birth defects, can be surgically repaired, as can many heart malformations.

The best time to seek genetic counseling is before becoming pregnant, when a counselor can help assess your risk factors. But even after you become pregnant, a meeting with a genetic counselor can still be helpful. A genetic counselor can help determine what testing is appropriate for your pregnancy.

Experts recommend that all pregnant women, regardless of age or circumstance, be offered genetic counseling and testing to screen for Down syndrome.

It's especially important to consider genetic counseling if any of the following risk factors apply to you:

- A standard prenatal screening test (such as the alpha fetoprotein test) yields an abnormal result.

- An amniocentesis yields an unexpected result (such as a chromosomal defect in the unborn baby).

- Either parent or a close relative has an inherited disease or birth defect.

- Either parent already has children with birth defects, intellectual disabilities, or genetic disorders.

- The mother-to-be has had two or more miscarriages or babies that died in infancy.

- The mother-to-be will be 35 or older when the baby is born. Chances of having a child with Down syndrome increase with the mother's age: a woman has about a 1 in 350 chance of conceiving a child with Down syndrome at age 35, a 1 in 110 chance at age 40, and a 1 in 30 chance at age 45.

- You are concerned about genetic defects that occur frequently in certain ethnic or racial groups. For example, couples of African descent are most at risk for having a child with sickle cell anemia; couples of central or Eastern European Ewish (Ashekenazi), Cajun, or Irish descent may be carriers of Tay-Sachs disease; and couples of Italian, Greek, Middle Eastern, Southern Asian, or African descent may carry the gene for thalassemia, a red blood cell disorder.

- Either parent is concerned about the effects of exposures they have had to radiation, medications, illegal drugs, infections, or chemicals.

Finding a Genetic Counselor

Working with a genetic counselor can be reassuring and informative, especially if you or your partner have known risk factors. Talk to your doctor if you feel you would benefit from genetic counseling. Many doctors have a list of local genetic counselors they work with.

Meeting with a Genetic Counselor

Before you meet with a genetic counselor in person, you may be asked to gather information about your family history. The counselor will want to know of any relatives with genetic disorders, multiple miscarriages, and early or unexplained deaths. The counselor will also want to look over your medical records, including any ultrasounds, prenatal test results, past pregnancies, and medications you may have taken before or during pregnancy.

When you meet with the counselor, you'll go over any gaps or potential problem areas in your family or medical history. The counselor can help you understand the inheritance patterns of any potential disorders and help assess your chances of having a child with those disorders.

The counselor will distinguish between risks that every pregnancy faces and risks that you personally face. Even if you discover you have a particular problem gene, science can't always predict the severity of the related disease. For instance, a child with cystic fibrosis can have debilitating lung problems or, less commonly, milder respiratory symptoms.

If more tests are necessary, the counselor will help you set up those appointments and track the paperwork. When the results come in, the counselor will call you with the news and may ask you to come in for another discussion.

After Counseling

Genetic counselors can help you understand your options and adjust to any uncertainties you face, but you and your family will have to decide what to do next.

If you've learned before conception that you and/or your partner are at high risk for having a child with a severe or fatal defect, your options might include:

- Pre-implantation diagnosis—when eggs that have been fertilized in vitro (in a laboratory, outside of the womb) are tested for defects at the 8-cell (blastocyst) stage, and only nonaffected blastocysts are implanted in the uterus to establish a pregnancy.

- Using donor sperm or donor eggs.

- Adoption

- Taking the risk and having a child.

- Establishing pregnancy and have specific prenatal testing.

If you've received a diagnosis of a severe or fatal defect after conception, your options might include:

- Preparing yourself for the challenges you'll face when you have your baby.

- Fetal surgery to repair the defect before birth (surgery can only be used to treat some defects, such as spina bifida or congenital diaphragmatic hernia, a hole in the diaphragm that can cause severely underdeveloped lungs. Most defects cannot be surgically repaired.)

- Ending the pregnancy.

For some families, knowing that they'll have an infant with a severe or fatal genetic condition seems too much to bear. Other families are able to adapt to the news—and to the birth—remarkably well.

Genetic counselors can share the experiences they've had with other families in your situation. But they will not suggest a particular course of action. A genetic counselor understands that what is right for one family may not be right for another.

Genetic counselors can, however, refer you to specialists for further help. For instance, many babies with Down syndrome are born with heart defects. Your counselor might encourage you to meet with a cardiologist to discuss heart surgery, and a neonatologist to discuss the care of a post-operative newborn. Genetic counselors can also refer you to social workers, support groups, or mental health professionals to help you adjust to and prepare for your complex new reality.

Chapter 12

Genetic Testing

What Is Genetic Testing?

Genetic testing is a type of medical test that identifies changes in chromosomes, genes, or proteins. The results of a genetic test can confirm or rule out a suspected genetic condition or help determine a person's chance of developing or passing on a genetic disorder. More than 1,000 genetic tests are currently in use, and more are being developed.

Several methods can be used for genetic testing:

- Molecular genetic tests (or gene tests) study single genes or short lengths of DNA to identify variations or mutations that lead to a genetic disorder.

- Chromosomal genetic tests analyze whole chromosomes or long lengths of DNA to see if there are large genetic changes, such as an extra copy of a chromosome, that cause a genetic condition.

- Biochemical genetic tests study the amount or activity level of proteins; abnormalities in either can indicate changes to the DNA that result in a genetic disorder.

Genetic testing is voluntary. Because testing has benefits as well as limitations and risks, the decision about whether to be tested is a

This chapter includes text excerpted from "Genetic Testing," Genetics Home Reference (GHR), National Institutes of Health (NIH), October 4, 2016.

personal and complex one. A geneticist or genetic counselor can help by providing information about the pros and cons of the test and discussing the social and emotional aspects of testing.

What Are the Types of Genetic Tests?

Genetic testing can provide information about a person's genes and chromosomes. Available types of testing include:

Newborn Screening

Newborn screening is used just after birth to identify genetic disorders that can be treated early in life. Millions of babies are tested each year in the United States. All states currently test infants for phenylketonuria (a genetic disorder that causes intellectual disability if left untreated) and congenital hypothyroidism (a disorder of the thyroid gland). Most states also test for other genetic disorders.

Diagnostic Testing

Diagnostic testing is used to identify or rule out a specific genetic or chromosomal condition. In many cases, genetic testing is used to confirm a diagnosis when a particular condition is suspected based on physical signs and symptoms. Diagnostic testing can be performed before birth or at any time during a person's life, but is not available for all genes or all genetic conditions. The results of a diagnostic test can influence a person's choices about healthcare and the management of the disorder.

Carrier Testing

Carrier testing is used to identify people who carry one copy of a gene mutation that, when present in two copies, causes a genetic disorder. This type of testing is offered to individuals who have a family history of a genetic disorder and to people in certain ethnic groups with an increased risk of specific genetic conditions. If both parents are tested, the test can provide information about a couple's risk of having a child with a genetic condition.

Prenatal Testing

Prenatal testing is used to detect changes in a fetus's genes or chromosomes before birth. This type of testing is offered during pregnancy if there is an increased risk that the baby will have a genetic or chromosomal disorder. In some cases, prenatal testing can lessen a couple's uncertainty or help them make decisions about a pregnancy. It cannot identify all possible inherited disorders and birth defects, however.

Preimplantation Testing

Preimplantation testing, also called preimplantation genetic diagnosis (PGD), is a specialized technique that can reduce the risk of having a child with a particular genetic or chromosomal disorder. It is used to detect genetic changes in embryos that were created using assisted reproductive techniques such as in-vitro fertilization. In-vitro fertilization involves removing egg cells from a woman's ovaries and fertilizing them with sperm cells outside the body. To perform preimplantation testing, a small number of cells are taken from these embryos and tested for certain genetic changes. Only embryos without these changes are implanted in the uterus to initiate a pregnancy.

Predictive and Presymptomatic Testing

Predictive and presymptomatic types of testing are used to detect gene mutations associated with disorders that appear after birth, often later in life. These tests can be helpful to people who have a family member with a genetic disorder, but who have no features of the disorder themselves at the time of testing. Predictive testing can identify mutations that increase a person's risk of developing disorders with a genetic basis, such as certain types of cancer. Presymptomatic testing can determine whether a person will develop a genetic disorder, such as hereditary hemochromatosis (an iron overload disorder), before any signs or symptoms appear. The results of predictive and presymptomatic testing can provide information about a person's risk of developing a specific disorder and help with making decisions about medical care.

Forensic Testing

Forensic testing uses DNA sequences to identify an individual for legal purposes. Unlike the tests described above, forensic testing is not used to detect gene mutations associated with disease. This type of testing can identify crime or catastrophe victims, rule out or implicate a crime suspect, or establish biological relationships between people (for example, paternity).

How Is Genetic Testing Done?

Once a person decides to proceed with genetic testing, a medical geneticist, primary care doctor, specialist, or nurse practitioner can order the test. Genetic testing is often done as part of a genetic consultation.

Genetic tests are performed on a sample of blood, hair, skin, amniotic fluid (the fluid that surrounds a fetus during pregnancy), or other tissue. For example, a procedure called a buccal smear uses a small brush or cotton swab to collect a sample of cells from the inside surface of the cheek. The sample is sent to a laboratory where technicians look for specific changes in chromosomes, DNA, or proteins, depending on the suspected disorder. The laboratory reports the test results in writing to a person's doctor or genetic counselor, or directly to the patient if requested.

Newborn screening tests are done on a small blood sample, which is taken by pricking the baby's heel. Unlike other types of genetic testing, a parent will usually only receive the result if it is positive. If the test result is positive, additional testing is needed to determine whether the baby has a genetic disorder.

Before a person has a genetic test, it is important that he or she understands the testing procedure, the benefits and limitations of the test, and the possible consequences of the test results. The process of educating a person about the test and obtaining permission is called informed consent.

What Are the Benefits of Genetic Testing?

Genetic testing has potential benefits whether the results are positive or negative for a gene mutation. Test results can provide a sense of relief from uncertainty and help people make informed decisions about managing their healthcare. For example, a negative result can eliminate the need for unnecessary checkups and screening tests in some cases. A positive result can direct a person toward available prevention, monitoring, and treatment options. Some test results can also help people make decisions about having children. Newborn screening can identify genetic disorders early in life so treatment can be started as early as possible.

What Are the Risks and Limitations of Genetic Testing?

The physical risks associated with most genetic tests are very small, particularly for those tests that require only a blood sample or buccal smear (a procedure that samples cells from the inside surface of the cheek). The procedures used for prenatal testing carry a small but real risk of losing the pregnancy (miscarriage) because they require a sample of amniotic fluid or tissue from around the fetus.

Many of the risks associated with genetic testing involve the emotional, social, or financial consequences of the test results. People may feel angry, depressed, anxious, or guilty about their results. In some cases, genetic testing creates tension within a family because the results can reveal information about other family members in addition to the person who is tested. The possibility of genetic discrimination in employment or insurance is also a concern.

Genetic testing can provide only limited information about an inherited condition. The test often can't determine if a person will show symptoms of a disorder, how severe the symptoms will be, or whether the disorder will progress over time. Another major limitation is the lack of treatment strategies for many genetic disorders once they are diagnosed.

A genetics professional can explain in detail the benefits, risks, and limitations of a particular test. It is important that any person who is considering genetic testing understand and weigh these factors before making a decision.

Part Two

The Pituitary Gland and Growth Disorders

Chapter 13

Growth Disorders in Children

Lately, it seems as though your child is looking up to classmates— literally. The other kids in the class have been getting taller and developing into young adults, but your child's growth seems to be lagging behind. Classmates now tower over your child.

Is something wrong? Maybe, maybe not. Some kids just grow more slowly than others because their parents did, too. But others may have an actual growth disorder, which is any type of problem that prevents kids from meeting realistic expectations of growth, from failure to gain height and weight in young children to short stature or delayed sexual development in teens.

Variations of Normal Growth Patterns

A couple of differences seen in the growth patterns of normal children include these common conditions, which are not growth disorders:

Constitutional growth delay: This condition describes children who are small for their ages but who are growing at a normal rate. They usually have a delayed "bone age," which means that their skeletal maturation is younger than their age in years. (Bone age is measured by taking an X-ray of the hand and wrist and comparing it with standard X-ray findings seen in kids the same age.)

These children don't have any signs or symptoms of diseases that affect growth. They tend to reach puberty later than their peers do,

---

Text in this chapter is excerpted from "What Is a Growth Disorder?" © 1995– 2016. The Nemours Foundation/KidsHealth®. Reprinted with permission.

with delay in the onset of sexual development and the pubertal growth spurt. But because they continue to grow until an older age, they tend to catch up to their peers when they reach adult height. One or both parents or other close relatives often had a similar "late-bloomer" growth pattern.

Familial (or genetic) short stature: This is a condition in which shorter parents tend to have shorter children. This term applies to short children who don't have any symptoms of diseases that affect their growth. Kids with familial short stature still have growth spurts and enter puberty at normal ages, but they usually will only reach a height similar to that of their parents.

With both constitutional growth delay and familial short stature, kids and families need to be reassured that the child does not have a disease or medical condition that poses a threat to health or that requires treatment.

However, because they may be short or may not enter puberty when their classmates do, some may need extra help coping with teasing or reassurance that they will go through full sexual development eventually. In a few children who are very short or very late entering puberty, hormone treatment may be helpful.

Growth Disorders

Diseases of the kidneys, heart, gastrointestinal tract, lungs, bones, or other body systems might affect growth. Other symptoms or physical signs in kids with these illnesses usually give clues as to the disease causing the growth delay. However, poor growth can be the first sign of a problem in some.

Growth disorders include:

Failure to thrive, which isn't a specific growth disorder itself, but can be a sign of an underlying condition causing growth problems. Although it's common for newborns to lose a little weight in the first few days, failure to thrive is a condition in which some infants continue to show slower-than-expected weight gain and growth. Usually caused by inadequate nutrition or a feeding problem, it's most common in kids younger than age 3. It may also be a symptom of another problem, such as an infection, a digestive problem, or child neglect or abuse.

Endocrine diseases (diseases involving hormones, the chemical messengers of the body) involve a deficiency or excess of hormones and can be responsible for growth failure during childhood and adolescence. Growth hormone deficiency is a disorder that involves the pituitary gland (the small gland at the base of the brain that secretes several hormones, including growth hormone). A damaged or malfunctioning pituitary gland may not produce enough hormones for normal growth. Hypothyroidism is a condition in which the thyroid gland fails to make enough thyroid hormone, which is essential for normal bone growth.

Turner syndrome, one of the most common genetic growth disorders, occurs in girls and is a syndrome in which there's a missing or abnormal X chromosome. In addition to short stature, girls with Turner syndrome usually don't undergo normal sexual development because their ovaries (the sex organs that produce eggs and female hormones) fail to mature and function normally.

Diagnosing a Growth Disorder

The tests a doctor may recommend to detect a growth disorder depend on the findings at each step of evaluation. A short child who's healthy and growing at a normal rate may just be observed throughout childhood, but one who has stopped growing or is growing more slowly than expected will often need additional testing.

Your doctor or an endocrinologist will look for signs of the many possible causes of short stature and growth failure. Blood tests may be done to look for hormone and chromosome abnormalities and to rule out other diseases associated with growth failure. A bone age X-ray might be done and special scans (such as an MRI) can check the pituitary gland for abnormalities.

To measure the ability of the pituitary gland to produce growth hormone, the doctor (usually a pediatric endocrinologist) may do a growth hormone stimulation test. This involves giving the child medications that cause the pituitary gland to secrete growth hormone, then drawing several small blood samples over time to check growth hormone levels.

Treating a Growth Disorder

Although the treatment of a growth problem usually isn't urgent, earlier diagnosis and treatment can help some kids catch up with peers and increase their final height.

If an underlying medical condition is identified, specific treatment may result in improved growth. Growth failure due to hypothyroidism, for example, is usually treated with thyroid hormone replacement pills.

Growth hormone injections for children with growth hormone deficiency, Turner syndrome, and chronic kidney failure may help kids reach a more normal height. Human growth hormone is generally considered safe and effective, although full treatment may take many years and not all kids will have a good response. And the treatment can be costly (about $20,000 to $30,000 per year), although many health insurance plans cover it.

What about growth hormone treatment for short children who aren't growth hormone deficient when tested? The U.S. Food and Drug Administration (FDA) has approved its use in such children if they're predicted to reach a very short final height (under 4 feet 11 inches [150 centimeters] for a girl; under 5 feet 4 inches [163 centimeters] for a boy).

Talk with your doctor for more information about treatment options if you're concerned.

Helping Your Child

You can boost your child's self-esteem by providing positive reinforcement and emphasizing other characteristics, like intelligence, personality, and talents. Try to take the focus off of height as a measure of social acceptance.

Kids who are very self-conscious about their size might need help in coping. In some cases, evaluation and treatment by a mental health professional may be needed.

If You Suspect a Problem

If you're concerned about your child's growth, speak with your doctor, who may refer you to a pediatric endocrinologist, who can help diagnose and treat specific growth disorders.

It's also important to watch for the social and emotional problems that kids with growth disorders face. It's not easy being the shortest kid in the class and it's never any fun being teased. Helping your child build self-esteem and emphasizing strengths—regardless of how tall he or she may grow—might be just what the doctor ordered.

Chapter 14

Isolated Growth Hormone Deficiency

What Is Isolated Growth Hormone Deficiency?

Isolated growth hormone deficiency is a condition caused by a severe shortage or absence of growth hormone. Growth hormone is a protein that is necessary for the normal growth of the body's bones and tissues. Because they do not have enough of this hormone, people with isolated growth hormone deficiency commonly experience a failure to grow at the expected rate and have unusually short stature. This condition is usually apparent by early childhood.

There are four types of isolated growth hormone deficiency differentiated by the severity of the condition, the gene involved, and the inheritance pattern.

1. Isolated growth hormone deficiency type IA is caused by an absence of growth hormone and is the most severe of all the types. In people with type IA, growth failure is evident in infancy as affected babies are shorter than normal at birth.

2. People with isolated growth hormone deficiency type IB produce very low levels of growth hormone. As a result, type IB is characterized by short stature, but this growth failure is

---

This chapter includes text excerpted from "Isolated Growth Hormone Deficiency," Genetics Home Reference (GHR), National Institutes of Health (NIH), October 4, 2016.

typically not as severe as in type IA. Growth failure in people with type IB is usually apparent in early to mid-childhood.

3. Individuals with isolated growth hormone deficiency type II have very low levels of growth hormone and short stature that varies in severity. Growth failure in these individuals is usually evident in early to mid-childhood. It is estimated that nearly half of the individuals with type II have underdevelopment of the pituitary gland (pituitary hypoplasia). The pituitary gland is located at the base of the brain and produces many hormones, including growth hormone.

4. Isolated growth hormone deficiency type III is similar to type II in that affected individuals have very low levels of growth hormone and short stature that varies in severity. Growth failure in type III is usually evident in early to mid-childhood. People with type III may also have a weakened immune system and are prone to frequent infections. They produce very few B cells, which are specialized white blood cells that help protect the body against infection (agammaglobulinemia).

Frequency

The incidence of isolated growth hormone deficiency is estimated to be 1 in 4,000 to 10,000 individuals worldwide.

Genetic Changes

Isolated growth hormone deficiency is caused by mutations in one of at least three genes. Isolated growth hormone deficiency types IA and II are caused by mutations in the *GH1* gene. Type IB is caused by mutations in either the *GH1* or *GHRHR* gene. Type III is caused by mutations in the *BTK* gene.

The *GH1* gene provides instructions for making the growth hormone protein. Growth hormone is produced in the pituitary gland and plays a major role in promoting the body's growth. Growth hormone also plays a role in various chemical reactions (metabolic processes) in the body. Mutations in the *GH1* gene prevent or impair the production of growth hormone. Without sufficient growth hormone, the body fails to grow at its normal rate, resulting in slow growth and short stature as seen in isolated growth hormone deficiency types IA, IB, and II.

The *GHRHR* gene provides instructions for making a protein called the growth hormone releasing hormone receptor (GHRHR).

This receptor attaches (binds) to a molecule called growth hormone releasing hormone. The binding of growth hormone releasing hormone to the receptor triggers the production of growth hormone and its release from the pituitary gland. Mutations in the *GHRHR* gene impair the production or release of growth hormone. The resulting shortage of growth hormone prevents the body from growing at the expected rate. Decreased growth hormone activity due to *GHRHR* gene mutations is responsible for many cases of isolated growth hormone deficiency type IB.

The *BTK* gene provides instructions for making a protein called Bruton tyrosine kinase (BTK), which is essential for the development and maturation of immune system cells called B cells. The BTK protein transmits important chemical signals that instruct B cells to mature and produce special proteins called antibodies. Antibodies attach to specific foreign particles and germs, marking them for destruction. It is unknown how mutations in the *BTK* gene contribute to short stature in people with isolated growth hormone deficiency type III.

Some people with isolated growth hormone deficiency do not have mutations in the *GH1*, *GHRHR*, or *BTK* genes. In these individuals, the cause of the condition is unknown. When this condition does not have an identified genetic cause, it is known as idiopathic isolated growth hormone deficiency.

Inheritance Pattern

Isolated growth hormone deficiency can have different inheritance patterns depending on the type of the condition.

Isolated growth hormone deficiency types IA and IB are inherited in an autosomal recessive pattern, which means both copies of the *GH1* or *GHRHR* gene in each cell have mutations. The parents of an individual with an autosomal recessive condition each carry one copy of the mutated gene, but they typically do not show signs and symptoms of the condition.

Isolated growth hormone deficiency type II can be inherited in an autosomal dominant pattern, which means a mutation in one copy of the *GH1* gene in each cell is sufficient to cause the disorder. This condition can also result from new mutations in the *GH1* gene and occur in people with no history of the disorder in their family.

Isolated growth hormone deficiency type III, caused by mutations in the *BTK* gene, is inherited in an X-linked recessive pattern. The *BTK* gene is located on the X chromosome, which is one of the two sex chromosomes. In males (who have only one X chromosome), one altered copy of the gene in each cell is sufficient to cause the condition. In females (who have two X chromosomes), a mutation would have to occur in both copies of the gene to cause the disorder. Because it is unlikely that females will have two altered copies of this gene, males are affected by X-linked recessive disorders much more frequently than females. A characteristic of X-linked inheritance is that fathers cannot pass X-linked traits to their sons.

Other Names for This Condition

- Dwarfism, growth hormone deficiency

- Dwarfism, pituitary

- Growth hormone deficiency dwarfism

- Isolated GH deficiency

- Isolated HGH deficiency

- Isolated human growth hormone deficiency

- Isolated somatotropin deficiency

- Isolated somatotropin deficiency disorder

Chapter 15

Growth Hormone Evaluation Process

Growth hormone (GH), sometimes called human growth hormone (hGH) or somatotropin, is a substance secreted by the pituitary gland that controls such functions as growth, cell reproduction, cell regeneration, and a healthy balance of fat, muscle, and bone. In children, too little GH can cause abnormal shortness, and too much can cause gigantism (acromegaly). In adults, an excess of GH can cause bones to thicken, those in the extremities and face to increase in size, and the person's appearance to change significantly, while a GH deficiency can result in such issues as excess fat in the abdomen, weakened muscle tone, osteoporosis, and high cholesterol levels. Of the two disorders, GH deficiency is by far the more common, and acromegaly is very rare in children.

GH disorders in children are usually the result of a problem with the hypothalamus—the part of the brain that, among other functions, controls the endocrine system—causing it to fail to stimulate the pituitary gland. An underactive hypothalamus is also possible in adults, but it is quite rare. More commonly, GH abnormalities in adults are caused by damage to the pituitary gland, such as might be caused by brain surgery, radiation treatment for a brain tumor, surgery to remove a pituitary tumor, or a traumatic head injury.

Testing for GH disorders primarily measures pituitary gland function and blood hormone levels. The examinations and test procedures, which are similar for children and adults, typically begin with a physical exam, in which the doctor will evaluate the patient's height, weight, and overall body proportions. If a visual examination raises concerns, measurements may be taken and compared to age-appropriate standards. But the primary way GH is tested is through a variety of blood tests and other evaluative procedures that are usually overseen by an endocrinologist, a physician who specializes in the endocrine system, which controls hormones.

Blood Tests for Growth Hormone Levels

Blood for GH testing is generally drawn in a doctor's office or clinic. No special preparation is normally required, although, depending on the specific tests, the patient may be asked to fast prior to the test or to stop taking regularly prescribed medication for a certain period beforehand. GH blood tests can include:

- **GH stimulation test.** This test, done after a 10–12-hour fast, checks for growth hormone deficiency by measuring the level of GH in the blood after the injection of substances, such as arginine, clonidine, and glucagon, which trigger the pituitary gland to release GH. By taking blood samples at timed intervals over several hours before, during, and after these injections are given, medical professionals are able to test accurately for GH levels.

- **GH suppression test.** Used to diagnose acromegaly, or an excess of GH, this test entails taking a blood sample after the patient has fasted for 10–12 hours. He or she is then given a large amount of glucose (sugar) solution, and blood samples are drawn at intervals. When tested for GH levels, these can help determine how much the pituitary gland has been suppressed from producing growth hormone.

- **Binding protein levels tests.** Generally done prior to GH testing, these tests (IGF-1 and IGFBP-3) evaluate pituitary function by measuring the amount of insulin-like growth factor (IGF) in the blood. Fasting is not required, and samples can be taken in a single blood draw. Unlike GH, whose levels fluctuate throughout the day, IGF tends to remain stable, making it reliable for gauging average GH levels. Low readings indicate GH deficiency and high levels are an indication of GH overproduction.

- **Insulin tolerance test.** Used in GH evaluation to measure pituitary function, this test involves injecting the patient with insulin through an IV to induce hypoglycemia, or low blood sugar. In response to this condition, among other bodily reactions, the pituitary gland releases GH. Measuring this response, facilitated by drawing blood at intervals, provides a means of assessing the gland's health. Note that hypoglycemia carries some risk, so this test is generally performed in a hospital setting so the patient can be monitored continuously and treated if necessary.

A number of other blood tests may be performed to evaluate the function of the pituitary and thyroid glands. Most of these are done before GH testing is ordered and may include checking the levels of various hormones, such as free LH, T4, TSH, cortisol, and testosterone. If abnormalities are found, the conditions indicated by these tests are normally treated with medication prior to proceeding to GH testing.

Other Tests Used to Evaluate Growth Hormone Issues

Although blood testing is the most common way to evaluate GH disorders, a number of other tests may be ordered help in the diagnosis or to rule out other conditions. These may include:

- **Head X-Rays.** By X-raying the patient's head, a doctor may be able to detect any problems related to growth of the skull, such as enlarged sinuses, thickening of the calvaria (skull cap), or enlarged sella turcica (the skull cavity that holds the pituitary gland).

- **Hand X-Rays.** X-rays of the hand can reveal bone-development issues. By comparing hand and wrist radiographs to established standards, and comparing apparent bone age to the patient's chronological age, the doctor may be able to begin the diagnosis of GH problems or other disorders.

- **Brain MRI or CT scan.** A clear picture of the brain can help the doctor assess abnormalities in the pituitary gland and hypothalamus. An MRI (magnetic resonance imaging) does this with a magnetic field, radio waves, and a computer, while a CT (computerized tomography) scan creates pictures using X-ray images and a computer.

- **DXA.** Dual X-ray absorptometry (DXA) is a method of measuring bone density, which can be an indication of GH disorders. It works by scanning the patient with two X-ray beams, one high energy and one low energy. By comparing the level of radiation that passes through the bone from each beam, an accurate determination of bone density can be made.

Risks

There are very few risks associated with most tests for GH disorders. And scans, such as X-rays, MRIs, and CTs, carry virtually no risk and generally cause no discomfort to the patient. There are, however, some slight risks with blood testing that may include:

- **Minor discomfort.** An injection or the insertion of an IV needle may cause discomfort in some patients. This is especially true in cases in which the medical professional has difficulty locating a suitable blood vessel.

- **Bruising.** Some patients experience bruising, or hematoma, at the site of the injection or IV. This can be minimized by keeping pressure on the site for a short time.

- **Fainting.** Occasionally patients may faint or feel light-headed during the testing procedures. Lying quietly for several minutes usually provides relief.

- **Excessive bleeding.** Certain blood-thinning medications, such as aspirin and warfarin, can increase the risk of bleeding. If a patient is taking such medicine, or if he or she has a bleeding disorder, the doctor should be informed prior to the blood draw.

- **Infection.** Any time the skin is broken, as when a needle is inserted for blood testing, there is at least a slight risk of infection. The individual administering the test will take appropriate precautions, but patients should be made aware of proper after-care procedures to guard against infection.

- **Phlebitis.** This is the inflammation of a vein caused by a blood clot. In rare instances, this can occur after a blood draw. It can usually be treated with warm compresses, although in some cases the doctor may prescribe anti-inflammatory medication to help relieve the symptoms.

- **Medication issues.** Some of the drugs in testing, such as those used to stimulate the pituitary, can cause side effects. For instance, the medication used in the insulin tolerance may, in very rare cases, cause heart palpitations or even loss of consciousness. In addition, some prescription drugs can interfere with GH test results. Examples include dopamine and estrogens, which can increase GH levels, and corticosteroids and phenothiazines, which can decrease levels.

References

1. Carmichael, Kim A., MD, FACP. "Growth Hormone Testing," Mount Sinai Hospital, December 2014.

2. Cook, David, MD. "Adult Growth Hormone Deficiency," The Magic Foundation, n.d.

3. Gentile, Julie M. "Growth Hormone Deficiency Diagnosis," EndocrineWeb.com, May 27, 2014.

4. "Growth Hormone," American Association for Clinical Chemistry, March 23, 2015.

5. Romito, Kathleen, MD. "Growth Hormone," WebMD.com, November 20, 2015.

Chapter 16

Acromegaly

What Is Acromegaly?

Acromegaly is a hormonal disorder that results from too much growth hormone (GH) in the body. The pituitary, a small gland in the brain, makes GH. In acromegaly, the pituitary produces excessive amounts of GH. Usually the excess GH comes from benign, or non-cancerous, tumors on the pituitary. These benign tumors are called adenomas.

Acromegaly is most often diagnosed in middle-aged adults, although symptoms can appear at any age. If not treated, acromegaly can result in serious illness and premature death. Acromegaly is treatable in most patients, but because of its slow and often "sneaky" onset, it often is not diagnosed early or correctly. The most serious health consequences of acromegaly are type 2 diabetes, high blood pressure, increased risk of cardiovascular disease, and arthritis. Patients with acromegaly are also at increased risk for colon polyps, which may develop into colon cancer if not removed.

When GH-producing tumors occur in childhood, the disease that results is called gigantism rather than acromegaly. A child's height is determined by the length of the so-called long bones in the legs. In response to GH, these bones grow in length at the growth plates—areas near either end of the bone. Growth plates fuse after puberty, so the

This chapter includes text excerpted from "Acromegaly," National Institute of Diabetes and Digestive and Kidney Diseases (NIDDK), April 2012. Reviewed October 2016.

excessive GH production in adults does not result in increased height. However, prolonged exposure to excess GH before the growth plates fuse causes increased growth of the long bones and thus increased height. Pediatricians may become concerned about this possibility if a child's growth rate suddenly and markedly increases beyond what would be predicted by previous growth and how tall the child's parents are.

What Are the Symptoms of Acromegaly?

The name acromegaly comes from the Greek words for "extremities" and "enlargement," reflecting one of its most common symptoms—the abnormal growth of the hands and feet. Swelling of the hands and feet is often an early feature, with patients noticing a change in ring or shoe size, particularly shoe width. Gradually, bone changes alter the patient's facial features: The brow and lower jaw protrude, the nasal bone enlarges, and the teeth space out.

Overgrowth of bone and cartilage often leads to arthritis. When tissue thickens, it may trap nerves, causing carpal tunnel syndrome, which results in numbness and weakness of the hands. Body organs, including the heart, may enlarge.

Other symptoms of acromegaly include:

- joint aches

- thick, coarse, oily skin

- skin tags

- enlarged lips, nose, and tongue

- deepening of the voice due to enlarged sinuses and vocal cords

- sleep apnea-breaks in breathing during sleep due to obstruction of the airway

- excessive sweating and skin odor

- fatigue and weakness

- headaches

- impaired vision

- abnormalities of the menstrual cycle and sometimes breast discharge in women

- erectile dysfunction in men

- decreased libido

What Causes Acromegaly?

Acromegaly is caused by prolonged overproduction of GH by the pituitary gland. The pituitary produces several important hormones that control body functions such as growth and development, reproduction, and metabolism. But hormones never seem to act simply and directly. They usually "cascade" or flow in a series, affecting each other's production or release into the bloodstream.

GH is part of a cascade of hormones that, as the name implies, regulates the physical growth of the body. This cascade begins in a part of the brain called the hypothalamus. The hypothalamus makes hormones that regulate the pituitary. One of the hormones in the GH series, or "axis," is growth hormone-releasing hormone (GHRH), which stimulates the pituitary gland to produce GH.

Secretion of GH by the pituitary into the bloodstream stimulates the liver to produce another hormone called insulin-like growth factor I (IGF-I). IGF-I is what actually causes tissue growth in the body. High levels of IGF-I, in turn, signal the pituitary to reduce GH production.

The hypothalamus makes another hormone called somatostatin, which inhibits GH production and release. Normally, GHRH, somatostatin, GH, and IGF-I levels in the body are tightly regulated by each other and by sleep, exercise, stress, food intake, and blood sugar levels. If the pituitary continues to make GH independent of the normal regulatory mechanisms, the level of IGF-I continues to rise, leading to bone overgrowth and organ enlargement. High levels of IGF-I also cause changes in glucose (sugar) and lipid (fat) metabolism and can lead to diabetes, high blood pressure, and heart disease.

Pituitary Tumors

In more than 95 percent of people with acromegaly, a benign tumor of the pituitary gland, called an adenoma, produces excess GH. Pituitary tumors are labeled either micro- or macro-adenomas, depending on their size. Most GH-secreting tumors are macro-adenomas, meaning they are larger than 1 centimeter. Depending on their location, these larger tumors may compress surrounding brain structures. For example, a tumor growing upward may affect the optic chiasm-where the optic nerves cross—leading to visual problems and vision loss. If the tumor grows to the side, it may enter an area of the brain called the cavernous sinus where there are many nerves, potentially damaging them.

Compression of the surrounding normal pituitary tissue can alter production of other hormones. These hormonal shifts can lead to changes in menstruation and breast discharge in women and erectile dysfunction in men. If the tumor affects the part of the pituitary that controls the thyroid—another hormone-producing gland—then thyroid hormones may decrease. Too little thyroid hormone can cause weight gain, fatigue, and hair and skin changes. If the tumor affects the part of the pituitary that controls the adrenal gland, the hormone cortisol may decrease. Too little cortisol can cause weight loss, dizziness, fatigue, low blood pressure, and nausea.

Some GH-secreting tumors may also secrete too much of other pituitary hormones. For example, they may produce prolactin, the hormone that stimulates the mammary glands to produce milk. Rarely, adenomas may produce thyroid-stimulating hormone. Doctors should assess all pituitary hormones in people with acromegaly.

Rates of GH production and the aggressiveness of the tumor vary greatly among people with adenomas. Some adenomas grow slowly and symptoms of GH excess are often not noticed for many years. Other adenomas grow more rapidly and invade surrounding brain areas or the venous sinuses, which are located near the pituitary gland. Younger patients tend to have more aggressive tumors. Regardless of size, these tumors are always benign.

Most pituitary tumors develop spontaneously and are not genetically inherited. They are the result of a genetic alteration in a single pituitary cell, which leads to increased cell division and tumor formation. This genetic change, or mutation, is not present at birth, but happens later in life. The mutation occurs in a gene that regulates the transmission of chemical signals within pituitary cells. It permanently switches on the signal that tells the cell to divide and secrete GH. The events within the cell that cause disordered pituitary cell growth and GH oversecretion currently are the subject of intensive research.

Nonpituitary Tumors

Rarely, acromegaly is caused not by pituitary tumors but by tumors of the pancreas, lungs, and other parts of the brain. These tumors also lead to excess GH, either because they produce GH themselves or, more frequently, because they produce GHRH, the hormone that stimulates the pituitary to make GH. When these non-pituitary tumors are surgically removed, GH levels fall and the symptoms of acromegaly improve.

In patients with GHRH-producing, non-pituitary tumors, the pituitary still may be enlarged and may be mistaken for a tumor. Physicians should carefully analyze all "pituitary tumors" removed from patients with acromegaly so they do not overlook the rare possibility that a tumor elsewhere in the body is causing the disorder.

How Common Is Acromegaly?

Small pituitary adenomas are common, affecting about 17 percent of the population. However, research suggests most of these tumors do not cause symptoms and rarely produce excess GH. Scientists estimate that three to four out of every million people develop acromegaly each year and about 60 out of every million people suffer from the disease at any time. Because the clinical diagnosis of acromegaly is often missed, these numbers probably underestimate the frequency of the disease.

How Is Acromegaly Diagnosed?

Blood Tests

If acromegaly is suspected, a doctor must measure the GH level in a person's blood to determine if it is elevated. However, a single measurement of an elevated blood GH level is not enough to diagnose acromegaly: Because GH is secreted by the pituitary in impulses, or spurts, its concentration in the blood can vary widely from minute to minute. At a given moment, a person with acromegaly may have a normal GH level, whereas a GH level in a healthy person may even be five times higher.

More accurate information is obtained when GH is measured under conditions that normally suppress GH secretion. Healthcare professionals often use the oral glucose tolerance test to diagnose acromegaly because drinking 75 to 100 grams of glucose solution lowers blood GH levels to less than 1 nanogram per milliliter (ng/ml) in healthy people. In people with GH overproduction, this suppression does not occur. The oral glucose tolerance test is a highly reliable method for confirming a diagnosis of acromegaly.

Physicians also can measure IGF-I levels, which increase as GH levels go up, in people with suspected acromegaly. Because IGF-I levels are much more stable than GH levels over the course of the day, they are often a more practical and reliable screening measure. Elevated IGF-I levels almost always indicate acromegaly. However, a pregnant woman's IGF-I levels are two to three times higher than normal. In addition, physicians must be aware that IGF-I levels decline with age and may also be abnormally low in people with poorly controlled diabetes or liver or kidney disease.

Imaging

After acromegaly has been diagnosed by measuring GH or IGF-I levels, a magnetic resonance imaging (MRI) scan of the pituitary is used to locate and detect the size of the tumor causing GH overproduction. MRI is the most sensitive imaging technique, but computerized tomography (CT) scans can be used if the patient should not have MRI.

If a head scan fails to detect a pituitary tumor, the physician should look for non-pituitary "ectopic" tumors in the chest, abdomen, or pelvis as the cause of excess GH. The presence of such tumors usually can be diagnosed by measuring GHRH in the blood and by a CT scan of possible tumor sites.

Rarely, a pituitary tumor secreting GH may be too tiny to detect even with a sensitive MRI scan.

How Is Acromegaly Treated?

The treatment options include:

- Surgical removal of the tumor
- Medical therapy
- Somatostatin analogs (SSAs)
- GH receptor antagonists (GHRAs)
- Dopamine agonists
- Radiation therapy of the pituitary
- Conventional radiation delivery
- Stereotactic delivery

Goals of treatment are to

- reduce excess hormone production to normal levels
- relieve the pressure that the growing pituitary tumor may be exerting on the surrounding brain areas
- preserve normal pituitary function or treat hormone deficiencies
- improve the symptoms of acromegaly

Which Treatment for Acromegaly Is Most Effective?

No single treatment is effective for all patients. Treatment should be individualized, and often combined, depending on patient characteristics such as age and tumor size.

If the tumor has not yet invaded surrounding nonpituitary tissues, removal of the pituitary adenoma by an experienced neurosurgeon is usually the first choice. Even if a cure is not possible, surgery may be performed if the patient has symptoms of neurological problems such as loss of peripheral vision or cranial nerve problems. After surgery, hormone levels are measured to determine whether a cure has been achieved. This determination can take up to 8 weeks because IGF-I lasts a long time in the body's circulation. If cured, a patient must be monitored for a long time for increasing GH levels.

If surgery does not normalize hormone levels or a relapse occurs, an endocrinologist should recommend additional drug therapy. With each medication, long-term therapy is necessary because their withdrawal can lead to rising GH levels and tumor re-expansion.

Radiation therapy is generally reserved for patients whose tumors are not completely removed by surgery, who are not good candidates for surgery because of other health problems, or who do not respond adequately to surgery and medication.

Chapter 17

Pituitary Cushing Disease

What Is Cushing Disease?

Cushing disease is caused by elevated levels of a hormone called cortisol, which leads to a wide variety of signs and symptoms. This condition usually occurs in adults between the ages of 20 and 50; however, children may also be affected. The first sign of this condition is usually weight gain around the trunk and in the face. Affected individuals may get stretch marks (striae) on their thighs and abdomen and bruise easily. Individuals with Cushing disease can develop a hump on their upper back caused by abnormal deposits of fat. People with this condition can have muscle weakness, severe tiredness, and progressively thin and brittle bones that are prone to fracture (osteoporosis). They also have a weakened immune system and are at an increased risk of infections. Cushing disease can cause mood disorders such as anxiety, irritability, and depression. This condition can also affect a person's concentration and memory. People with Cushing disease have an increased chance of developing high blood pressure (hypertension) and diabetes. Women with Cushing disease may experience irregular menstruation and have excessive hair growth (hirsutism) on their face, abdomen, and legs. Men with Cushing disease may have erectile dysfunction. Children with Cushing disease typically experience slow growth.

This chapter includes text excerpted from "Cushing Disease," Genetics Home Reference (GHR), National Institutes of Health (NIH), September 20, 2016.

Frequency

Cushing disease is estimated to occur in 10 to 15 per million people worldwide. For reasons that are unclear, Cushing disease affects females more often than males.

Genetic Changes

The genetic cause of Cushing disease is often unknown. In only a few instances, mutations in certain genes have been found to lead to Cushing disease. These genetic changes are called somatic mutations. They are acquired during a person's lifetime and are present only in certain cells. The genes involved often play a role in regulating the activity of hormones.

Cushing disease is caused by an increase in the hormone cortisol, which helps maintain blood sugar levels, protects the body from stress, and stops (suppresses) inflammation. Cortisol is produced by the adrenal glands, which are small glands located at the top of each kidney. The production of cortisol is triggered by the release of a hormone called adrenocorticotropic hormone (ACTH) from the pituitary gland, located at the base of the brain. The adrenal and pituitary glands are part of the hormone-producing (endocrine) system in the body that regulates development, metabolism, mood, and many other processes.

Cushing disease occurs when a noncancerous (benign) tumor called an adenoma forms in the pituitary gland, causing excessive release of ACTH and, subsequently, elevated production of cortisol. Prolonged exposure to increased cortisol levels results in the signs and symptoms of Cushing disease: changes to the amount and distribution of body fat, decreased muscle mass leading to weakness and reduced stamina, thinning skin causing stretch marks and easy bruising, thinning of the bones resulting in osteoporosis, increased blood pressure, impaired regulation of blood sugar leading to diabetes, a weakened immune system, neurological problems, irregular menstruation in women, and slow growth in children. The overactive adrenal glands that produce cortisol may also produce increased amounts of male sex hormones (androgens), leading to hirsutism in females. The effect of the excess androgens on males is unclear.

Most often, Cushing disease occurs alone, but rarely, it appears as a symptom of genetic syndromes that have pituitary adenomas as a feature, such as multiple endocrine neoplasia type 1 (MEN1) or familial isolated pituitary adenoma (FIPA).

Cushing disease is a subset of a larger condition called Cushing syndrome, which results when cortisol levels are increased by one of a number of possible causes. Sometimes adenomas that occur in organs or tissues other than the pituitary gland, such as adrenal gland adenomas, can also increase cortisol production, causing Cushing syndrome. Certain prescription drugs can result in an increase in cortisol production and lead to Cushing syndrome. Sometimes prolonged periods of stress or depression can cause an increase in cortisol levels; when this occurs, the condition is known as pseudo-Cushing syndrome. Not accounting for increases in cortisol due to prescription drugs, pituitary adenomas cause the vast majority of Cushing syndrome in adults and children.

Inheritance Pattern

Most cases of Cushing disease are sporadic, which means they occur in people with no history of the disorder in their family. Rarely, the condition has been reported to run in families; however, it does not have a clear pattern of inheritance.

The various syndromes that have Cushing disease as a feature can have different inheritance patterns. Most of these disorders are inherited in an autosomal dominant pattern, which means one copy of the altered gene in each cell is sufficient to cause the disorder.

Other Names for This Condition

- Hypercortisolism

- Pituitary ACTH hypersecretion

- Pituitary cushing syndrome

- Pituitary-dependant cushing syndrome

- Pituitary-dependant hypercortisolism

- Pituitary-dependant hypercortisolism disorder

Chapter 18

Diabetes Insipidus

What Is Diabetes Insipidus?

Diabetes insipidus is a rare disorder that occurs when a person's kidneys pass an abnormally large volume of urine that is insipid—dilute and odorless. In most people, the kidneys pass about 1 to 2 quarts of urine a day. In people with diabetes insipidus, the kidneys can pass 3 to 20 quarts of urine a day. As a result, a person with diabetes insipidus may feel the need to drink large amounts of liquids.

Diabetes insipidus and diabetes mellitus—which includes both type 1 and type 2 diabetes—are unrelated, although both conditions cause frequent urination and constant thirst. Diabetes mellitus causes high blood glucose, or blood sugar, resulting from the body's inability to use blood glucose for energy. People with diabetes insipidus have normal blood glucose levels; however, their kidneys cannot balance fluid in the body.

What Are the Kidneys and What Do They Do?

The kidneys are two bean-shaped organs, each about the size of a fist. They are located just below the rib cage, one on each side of the spine. Every day, the kidneys normally filter about 120 to 150 quarts of blood to produce about 1 to 2 quarts of urine, composed of wastes and extra fluid. The urine flows from the kidneys to the bladder through

This chapter includes text excerpted from "Diabetes Insipidus (DI)," National Institute of Diabetes and Digestive and Kidney Diseases (NIDDK), October 2015.

tubes called ureters. The bladder stores urine. When the bladder empties, urine flows out of the body through a tube called the urethra, located at the bottom of the bladder.

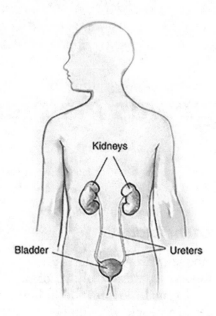

Figure 18.1. *Function of Kidneys*

Every day, the kidneys normally filter about 120 to 150 quarts of blood to produce about 1 to 2 quarts of urine.

How Is Fluid Regulated in the Body?

A person's body regulates fluid by balancing liquid intake and removing extra fluid. Thirst usually controls a person's rate of liquid intake, while urination removes most fluid, although people also lose fluid through sweating, breathing, or diarrhea. The hormone vasopressin, also called antidiuretic hormone, controls the fluid removal rate through urination. The hypothalamus, a small gland located at the base of the brain, produces vasopressin. The nearby pituitary gland stores the vasopressin and releases it into the bloodstream when the body has a low fluid level. Vasopressin signals the kidneys to absorb less fluid from the bloodstream, resulting in less urine. When the body has extra fluid, the pituitary gland releases smaller amounts of vasopressin, and sometimes none, so the kidneys remove more fluid from the bloodstream and produce more urine.

What Are the Types of Diabetes Insipidus?

The types of diabetes insipidus include:

- Central
- Dipsogenic
- Gestational
- Nephrogenic

Each type of diabetes insipidus has a different cause.

Central Diabetes Insipidus

Central diabetes insipidus happens when damage to a person's hypothalamus or pituitary gland causes disruptions in the normal production, storage, and release of vasopressin. The disruption of vasopressin causes the kidneys to remove too much fluid from the body, leading to an increase in urination. Damage to the hypothalamus or pituitary gland can result from the following:

- A tumor
- Head injury
- Infection
- Inflammation
- Surgery

Central diabetes insipidus can also result from an inherited defect in the gene that produces vasopressin, although this cause is rare. In some cases, the cause is unknown.

Nephrogenic Diabetes Insipidus

Nephrogenic diabetes insipidus occurs when the kidneys do not respond normally to vasopressin and continue to remove too much fluid from a person's bloodstream. Nephrogenic diabetes insipidus can result from inherited gene changes, or mutations, that prevent the kidneys from responding to vasopressin. Other causes of nephrogenic diabetes insipidus include:

- Blockage of the urinary tract
- Certain medications, particularly lithium

- Chronic kidney disease
- High calcium levels in the blood
- Low potassium levels in the blood

The causes of nephrogenic diabetes insipidus can also be unknown.

Dipsogenic Diabetes Insipidus

A defect in the thirst mechanism, located in a person's hypothalamus, causes dipsogenic diabetes insipidus. This defect results in an abnormal increase in thirst and liquid intake that suppresses vasopressin secretion and increases urine output. The same events and conditions that damage the hypothalamus or pituitary—surgery, infection, inflammation, a tumor, head injury—can also damage the thirst mechanism. Certain medications or mental health problems may predispose a person to dipsogenic diabetes insipidus.

Gestational Diabetes Insipidus

Gestational diabetes insipidus occurs only during pregnancy. In some cases, an enzyme made by the placenta—a temporary organ joining mother and baby—breaks down the mother's vasopressin. In other cases, pregnant women produce more prostaglandin, a hormone-like chemical that reduces kidney sensitivity to vasopressin. Most pregnant women who develop gestational diabetes insipidus have a mild case that does not cause noticeable symptoms. Gestational diabetes insipidus usually goes away after the mother delivers the baby; however, it may return if the mother becomes pregnant again.

What Are the Complications of Diabetes Insipidus?

The main complication of diabetes insipidus is dehydration if fluid loss is greater than liquid intake. Signs of dehydration include:

- Confusion
- Dizziness
- Dry skin
- Fatigue
- Nausea
- Sluggishness
- Thirst

Severe dehydration can lead to seizures, permanent brain damage, and even death.

How Is Diabetes Insipidus Diagnosed?

A healthcare provider can diagnose a person with diabetes insipidus based on the following:

- Blood tests
- Fluid deprivation test
- Magnetic resonance imaging (MRI)
- Medical and family history
- Physical exam
- Urinalysis

How Is Diabetes Insipidus Treated?

The primary treatment for diabetes insipidus involves drinking enough liquid to prevent dehydration. A healthcare provider may refer a person with diabetes insipidus to a nephrologist—a doctor who specializes in treating kidney problems—or to an endocrinologist—a doctor who specializes in treating disorders of the hormone-producing glands. Treatment for frequent urination or constant thirst depends on the patient's type of diabetes insipidus:

- **Central diabetes insipidus.** A synthetic, or man-made, hormone called desmopressin treats central diabetes insipidus. The medication comes as an injection, a nasal spray, or a pill. The medication works by replacing the vasopressin that a patient's body normally produces. This treatment helps a patient manage symptoms of central diabetes insipidus; however, it does not cure the disease.

- **Nephrogenic diabetes insipidus.** In some cases, nephrogenic diabetes insipidus goes away after treatment of the cause. For example, switching medications or taking steps to balance the amount of calcium or potassium in the patient's body may resolve the problem. Medications for nephrogenic diabetes insipidus include diuretics, either alone or combined with aspirin or ibuprofen. Healthcare providers commonly prescribe diuretics to help patients' kidneys remove fluid from the body. Paradoxically, in people with nephrogenic diabetes insipidus, a class of diuretics called thiazides reduces urine production and helps patients' kidneys concentrate urine. Aspirin or ibuprofen also helps reduce urine volume.

- **Dipsogenic diabetes insipidus.** Researchers have not yet found an effective treatment for dipsogenic diabetes insipidus. People can try sucking on ice chips or sour candies to moisten their mouths and increase saliva flow, which may reduce the desire to drink. For a person who wakes multiple times at night to urinate because of dipsogenic diabetes insipidus, taking a small dose of desmopressin at bedtime may help. Initially, the healthcare provider will monitor the patient's blood sodium levels to prevent hyponatremia, or low sodium levels in the blood.

- **Gestational diabetes insipidus.** A healthcare provider can prescribe desmopressin for women with gestational diabetes insipidus. An expecting mother's placenta does not destroy desmopressin as it does vasopressin. Most women will not need treatment after delivery.

Most people with diabetes insipidus can prevent serious problems and live a normal life if they follow the healthcare provider's recommendations and keep their symptoms under control.

Chapter 19

Prolactinomas

What Is a Prolactinoma?

A prolactinoma is a benign noncancerous tumor of the pituitary gland that produces a hormone called prolactin. Prolactinomas are the most common type of pituitary tumor. Symptoms of prolactinoma are caused by hyperprolactinemia—too much prolactin in the blood—or by pressure of the tumor on surrounding tissues.

Prolactin stimulates the breast to produce milk during pregnancy. After giving birth, a mother's prolactin levels fall unless she breast-feeds her infant. Each time the baby nurses, prolactin levels rise to maintain milk production.

What Is the Pituitary Gland?

The pituitary gland, sometimes called the master gland, plays a critical role in regulating growth and development, metabolism, and reproduction. It produces prolactin and other key hormones including

- Growth hormone, which regulates growth.

- Adrenocorticotropin (ACTH), which stimulates the adrenal glands to produce cortisol, a hormone important in metabolism and the body's response to stress.

This chapter includes text excerpted from "Prolactinomas," National Institute of Diabetes and Digestive and Kidney Diseases (NIDDK), April 2012. Reviewed October 2016.

- Thyrotropin, which signals the thyroid gland to produce thyroid hormone, also involved in metabolism and growth.

- Luteinizing hormone and follicle-stimulating hormone, which regulate ovulation and estrogen and progesterone production in women and sperm formation and testosterone production in men.

The pituitary gland sits in the middle of the head in a bony box called the *sella turcica*. The optic nerves sit directly above the pituitary gland. Enlargement of the gland can cause symptoms such as headaches or visual disturbances. Pituitary tumors may also impair production of one or more pituitary hormones, causing reduced pituitary function, also called hypopituitarism.

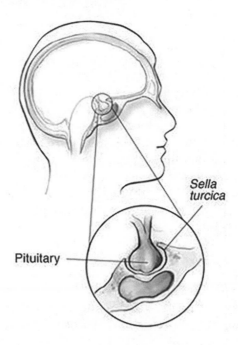

Figure 19.1. *Pituitary Gland*

How Common Is Prolactinoma?

Although small benign pituitary tumors are fairly common in the general population, symptomatic prolactinomas are uncommon. Prolactinomas occur more often in women than men and rarely occur in children.

What Are the Symptoms of Prolactinoma?

In women, high levels of prolactin in the blood often cause infertility and changes in menstruation. In some women, periods may stop. In others, periods may become irregular or menstrual flow may change. Women who are not pregnant or nursing may begin producing breast milk. Some women may experience a loss of libido-interest in sex. Intercourse may become painful because of vaginal dryness.

In men, the most common symptom of prolactinoma is erectile dysfunction. Because men have no reliable indicator such as changes in menstruation to signal a problem, many men delay going to the doctor until they have headaches or eye problems caused by the enlarged pituitary pressing against nearby optic nerves. They may not recognize a gradual loss of sexual function or libido. Only after treatment do some men realize they had a problem with sexual function.

What Causes Prolactinoma?

The cause of pituitary tumors remains largely unknown. Most pituitary tumors are sporadic, meaning they are not genetically passed from parents to their children.

What Else Causes Prolactin to Rise?

In some people, high blood levels of prolactin can be traced to causes other than prolactinoma.

Prescription drugs. Prolactin secretion in the pituitary is normally suppressed by the brain chemical dopamine. Drugs that block the effects of dopamine at the pituitary or deplete dopamine stores in the brain may cause the pituitary to secrete prolactin. These drugs include older antipsychotic medications such as trifluoperazine (Stelazine) and haloperidol (Haldol); the newer antipsychotic drugs risperidone (Risperdal) and molindone (Moban); metoclopramide (Reglan), used to treat gastroesophageal reflux and the nausea caused by certain cancer drugs; and less often, verapamil, alpha-methyldopa (Aldochlor, Aldoril), and reserpine (Serpalan, Serpasil), used to control high blood pressure. Some antidepressants may cause hyperprolactinemia, but further research is needed.

Other pituitary tumors. Other tumors arising in or near the pituitary may block the flow of dopamine from the brain to the prolactin-secreting cells. Such tumors include those that cause acromegaly, a condition caused by too much growth hormone, and Cushing syndrome, caused by too much cortisol. Other pituitary tumors that do not result in excess hormone production may also block the flow of dopamine.

Hypothyroidism. Increased prolactin levels are often seen in people with hypothyroidism, a condition in which the thyroid does not produce enough thyroid hormone. Doctors routinely test people with hyperprolactinemia for hypothyroidism.

Chest involvement. Nipple stimulation also can cause a modest increase in the amount of prolactin in the blood. Similarly, chest wall injury or shingles involving the chest wall may also cause hyperprolactinemia.

How Is Prolactinoma Diagnosed?

A doctor will test for prolactin blood levels in women with unexplained milk secretion, called galactorrhea, or with irregular menses or infertility and in men with impaired sexual function and, in rare cases, milk secretion. If prolactin levels are high, a doctor will test thyroid function and ask first about other conditions and medications known to raise prolactin secretion. The doctor may also request magnetic resonance imaging (MRI), which is the most sensitive test for detecting pituitary tumors and determining their size. MRI scans may be repeated periodically to assess tumor progression and the effects of therapy. Computerized tomography (CT) scan also gives an image of the pituitary but is less precise than the MRI.

The doctor will also look for damage to surrounding tissues and perform tests to assess whether production of other pituitary hormones is normal. Depending on the size of the tumor, the doctor may request an eye exam with measurement of visual fields.

How Is Prolactinoma Treated?

The goals of treatment are to return prolactin secretion to normal, reduce tumor size, correct any visual abnormalities, and restore normal pituitary function. In the case of large tumors, only partial achievement of these goals may be possible.

Medical Treatment

Because dopamine is the chemical that normally inhibits prolactin secretion, doctors may treat prolactinoma with the dopamine agonists bromocriptine (Parlodel) or cabergoline (Dostinex). Agonists are drugs that act like a naturally occurring substance. These drugs shrink the tumor and return prolactin levels to normal in approximately 80 percent of patients. Both drugs have been approved by the U.S. Food and Drug Administration (FDA) for the treatment of hyperprolactinemia. Bromocriptine is the only dopamine agonist approved for the treatment of infertility. This drug has been in use longer than cabergoline and has a well-established safety record.

Nausea and dizziness are possible side effects of bromocriptine. To avoid these side effects, bromocriptine treatment must be started slowly. A typical starting dose is one-quarter to one-half of a 2.5 milligram (mg) tablet taken at bedtime with a snack. The dose is gradually increased every 3 to 7 days as needed and taken in divided doses with meals or at bedtime with a snack. Most people are successfully treated with 7.5 mg a day or less, although some people need 15 mg or more each day. Because bromocriptine is short acting, it should be taken either twice or three times daily.

Cabergoline is a newer drug that may be more effective than bromocriptine in normalizing prolactin levels and shrinking tumor size. Cabergoline also has less frequent and less severe side effects. Cabergoline is more expensive than bromocriptine and, being newer on the market, its long-term safety record is less well defined. As with bromocriptine therapy, nausea and dizziness are possible side effects but may be avoided if treatment is started slowly. The usual starting dose is. 25 mg twice a week. The dose may be increased every 4 weeks as needed, up to 1 mg two times a week. Cabergoline should not be stopped without consulting a qualified endocrinologist.

Surgery

Surgery to remove all or part of the tumor should only be considered if medical therapy cannot be tolerated or if it fails to reduce prolactin levels, restore normal reproduction and pituitary function, and reduce tumor size. If medical therapy is only partially successful, it should be continued, possibly combined with surgery or radiation.

Most often, the tumor is removed through the nasal cavity. Rarely, if the tumor is large or has spread to nearby brain tissue, the surgeon will access the tumor through an opening in the skull.

The results of surgery depend a great deal on tumor size and prolactin levels as well as the skill and experience of the neurosurgeon. The higher the prolactin level before surgery, the lower the chance of normalizing serum prolactin. Serum is the portion of the blood used in measuring prolactin levels. In the best medical centers, surgery corrects prolactin levels in about 80 percent of patients with small tumors and a serum prolactin less than 200 nanograms per milliliter (ng/ml). A surgical cure for large tumors is lower, at 30 to 40 percent. Even in patients with large tumors that cannot be completely removed, drug therapy may be able to return serum prolactin to the normal range-20 ng/ml or less-after surgery.

Radiation

Rarely, radiation therapy is used if medical therapy and surgery fail to reduce prolactin levels. Depending on the size and location of the tumor, radiation is delivered in low doses over the course of 5 to 6 weeks or in a single high dose. Radiation therapy is effective about 30 percent of the time.

How Does Prolactinoma Affect Pregnancy?

If a woman has a small prolactinoma, she can usually conceive and have a normal pregnancy after effective medical therapy. If she had a successful pregnancy before, the chance of her having more successful pregnancies is high.

A woman with prolactinoma should discuss her plans to conceive with her physician so she can be carefully evaluated prior to becoming pregnant. This evaluation will include an MRI scan to assess the size of the tumor and an eye examination with measurement of visual fields. As soon as a woman is pregnant, her doctor will usually advise her to stop taking bromocriptine or cabergoline. Although these drugs are safe for the fetus in early pregnancy, their safety throughout an entire pregnancy has not been established. Many doctors prefer to use bromocriptine in patients who plan to become pregnant because it has a longer record of safety in early pregnancy than cabergoline.

The pituitary enlarges and prolactin production increases during pregnancy in women without pituitary disorders. Women with prolactin-secreting tumors may experience further pituitary enlargement and must be closely monitored during pregnancy. Less than 3 percent of pregnant women with small prolactinomas have symptoms of tumor growth such as headaches or vision problems. In women with large prolactinomas, the risk of symptomatic tumor growth is greater, and may be as high as 30 percent.

Most endocrinologists see patients every 2 months throughout the pregnancy. A woman should consult her endocrinologist promptly if she develops symptoms of tumor growth—particularly headaches, vision changes, nausea, vomiting, excessive thirst or urination, or extreme lethargy. Bromocriptine or, less often, cabergoline treatment may be reinitiated and additional treatment may be required if the woman develops symptoms during pregnancy.

How Do Oral Contraceptives and Hormone Replacement Therapy Affect Prolactinoma?

Oral contraceptives are not thought to contribute to the development of prolactinomas, although some studies have found increased prolactin levels in women taking these medications. Because oral contraceptives may produce regular menstrual bleeding in women who would otherwise have irregular menses due to hyperprolactinemia, prolactinoma may not be diagnosed until women stop oral contraceptives and find their menses are absent or irregular. Women with prolactinoma treated with bromocriptine or cabergoline may safely take oral contraceptives. Similarly, postmenopausal women treated with medical therapy or surgery for prolactinoma may be candidates for estrogen replacement therapy.

Is Osteoporosis a Risk in Women with High Prolactin Levels?

Women whose ovaries produce inadequate estrogen are at increased risk for osteoporosis. Hyperprolactinemia can reduce estrogen production. Although estrogen production may be restored after treatment for hyperprolactinemia, even a year or 2 without estrogen can compromise bone strength. Women should protect themselves from osteoporosis by increasing exercise and calcium intake through diet or supplements and by not smoking. Women treated for hyperprolactinemia may want to have periodic bone density measurements and discuss estrogen replacement therapy or other bone-strengthening medications with their doctor.

Chapter 20

Pituitary Tumors and Treatment Options

A Pituitary Tumor Is a Growth of Abnormal Cells in the Tissues of the Pituitary Gland

Pituitary tumors form in the pituitary gland, a pea-sized organ in the center of the brain, just above the back of the nose. The pituitary gland is sometimes called the "master endocrine gland" because it makes hormones that affect the way many parts of the body work. It also controls hormones made by many other glands in the body.

Pituitary tumors are divided into three groups:

- Benign pituitary adenomas: Tumors that are not cancer. These tumors grow very slowly and do not spread from the pituitary gland to other parts of the body.

- Invasive pituitary adenomas: Benign tumors that may spread to bones of the skull or the sinus cavity below the pituitary gland.

- Pituitary carcinomas: Tumors that are malignant (cancer). These pituitary tumors spread into other areas of the central nervous system (brain and spinal cord) or outside of the central nervous system. Very few pituitary tumors are malignant.

This chapter includes text excerpted from "Pituitary Tumors Treatment (PDQ®)—Patient Version," National Cancer Institute (NCI), May 27, 2016.

Pituitary tumors may be either non-functioning or functioning.

- Non-functioning pituitary tumors do not make extra amounts of hormones.

- Functioning pituitary tumors make more than the normal amount of one or more hormones. Most pituitary tumors are functioning tumors. The extra hormones made by pituitary tumors may cause certain signs or symptoms of disease.

The Pituitary Gland Hormones Control Many Other Glands in the Body

Hormones made by the pituitary gland include:

- Prolactin: A hormone that causes a woman's breasts to make milk during and after pregnancy.

- Adrenocorticotropic hormone (ACTH): A hormone that causes the adrenal glands to make a hormone called cortisol. Cortisol helps control the use of sugar, protein, and fats in the body and helps the body deal with stress.

- Growth hormone: A hormone that helps control body growth and the use of sugar and fat in the body. Growth hormone is also called somatotropin.

- Thyroid-stimulating hormone: A hormone that causes the thyroid gland to make other hormones that control growth, body temperature, and heart rate. Thyroid-stimulating hormone is also called thyrotropin.

- Luteinizing hormone (LH) and follicle-stimulating hormone (FSH): Hormones that control the menstrual cycle in women and the making of sperm in men.

Having Certain Genetic Conditions Increases the Risk of Developing a Pituitary Tumor

Anything that increases your risk of getting a disease is called a risk factor. Having a risk factor does not mean that you will get cancer; not having risk factors doesn't mean that you will not get cancer. Talk with your doctor if you think you may be at risk. Risk factors for pituitary tumors include having the following hereditary diseases:

- multiple endocrine neoplasia type 1 (MEN1) syndrome

- carney complex
- isolated familial acromegaly

Signs of a Pituitary Tumor Include Problems with Vision and Certain Physical Changes

Signs and symptoms can be caused by the growth of the tumor and/ or by hormones the tumor makes or by other conditions. Some tumors may not cause signs or symptoms. Check with your doctor if you have any of these problems.

Signs and Symptoms of a Non-Functioning Pituitary Tumor

Sometimes, a pituitary tumor may press on or damage parts of the pituitary gland, causing it to stop making one or more hormones. Too little of a certain hormone will affect the work of the gland or organ that the hormone controls. The following signs and symptoms may occur:

- headache
- some loss of vision
- loss of body hair
- in women, less frequent or no menstrual periods or no milk from the breasts
- in men, loss of facial hair, growth of breast tissue, and impotence
- in women and men, lower sex drive
- in children, slowed growth and sexual development

Most of the tumors that make LH and FSH do not make enough extra hormone to cause signs and symptoms. These tumors are considered to be non-functioning tumors.

Signs and Symptoms of a Functioning Pituitary Tumor

When a functioning pituitary tumor makes extra hormones, the signs and symptoms will depend on the type of hormone being made. **Too much prolactin may cause:**

- headache
- some loss of vision

131

- less frequent or no menstrual periods or menstrual periods with a very light flow

- trouble becoming pregnant or an inability to become pregnant

- impotence in men

- lower sex drive

- flow of breast milk in a woman who is not pregnant or breast-feeding

Too much ACTH may cause:

- headache

- some loss of vision

- weight gain in the face, neck, and trunk of the body, and thin arms and legs

- a lump of fat on the back of the neck

- thin skin that may have purple or pink stretch marks on the chest or abdomen

- easy bruising

- growth of fine hair on the face, upper back, or arms

- bones that break easily

- anxiety, irritability, and depression

Too much growth hormone may cause:

- headache

- some loss of vision

- In adults, acromegaly (growth of the bones in the face, hands, and feet). In children, the whole body may grow much taller and larger than normal.

- tingling or numbness in the hands and fingers

- snoring or pauses in breathing during sleep

- joint pain

- sweating more than usual

- dysmorphophobia (extreme dislike of or concern about one or more parts of the body)

Too much thyroid-stimulating hormone may cause:

- irregular heartbeat
- shakiness
- weight loss
- trouble sleeping
- frequent bowel movements
- sweating

Other general signs and symptoms of pituitary tumors:

- nausea and vomiting
- confusion
- dizziness
- seizures
- runny or "drippy" nose (cerebrospinal fluid that surrounds the brain and spinal cord leaks into the nose)

Imaging Studies and Tests That Examine the Blood and Urine Are Used to Detect (Find) and Diagnose a Pituitary Tumor

The following tests and procedures may be used:

- physical exam and history
- eye exam
- visual field exam
- neurological exam
- MRI (magnetic resonance imaging) with gadolinium
- blood chemistry study
- blood tests
- twenty-four-hour urine test
- high-dose dexamethasone suppression test
- low-dose dexamethasone suppression test
- venous sampling for pituitary tumors

- biopsy

- immunohistochemistry

- immunocytochemistry

- light and electron microscopy

Certain Factors Affect Prognosis (Chance of Recovery) and Treatment Options

The prognosis (chance of recovery) depends on the type of tumor and whether the tumor has spread into other areas of the central nervous system (brain and spinal cord) or outside of the central nervous system to other parts of the body.

Treatment options depend on the following:

- The type and size of the tumor.

- Whether the tumor is making hormones.

- Whether the tumor is causing problems with vision or other signs or symptoms.

- Whether the tumor has spread into the brain around the pituitary gland or to other parts of the body.

- Whether the tumor has just been diagnosed or has recurred (come back).

Treatment Option Overview

There Are Different Types of Treatment for Patients with Pituitary Tumors

Different types of treatments are available for patients with pituitary tumors. Some treatments are standard (the currently used treatment), and some are being tested in clinical trials. A treatment clinical trial is a research study meant to help improve current treatments or obtain information on new treatments for patients with cancer. When clinical trials show that a new treatment is better than the standard treatment, the new treatment may become the standard treatment. Patients may want to think about taking part in a clinical trial. Some clinical trials are open only to patients who have not started treatment.

Four types of standard treatment are used:

1. Surgery

- Transsphenoidal surgery
- Endoscopic transsphenoidal surgery
- Craniotomy

2. Radiation therapy
   - External radiation therapy
   - Stereotactic radiosurgery
   - Internal radiation therapy

3. Drug therapy

4. Chemotherapy
   - Systemic chemotherapy
   - Regional chemotherapy

Treatment Options for Pituitary Tumors

Non-functioning Pituitary Tumors

Treatment may include the following:

- Surgery (transsphenoidal surgery, if possible). Radiation therapy is given if the tumor comes back
- Radiation therapy alone

Prolactin-Producing Pituitary Tumors

Treatment may include the following:

- Drug therapy
- Surgery to remove the tumor (transsphenoidal surgery or craniotomy)
- Radiation therapy
- Surgery followed by radiation therapy

ACTH-Producing Pituitary Tumors

Treatment may include the following:

- Surgery (usually transsphenoidal surgery)
- Radiation therapy alone

- Drug therapy
- A clinical trial of stereotactic radiation surgery

Growth Hormone-Producing Pituitary Tumors

Treatment may include the following:

- Surgery (usually transsphenoidal or endoscopic transsphenoidal surgery)
- Drug therapy

Thyroid-Stimulating Hormone-Producing Tumors

Treatment may include the following:

- Surgery (usually transsphenoidal surgery)
- Drug therapy

Pituitary Carcinomas

Treatment of pituitary carcinomas is palliative, to relieve symptoms and improve the quality of life. Treatment may include the following:

- Surgery (transsphenoidal surgery or craniotomy)
- Drug therapy
- Chemotherapy

Recurrent Pituitary Tumors

Treatment may include the following:

- Radiation therapy
- A clinical trial of stereotactic radiation surgery

Part Three

Thyroid and Parathyroid Gland Disorders

Chapter 21

Thyroid Function

What Is the Thyroid?

The thyroid is a 2-inch-long, butterfly-shaped gland weighing less than 1 ounce. Located in the front of the neck below the larynx, or voice box, it has two lobes, one on either side of the windpipe.

The thyroid is one of the glands that make up the endocrine system. The glands of the endocrine system produce and store hormones and release them into the bloodstream. The hormones then travel through the body and direct the activity of the body's cells.

What Is the Role of Thyroid Hormones?

Thyroid hormones regulate metabolism—the way the body uses energy—and affect nearly every organ in the body. Thyroid hormones also affect brain development, breathing, heart and nervous system functions, body temperature, muscle strength, skin dryness, menstrual cycles, weight, and cholesterol levels.

The thyroid makes two thyroid hormones:

1. thyroxine (T_4)

2. triiodothyronine (T_3)

Only a small amount of T_3 in the blood comes from the thyroid. Most T_3 comes from cells all over the body, where it is made from T_4.

This chapter includes text excerpted from "Thyroid Tests," National Institute of Diabetes and Digestive and Kidney Diseases (NIDDK), February 2014.

Thyroid-stimulating hormone (TSH), which is made by the pituitary gland in the brain, regulates thyroid hormone production. When thyroid hormone levels in the blood are low, the pituitary releases more TSH. When thyroid hormone levels are high, the pituitary decreases TSH production.

Why Do Healthcare Providers Perform Thyroid Tests?

Healthcare providers perform thyroid tests to assess how well the thyroid is working. The tests are also used to diagnose and help find the cause of thyroid disorders such as hyperthyroidism and hypothyroidism:

- Hyperthyroidism is a disorder caused by too much thyroid hormone in the bloodstream, which increases the speed of bodily functions and leads to weight loss, sweating, rapid heart rate, and high blood pressure, among other symptoms.

- Hypothyroidism is a disorder that occurs when the thyroid doesn't make enough thyroid hormone for the body's needs. Without enough thyroid hormone, many of the body's functions slow down. People may have symptoms such as fatigue, weight gain, and cold intolerance.

What Blood Tests Do Healthcare Providers Use to Check a Person's Thyroid Function?

A healthcare provider may order several blood tests to check thyroid function, including the following:

- TSH test

- T_4 tests

- T_3 test

- thyroid-stimulating immunoglobulin (TSI) test

- antithyroid antibody test, also called the thyroid peroxidase antibody test (TPOab)

Blood tests assess thyroid function by measuring TSH and thyroid hormone levels, and by detecting certain autoantibodies present in autoimmune thyroid disease. Autoantibodies are molecules produced by a person's body that mistakenly attack the body's own tissues.

Many complex factors affect thyroid function and hormone levels. Healthcare providers take a patient's full medical history into account when interpreting thyroid function tests.

TSH Test

A healthcare provider usually performs the TSH blood test first to check how well the thyroid is working. The TSH test measures the amount of TSH a person's pituitary is secreting. The TSH test is the most accurate test for diagnosing both hyperthyroidism and hypothyroidism. Generally, a below-normal level of TSH suggests hyperthyroidism. An abnormally high TSH level suggests hypothyroidism.

The TSH test detects even tiny amounts of TSH in the blood. Normally, the pituitary boosts TSH production when thyroid hormone levels in the blood are low. The thyroid responds by making more hormone. Then, when the body has enough thyroid hormone circulating in the blood, TSH output drops. The cycle repeats continuously to maintain a healthy level of thyroid hormone in the body. In people whose thyroid produces too much thyroid hormone, the pituitary shuts down TSH production, leading to low or even undetectable TSH levels in the blood.

In people whose thyroid is not functioning normally and produces too little thyroid hormone, the thyroid cannot respond normally to TSH by producing thyroid hormone. As a result, the pituitary keeps making TSH, trying to get the thyroid to respond.

If results of the TSH test are abnormal, a person will need one or more additional tests to help find the cause of the problem.

T_4 Tests

The thyroid primarily secretes T_4 and only a small amount of T_3. T_4 exists in two forms:

1. T_4 that is bound to proteins in the blood and is kept in reserve until needed.

2. A small amount of unbound or "free" T_4 (FT_4), which is the active form of the hormone and is available to enter body tissues when needed.

A high level of total T_4—bound and FT_4 together—or FT_4 suggests hyperthyroidism, and a low level of total T_4 or FT_4 suggests hypothyroidism.

Both pregnancy and taking oral contraceptives increase levels of binding protein in the blood. In either of these cases, although a woman may have a high total T_4 level, she may not have hyperthyroidism. Severe illness or the use of corticosteroids—a class of medications that treat asthma, arthritis, and skin conditions, among other health problems—can decrease binding protein levels. Therefore, in these cases, the total T_4 level may be low, yet the person does not have hypothyroidism.

T_3 Test

If a healthcare provider suspects hyperthyroidism in a person who has a normal FT_4 level, a T_3 test can be useful to confirm the condition. In some cases of hyperthyroidism, FT_4 is normal yet free T_3 (FT_3) is elevated, so measuring both T_4 and T_3 can be useful if a healthcare provider suspects hyperthyroidism. The T_3 test is not useful in diagnosing hypothyroidism because levels are not reduced until the hypothyroidism is severe.

TSI Test

Thyroid-stimulating immunoglobulin (TSI) is an autoantibody present in Graves disease. TSI mimics TSH by stimulating the thyroid cells, causing the thyroid to secrete extra hormone. The TSI test detects TSI circulating in the blood and is usually measured

- in people with Graves disease when the diagnosis is obscure

- during pregnancy

- to find out if a person is in remission, or no longer has hyperthyroidism and its symptoms

Antithyroid Antibody Test

Antithyroid antibodies are markers in the blood that are extremely helpful in diagnosing Hashimoto disease. Two principal types of antithyroid antibodies are

1. Anti-thyroglobulin, or anti-TG antibodies, which attack a protein in the thyroid called thyroglobulin.

2. Anti-thyroperoxidase, or anti-TPO antibodies, which attack an enzyme in thyroid cells called thyroperoxidase.

What Do Thyroid Test Results Tell Healthcare Providers?

Healthcare providers look at thyroid test results in people with hyperthyroidism or hypothyroidism to find the underlying cause of their thyroid disorder.

What Imaging Tests Do Healthcare Providers Use to Diagnose and Find the Cause of Thyroid Disorders?

A healthcare provider may use one or a combination of imaging tests, to diagnose and find the cause of thyroid disorders.

- Ultrasound

- CT scan

- Nuclear medicine tests

  - Radioactive iodine uptake test

  - Thyroid scan

What Tests Do Healthcare Providers Use If a Thyroid Nodule Is Found?

If a healthcare provider feels a nodule in a patient's neck during a physical exam or detects one during imaging tests of the thyroid, a fine needle aspiration biopsy may be done to confirm whether the nodule is cancerous or benign.

Chapter 22

Hashimoto Thyroiditis

What Is Hashimoto Thyroiditis?

Hashimoto thyroiditis is a condition that affects the function of the thyroid, which is a butterfly-shaped gland in the lower neck. The thyroid makes hormones that help regulate a wide variety of critical body functions. For example, thyroid hormones influence growth and development, body temperature, heart rate, menstrual cycles, and weight. Hashimoto thyroiditis is a form of chronic inflammation that can damage the thyroid, reducing its ability to produce hormones.

One of the first signs of Hashimoto thyroiditis is an enlargement of the thyroid called a goiter. Depending on its size, the enlarged thyroid can cause the neck to look swollen and may interfere with breathing and swallowing. As damage to the thyroid continues, the gland can shrink over a period of years and the goiter may eventually disappear.

Other signs and symptoms resulting from an underactive thyroid can include excessive tiredness (fatigue), weight gain or difficulty losing weight, hair that is thin and dry, a slow heart rate, joint or muscle pain, and constipation. People with this condition may also have a pale, puffy face and feel cold even when others around them are warm. Affected women can have heavy or irregular menstrual periods and difficulty conceiving a child (impaired fertility). Difficulty

This chapter includes text excerpted from "Hashimoto Thyroiditis," Genetics Home Reference (GHR), National Institutes of Health (NIH), November 1, 2016.

concentrating and depression can also be signs of a shortage of thyroid hormones.

Hashimoto thyroiditis usually appears in mid-adulthood, although it can occur earlier or later in life. Its signs and symptoms tend to develop gradually over months or years.

Frequency

Hashimoto thyroiditis affects 1 to 2 percent of people in the United States. It occurs more often in women than in men, which may be related to hormonal factors. The condition is the most common cause of thyroid underactivity (hypothyroidism) in the United States.

Genetic Changes

Hashimoto thyroiditis is thought to result from a combination of genetic and environmental factors. Some of these factors have been identified, but many remain unknown.

Hashimoto thyroiditis is classified as an autoimmune disorder, one of a large group of conditions that occur when the immune system attacks the body's own tissues and organs. In people with Hashimoto thyroiditis, white blood cells called lymphocytes accumulate abnormally in the thyroid, which can damage it. The lymphocytes make immune system proteins called antibodies that attack and destroy thyroid cells. When too many thyroid cells become damaged or die, the thyroid can no longer make enough hormones to regulate body functions. This shortage of thyroid hormones underlies the signs and symptoms of Hashimoto thyroiditis. However, some people with thyroid antibodies never develop hypothyroidism or experience any related signs or symptoms.

People with Hashimoto thyroiditis have an increased risk of developing other autoimmune disorders, including vitiligo, rheumatoid arthritis, Addison disease, type 1 diabetes, multiple sclerosis, and pernicious anemia.

Variations in several genes have been studied as possible risk factors for Hashimoto thyroiditis. Some of these genes are part of a family called the human leukocyte antigen (HLA) complex. The HLA complex helps the immune system distinguish the body's own proteins from proteins made by foreign invaders (such as viruses and bacteria). Other genes that have been associated with Hashimoto thyroiditis help regulate the immune system or are involved in normal thyroid function. Most of the genetic variations that have been discovered are thought to have a small impact on a person's overall risk of developing this condition.

Other, nongenetic factors also play a role in Hashimoto thyroiditis. These factors may trigger the condition in people who are at risk, although the mechanism is unclear. Potential triggers include changes in sex hormones (particularly in women), viral infections, certain medications, exposure to ionizing radiation, and excess consumption of iodine (a substance involved in thyroid hormone production).

Inheritance Pattern

The inheritance pattern of Hashimoto thyroiditis is unclear because many genetic and environmental factors appear to be involved. However, the condition can cluster in families, and having a close relative with Hashimoto thyroiditis or another autoimmune disorder likely increases a person's risk of developing the condition.

Other Names for This Condition

- Autoimmune chronic lymphocytic thyroiditis
- Autoimmune thyroiditis
- Chronic lymphocytic thyroiditides
- Chronic lymphocytic thyroiditis
- Hashimoto disease
- Hashimoto struma
- Hashimoto syndrome
- Hashimoto disease
- Lymphocytic thyroiditis

Chapter 23

Hypothyroidism

What Is Hypothyroidism?

Hypothyroidism, also called underactive thyroid, is when the thyroid gland doesn't make enough thyroid hormones to meet your body's needs. The thyroid is a small, butterfly-shaped gland in the front of your neck. Thyroid hormones control the way the body uses energy, so they affect nearly every organ in your body, even the way your heart beats. Without enough thyroid hormones, many of your body's functions slow down.

How Common Is Hypothyroidism?

About 4.6 percent of the U.S. population ages 12 and older has hypothyroidism, although most cases are mild. That's almost 5 people out of 100.

Who Is More Likely to Develop Hypothyroidism?

Women are much more likely than men to develop hypothyroidism. The disease is also more common among people older than age 60.
You are more likely to have hypothyroidism if you:

* have had a thyroid problem before, such as a goiter

This chapter includes text excerpted from "Hypothyroidism," National Institute of Diabetes and Digestive and Kidney Diseases (NIDDK), July 2016.

- have had surgery to correct a thyroid problem
- have received radiation treatment to the thyroid, neck, or chest
- have a family history of thyroid disease
- were pregnant in the past 6 months
- have Turner syndrome, a genetic disorder that affects females
- have other health problems, including
  - Sjögren syndrome, a disease that causes dry eyes and mouth
  - pernicious anemia, a condition caused by a vitamin B12 deficiency
  - type 1 diabetes
  - rheumatoid arthritis, an autoimmune disease that affects the joints
  - lupus, a chronic inflammatory condition

Is Hypothyroidism during Pregnancy a Problem?

Hypothyroidism that isn't treated can affect both the mother and the baby. However, thyroid medicines can help prevent problems and are safe to take during pregnancy.

What Other Health Problems Could I Have Because of Hypothyroidism?

Hypothyroidism can contribute to high cholesterol, so people with high cholesterol should be tested for hypothyroidism. Rarely, severe, untreated hypothyroidism may lead to myxedema coma, an extreme form of hypothyroidism in which the body's functions slow to the point that it becomes life threatening. Myxedema coma requires immediate medical treatment.

What Are the Symptoms of Hypothyroidism?

Hypothyroidism has many symptoms that can vary from person to person. Some common symptoms of hypothyroidism include:

- constipation
- decreased sweating

- depression
- dry skin
- dry, thinning hair
- fatigue
- fertility problems
- goiter
- heavy or irregular menstrual periods
- joint and muscle pain
- a puffy face
- slowed heart rate
- trouble tolerating cold
- weight gain

Because hypothyroidism develops slowly, many people don't notice symptoms of the disease for months or even years.

Many of these symptoms, especially fatigue and weight gain, are common and don't always mean that someone has a thyroid problem.

What Causes Hypothyroidism?

Hypothyroidism has several causes, including

- Hashimoto disease
- thyroiditis, or inflammation of the thyroid
- congenital hypothyroidism, or hypothyroidism that is present at birth
- surgical removal of part or all of the thyroid
- radiation treatment of the thyroid
- some medicines

Less often, hypothyroidism is caused by too much or too little iodine in the diet or by pituitary disease.

Hashimoto Disease

Hashimoto disease is the most common cause of hypothyroidism. Hashimoto disease is an autoimmune disorder. With this disease, your immune system attacks the thyroid. The thyroid becomes inflamed and can't make enough thyroid hormones.

Thyroiditis

Thyroiditis is inflammation of your thyroid that causes stored thyroid hormone to leak out of your thyroid gland. At first, the leakage increases hormone levels in the blood, leading to hyperthyroidism, a condition in which thyroid hormone levels are too high. The hyperthyroidism may last for up to 3 months, after which your thyroid may become underactive. The resulting hypothyroidism usually lasts 12 to 18 months, but sometimes is permanent.

Several types of thyroiditis can cause hyperthyroidism and then cause hypothyroidism:

- Subacute thyroiditis

- Postpartum thyroiditis

- Silent thyroiditis

Congenital Hypothyroidism

Some babies are born with a thyroid that is not fully developed or does not function properly. If untreated, congenital hypothyroidism can lead to intellectual disability and growth failure—when a baby doesn't grow as expected. Early treatment can prevent these problems, which is why most newborns in the United States are tested for hypothyroidism.

Surgical Removal of Part or All of the Thyroid

When surgeons remove part of the thyroid, the remaining part may produce normal amounts of thyroid hormone, but some people who have this surgery develop hypothyroidism. Removal of the entire thyroid always results in hypothyroidism.

Surgeons may remove part or all of the thyroid as a treatment for

- hyperthyroidism

- a large goiter

- thyroid nodules, which are noncancerous tumors or lumps in the thyroid that can produce too much thyroid hormone

- thyroid cancer

Radiation Treatment of the Thyroid

Radioactive iodine, a common treatment for hyperthyroidism, gradually destroys the cells of the thyroid. Most people who receive radioactive iodine treatment eventually develop hypothyroidism. Doctors treat people with head or neck cancers with radiation, which can also damage the thyroid.

Medicines

Some medicines can interfere with thyroid hormone production and lead to hypothyroidism, including

- amiodarone, a heart medicine

- interferon alpha, a cancer medicine

- interleukin-2, a kidney cancer medicine

- lithium, a bipolar disorder medicine

How Do Doctors Diagnose Hypothyroidism?

Your doctor will take a medical history and do a physical exam, but also will need to do some tests to confirm a diagnosis of hypothyroidism. Many symptoms of hypothyroidism are the same as those of other diseases, so doctors usually can't diagnose hyperthyroidism based on symptoms alone.

Because hypothyroidism can cause fertility problems, women who have trouble getting pregnant often get tested for thyroid problems.

Your doctor may use several blood tests to confirm a diagnosis of hypothyroidism and find its cause.

How Is Hypothyroidism Treated?

Hypothyroidism is treated by replacing the hormone that your own thyroid can no longer make. You will take levothyroxine, a thyroid hormone medicine that is identical to a hormone the thyroid normally makes. Your doctor may recommend taking the medicine in the morning before eating.

Your doctor will give you a blood test about 6 to 8 weeks after you begin taking thyroid hormone and adjust your dose if needed. Each time your dose is adjusted, you'll have another blood test. Once you've reached a dose that's working for you, your healthcare provider will probably repeat the blood test in 6 months and then once a year.

Your hypothyroidism most likely can be completely controlled with thyroid hormone medicine, as long as you take the recommended dose as instructed. Never stop taking your medicine without talking with your healthcare provider first.

What Should I Eat or Avoid Eating If I Have Hypothyroidism?

The thyroid uses iodine to make thyroid hormones. However, people with Hashimoto disease or other types of autoimmune thyroid disorders may be sensitive to harmful side effects from iodine. Eating foods that have large amounts of iodine—such as kelp, dulse, or other kinds of seaweed—may cause or worsen hypothyroidism. Taking iodine supplements can have the same effect.

Talk with members of your healthcare team about what foods you should limit or avoid, and let them know if you take iodine supplements. Also, share information about any cough syrups that you take because they may contain iodine.

Women need more iodine when they are pregnant because the baby gets iodine from the mother's diet. If you are pregnant, talk with your healthcare provider about how much iodine you need.

Chapter 24

Congenital Hypothyroidism

What Is Congenital Hypothyroidism?

Congenital hypothyroidism is a partial or complete loss of function of the thyroid gland (hypothyroidism) that affects infants from birth (congenital). The thyroid gland is a butterfly-shaped tissue in the lower neck. It makes iodine-containing hormones that play an important role in regulating growth, brain development, and the rate of chemical reactions in the body (metabolism). People with congenital hypothyroidism have lower-than-normal levels of these important hormones.

Congenital hypothyroidism occurs when the thyroid gland fails to develop or function properly. In 80 to 85 percent of cases, the thyroid gland is absent, severely reduced in size (hypoplastic), or abnormally located. These cases are classified as thyroid dysgenesis. In the remainder of cases, a normal-sized or enlarged thyroid gland (goiter) is present, but production of thyroid hormones is decreased or absent. Most of these cases occur when one of several steps in the hormone synthesis process is impaired; these cases are classified as thyroid dyshormonogenesis. Less commonly, reduction or absence of thyroid hormone production is caused by impaired stimulation of the production process (which is normally done by a structure at the base of the brain called the pituitary gland), even though the process

This chapter includes text excerpted from "Congenital Hypothyroidism," Genetics Home Reference (GHR), National Institutes of Health (NIH), October 4, 2016.

itself is unimpaired. These cases are classified as central (or pituitary) hypothyroidism.

Signs and symptoms of congenital hypothyroidism result from the shortage of thyroid hormones. Affected babies may show no features of the condition, although some babies with congenital hypothyroidism are less active and sleep more than normal. They may have difficulty feeding and experience constipation. If untreated, congenital hypothyroidism can lead to intellectual disability and slow growth. In the United States, all hospitals test newborns for congenital hypothyroidism. If treatment begins in the first two weeks after birth, infants usually develop normally.

Congenital hypothyroidism can also occur as part of syndromes that affect other organs and tissues in the body. These forms of the condition are described as syndromic. Some common forms of syndromic hypothyroidism include Pendred syndrome, Bamforth-Lazarus syndrome, and brain-lung-thyroid syndrome.

Frequency

Congenital hypothyroidism affects an estimated 1 in 2,000 to 4,000 newborns. For reasons that remain unclear, congenital hypothyroidism affects more than twice as many females as males.

Genetic Changes

Congenital hypothyroidism can be caused by a variety of factors, only some of which are genetic. The most common cause worldwide is a shortage of iodine in the diet of the mother and the affected infant. Iodine is essential for the production of thyroid hormones. Genetic causes account for about 15 to 20 percent of cases of congenital hypothyroidism.

The cause of the most common type of congenital hypothyroidism, thyroid dysgenesis, is usually unknown. Studies suggest that 2 to 5 percent of cases are inherited. Two of the genes involved in this form of the condition are *PAX8* and *TSHR*. These genes play roles in the proper growth and development of the thyroid gland. Mutations in these genes prevent or disrupt normal development of the gland. The abnormal or missing gland cannot produce normal amounts of thyroid hormones.

Thyroid dyshormonogenesis results from mutations in one of several genes involved in the production of thyroid hormones. These genes include *DUOX2*, *SLC5A5*, *TG*, and *TPO*. Mutations in each of these genes disrupt a step in thyroid hormone synthesis, leading to abnormally low levels of these hormones. Mutations in the *TSHB* gene disrupt the synthesis of thyroid hormones by impairing the stimulation of hormone production. Changes in this gene are the primary cause of central hypothyroidism. The resulting shortage of thyroid hormones disrupts normal growth, brain development, and metabolism, leading to the features of congenital hypothyroidism.

Mutations in other genes that have not been as well characterized can also cause congenital hypothyroidism. Still other genes are involved in syndromic forms of the disorder.

Inheritance Pattern

Most cases of congenital hypothyroidism are sporadic, which means they occur in people with no history of the disorder in their family.

When inherited, the condition usually has an autosomal recessive inheritance pattern, which means both copies of the gene in each cell have mutations. Typically, the parents of an individual with an autosomal recessive condition each carry one copy of the mutated gene, but they do not show signs and symptoms of the condition.

When congenital hypothyroidism results from mutations in the *PAX8* gene or from certain mutations in the *TSHR* or *DUOX2* gene, the condition has an autosomal dominant pattern of inheritance, which means one copy of the altered gene in each cell is sufficient to cause the disorder. In some of these cases, an affected person inherits the mutation from one affected parent. Other cases result from new (de novo) mutations in the gene that occur during the formation of reproductive cells (eggs or sperm) or in early embryonic development. These cases occur in people with no history of the disorder in their family.

Other Names for This Condition

- CH
- CHT
- Congenital myxedema
- Cretinism

Chapter 25

Hyperthyroidism

What Is Hyperthyroidism?

Hyperthyroidism, also called overactive thyroid, is when the thyroid gland makes more thyroid hormones than your body needs. The thyroid is a small, butterfly-shaped gland in the front of your neck. Thyroid hormones control the way the body uses energy, so they affect nearly every organ in your body, even the way your heart beats.

If left untreated, hyperthyroidism can cause serious problems with the heart, bones, muscles, menstrual cycle, and fertility. During pregnancy, untreated hyperthyroidism can lead to health problems for the mother and baby.

How Common Is Hyperthyroidism?

About 1.2 percent of people in the United States have hyperthyroidism. That's a little more than 1 person out of 100.

Who Is More Likely to Develop Hyperthyroidism?

Women are 2 to 10 times more likely than men to develop hyperthyroidism. You are more likely to have hyperthyroidism if you

- have a family history of thyroid disease

This chapter includes text excerpted from "Hyperthyroidism," National Institute of Diabetes and Digestive and Kidney Diseases (NIDDK), July 2016.

- have other health problems, including

  - type 1 diabetes

  - pernicious anemia, a condition caused by a vitamin B12 deficiency

  - primary adrenal insufficiency, a hormonal disorder

- eat large amounts of food containing iodine, such as kelp, or use medicines that contain iodine, such as amiodarone, a heart medicine

- are older than age 60, especially if you are a woman

- were pregnant within the past 6 months

Is Hyperthyroidism during Pregnancy a Problem?

Thyroid hormone levels that are just a little high are usually not a problem in pregnancy. However, more severe hyperthyroidism that isn't treated can affect both the mother and the baby. If you have hyperthyroidism, be sure your disease is under control before becoming pregnant.

What Other Health Problems Could I Have Because of Hyperthyroidism?

If hyperthyroidism isn't treated, it can cause some serious health problems, including

- an irregular heartbeat that can lead to blood clots, stroke, heart failure, and other heart-related problems

- an eye disease called Graves ophthalmopathy that can cause double vision, light sensitivity, and eye pain, and rarely can lead to vision loss

- thinning bones and osteoporosis

What Are the Symptoms of Hyperthyroidism?

Symptoms of hyperthyroidism can vary from person to person and may include:

- Fatigue or muscle weakness

- Frequent bowel movements or diarrhea

- Goiter

- Mood swings

- Nervousness or irritability

- Rapid and irregular heartbeat

- Shaky hands

- Trouble sleeping

- Trouble tolerating heat

- Weight loss

In people over age 60, hyperthyroidism is sometimes mistaken for depression or dementia. Older adults may have different symptoms, such as loss of appetite or withdrawal from people, than younger adults with hyperthyroidism. You may want to ask your healthcare provider about hyperthyroidism if you or your loved one show these symptoms.

What Causes Hyperthyroidism?

Hyperthyroidism has several causes, including Graves disease, thyroid nodules, and thyroiditis—inflammation of the thyroid. Rarely, hyperthyroidism is caused by a noncancerous tumor of the pituitary gland located at the base of the brain. Consuming too much iodine or taking too much thyroid hormone medicine also may raise your thyroid hormone levels.

Graves Disease

Graves disease is the most common cause of hyperthyroidism. Graves disease is an autoimmune disorder. With this disease, your immune system attacks the thyroid and causes it to make too much thyroid hormone.

Overactive Thyroid Nodules

Thyroid nodules are lumps in your thyroid. Thyroid nodules are common and usually benign, meaning they are not cancerous. However, one or more nodules may become overactive and produce too much thyroid hormone. The presence of many overactive nodules occurs most often in older adults.

Thyroiditis

Thyroiditis is inflammation of your thyroid that causes stored thyroid hormone to leak out of your thyroid gland. The hyperthyroidism may last for up to 3 months, after which your thyroid may become underactive, a condition called hypothyroidism. The hypothyroidism usually lasts 12 to 18 months, but sometimes is permanent.

Several types of thyroiditis can cause hyperthyroidism and then cause hypothyroidism:

- Silent thyroiditis

- Subacute thyroiditis

- Postpartum thyroiditis

Too Much Iodine

Your thyroid uses iodine to make thyroid hormone. The amount of iodine you consume affects the amount of thyroid hormone your thyroid makes. In some people, consuming large amounts of iodine may cause the thyroid to make too much thyroid hormone.

Some medicines and cough syrups may contain a lot of iodine. One example is the heart medicine amiodarone. Seaweed and seaweed-based supplements also contain a lot of iodine.

Too Much Thyroid Hormone Medicine

Some people who take thyroid hormone medicine for hypothyroidism may take too much. If you take thyroid hormone medicine, you should see your doctor at least once a year to have your thyroid hormone levels checked. You may need to adjust your dose if your thyroid hormone level is too high.

Some other medicines may also interact with thyroid hormone medicine to raise hormone levels. If you take thyroid hormone medicine, ask your doctor about interactions when starting new medicines.

How Do Doctors Diagnose Hyperthyroidism?

Your doctor will take a medical history and do a physical exam, but also will need to do some tests to confirm a diagnosis of hyperthyroidism. Many symptoms of hyperthyroidism are the same as those of other diseases, so doctors usually can't diagnose hyperthyroidism based on symptoms alone.

Because hypothyroidism can cause fertility problems, women who have trouble getting pregnant often get tested for thyroid problems.

Your doctor may use several blood tests to confirm a diagnosis of hyperthyroidism and find its cause. Imaging tests, such as a thyroid scan, can also help diagnose and find the cause of hyperthyroidism.

What Are My Hyperthyroidism Treatment Options?

You may receive medicines, radioiodine therapy, or thyroid surgery to treat your hyperthyroidism. The aim of treatment is to bring thyroid hormone levels back to normal to prevent long-term health problems and to relieve uncomfortable symptoms. No single treatment works for everyone.

Treatment depends on the cause of your hyperthyroidism and how severe it is. When recommending a treatment, your doctor will consider your age, possible allergies to or side effects of the medicines, other conditions such as pregnancy or heart disease, and whether you have access to an experienced thyroid surgeon.

Medicines

Beta blockers. Beta blockers do not stop thyroid hormone production, but can reduce symptoms until other treatments take effect. Beta blockers act quickly to relieve many of the symptoms of hyperthyroidism, such as tremors, rapid heartbeat, and nervousness. Most people feel better within hours of taking beta blockers.

Antithyroid medicines. Antithyroid therapy is the simplest way to treat hyperthyroidism. Antithyroid medicines cause the thyroid to make less thyroid hormone. These medicines usually don't provide a permanent cure. Healthcare providers most often use the antithyroid medicine methimazole. Healthcare providers more often treat pregnant women with propylthiouracil during the first 3 months of pregnancy, however, because methimazole can harm the fetus, although this happens rarely.

Once treatment with antithyroid medicine begins, your thyroid hormone levels may not move into the normal range for several weeks or months. The total average treatment time is about 1 to 2 years, but treatment can continue for many years. Antithyroid medicines are not used to treat hyperthyroidism caused by thyroiditis.

Antithyroid medicines can cause side effects in some people, including

- a decrease in the number of white blood cells in your body, which can lower resistance to infection

- allergic reactions such as rashes and itching

- liver failure, in rare cases

Call your doctor right away if you have any of the following symptoms:

- constant sore throat

- dull pain in your abdomen

- easy bruising

- fatigue

- fever

- loss of appetite

- skin rash or itching

- weakness

- yellowing of your skin or whites of your eyes, called jaundice

Doctors usually treat pregnant and breastfeeding women with antithyroid medicine, since this treatment may be safer for the baby than other treatments.

Radioiodine Therapy

Radioactive iodine is a common and effective treatment for hyperthyroidism. In radioiodine therapy, you take radioactive iodine-131 by mouth as a capsule or liquid. The radioactive iodine slowly destroys the cells of the thyroid gland that produce thyroid hormone. Radioactive iodine does not affect other body tissues.

You may need more than one radioiodine treatment to bring your thyroid hormone levels into the normal range. In the meantime, treatment with beta blockers can control your symptoms.

Almost everyone who has radioactive iodine treatment later develops hypothyroidism because the thyroid hormone-producing cells have been destroyed. However, hypothyroidism is easier to treat and causes fewer long-term health problems than hyperthyroidism. People with hypothyroidism can completely control the condition with daily thyroid hormone medicine.

Doctors don't use radioiodine therapy in pregnant women or in women who are breastfeeding. Radioactive iodine can harm the fetus' thyroid and can be passed from mother to child in breast milk.

Thyroid Surgery

The least-used treatment for hyperthyroidism is surgery to remove part or most of the thyroid gland. Sometimes doctors use surgery to treat people with large goiters or pregnant women who cannot take antithyroid medicines.

Before surgery, your doctor may prescribe antithyroid medicines to bring your thyroid hormone levels into the normal range. This treatment prevents a condition called thyroid storm—a sudden, severe worsening of symptoms—that can occur when people with hyperthyroidism have general anesthesia.

When part of your thyroid is removed, your thyroid hormone levels may return to normal. You may still develop hypothyroidism after surgery and need to take thyroid hormone medicine. If your whole thyroid is removed, you will need to take thyroid hormone medicine for life. After surgery, your doctor will continue to check your thyroid hormone levels.

What Should I Avoid Eating If I Have Hyperthyroidism?

People with Graves disease or other type of autoimmune thyroid disorder may be sensitive to harmful side effects from iodine. Eating foods that have large amounts of iodine—such as kelp, dulse, or other kinds of seaweed—may cause or worsen hyperthyroidism. Taking iodine supplements can have the same effect. Talk with members of your healthcare team about what foods you should limit or avoid, and let them know if you take iodine supplements. Also, share information about any cough syrups or multivitamins that you take because they may contain iodine.

Chapter 26

Graves Disease

What Is Graves Disease?

Graves disease, also known as toxic diffuse goiter, is the most common cause of hyperthyroidism in the United States. Hyperthyroidism is a disorder that occurs when the thyroid gland makes more thyroid hormone than the body needs.

What Are the Symptoms of Graves Disease?

People with Graves disease may have common symptoms of hyperthyroidism such as:

- Fatigue or muscle weakness
- Frequent bowel movements or diarrhea
- Goiter, which is an enlarged thyroid that may cause the neck to look swollen and can interfere with normal breathing and swallowing
- Hand tremors
- Heat intolerance
- Nervousness or irritability
- Rapid and irregular heartbeat

This chapter includes text excerpted from "Graves' Disease," National Institute of Diabetes and Digestive and Kidney Diseases (NIDDK), August 2012. Reviewed October 2016.

- Trouble sleeping

- Weight loss

A small number of people with Graves disease also experience thickening and reddening of the skin on their shins. This usually painless problem is called pretibial myxedema or Graves dermopathy.

In addition, the eyes of people with Graves disease may appear enlarged because their eyelids are retracted—seem pulled back into the eye sockets—and their eyes bulge out from the eye sockets. This condition is called Graves ophthalmopathy (GO).

What Is Graves Ophthalmopathy?

Graves ophthalmopathy (GO) is a condition associated with Graves disease that occurs when cells from the immune system attack the muscles and other tissues around the eyes.

The result is inflammation and a buildup of tissue and fat behind the eye socket, causing the eyeballs to bulge out. Rarely, inflammation is severe enough to compress the optic nerve that leads to the eye, causing vision loss.

Other GO symptoms are:

- Double vision

- Dry, gritty, and irritated eyes

- Light sensitivity

- Pressure or pain in the eyes

- Puffy eyelids

- Trouble moving the eyes

About 25 to 30 percent of people with Graves disease develop mild GO, and 2 to 5 percent develop severe GO. This eye condition usually lasts 1 to 2 years and often improves on its own.

GO can occur before, at the same time as, or after other symptoms of hyperthyroidism develop and may even occur in people whose thyroid function is normal. Smoking makes GO worse.

Who Is Likely to Develop Graves Disease?

Scientists cannot predict who will develop Graves disease. However, factors such as age, sex, heredity, and emotional and environmental stress are likely involved.

Graves disease usually occurs in people younger than age 40 and is seven to eight times more common in women than men. Women are most often affected between ages 30 and 60. And a person's chance of developing Graves disease increases if other family members have the disease.

Researchers have not been able to find a specific gene that causes the disease to be passed from parent to child. While scientists know some people inherit an immune system that can make antibodies against healthy cells, predicting who will be affected is difficult.

People with other autoimmune diseases have an increased chance of developing Graves disease. Conditions associated with Graves disease include type 1 diabetes, rheumatoid arthritis, and vitiligo—a disorder in which some parts of the skin are not pigmented.

How Is Graves Disease Diagnosed?

Healthcare providers can sometimes diagnose Graves disease based only on a physical examination and a medical history. Blood tests and other diagnostic tests, such as the following, then confirm the diagnosis.

- Radioactive iodine uptake test
- T3 and T4 test
- Thyroid scan
- TSH test
- TSI test

How Is Graves Disease Treated?

People with Graves disease have three treatment options:

1. Radioiodine therapy
2. Medications
3. Thyroid surgery

Radioiodine Therapy

In radioiodine therapy, patients take radioactive iodine-131 by mouth. Because the thyroid gland collects iodine to make thyroid hormone, it will collect the radioactive iodine from the bloodstream in the same way. Iodine-131—stronger than the radioactive iodine used in diagnostic tests—gradually destroys the cells that make up the thyroid gland but does not affect other body tissues.

Many healthcare providers use a large enough dose of iodine-131 to shut down the thyroid completely, but some prefer smaller doses to try to bring hormone production into the normal range. More than one round of radioiodine therapy may be needed. Results take time and people undergoing this treatment may not notice improvement in symptoms for several weeks or months.

People with GO should talk with a healthcare provider about any risks associated with radioactive iodine treatments. Several studies suggest radioiodine therapy can worsen GO in some people. Other treatments, such as prescription steroids, may prevent this complication.

Although iodine-131 is not known to cause birth defects or infertility, radioiodine therapy is not used in pregnant women or women who are breastfeeding. Radioactive iodine can be harmful to the fetus thyroid and can be passed from mother to child in breast milk. Experts recommend that women wait a year after treatment before becoming pregnant.

Almost everyone who receives radioactive iodine treatment eventually develops hypothyroidism, which occurs when the thyroid does not make enough thyroid hormone. People with hypothyroidism must take synthetic thyroid hormone, a medication that replaces their natural thyroid hormone.

Medications

Beta blockers. Healthcare providers may prescribe a medication called a beta blocker to reduce many of the symptoms of hyperthyroidism, such as tremors, rapid heartbeat, and nervousness. But beta blockers do not stop thyroid hormone production.

Antithyroid medications. Healthcare providers sometimes prescribe antithyroid medications as the only treatment for Graves disease. Antithyroid medications interfere with thyroid hormone production but don't usually have permanent results. Use of these medications requires frequent monitoring by a healthcare provider. More often, antithyroid medications are used to pretreat patients before surgery or radioiodine therapy, or they are used as supplemental treatment after radioiodine therapy.

Antithyroid medications can cause side effects in some people, including:

- allergic reactions such as rashes and itching

- a decrease in the number of white blood cells in the body, which can lower a person's resistance to infection

- liver failure, in rare cases

In the United States, healthcare providers prescribe the antithyroid medication methimazole (Tapazole, Northyx) for most types of hyperthyroidism.

Antithyroid medications and pregnancy. Because pregnant and breastfeeding women cannot receive radioiodine therapy, they are usually treated with an antithyroid medication instead. However, experts agree that women in their first trimester of pregnancy should probably not take methimazole due to the rare occurrence of damage to the fetus.

Another antithyroid medication, propylthiouracil (PTU), is available for women in this stage of pregnancy or for women who are allergic to or intolerant of methimazole and have no other treatment options. Healthcare providers may prescribe PTU for the first trimester of pregnancy and switch to methimazole for the second and third trimesters.

Some women are able to stop taking antithyroid medications in the last 4 to 8 weeks of pregnancy due to the remission of hyperthyroidism that occurs during pregnancy. However, these women should continue to be monitored for recurrence of thyroid problems following delivery.

Studies have shown that mothers taking antithyroid medications may safely breastfeed. However, they should take only moderate doses, less than 10–20 milligrams daily, of the antithyroid medication methimazole. Doses should be divided and taken after feedings, and the infants should be monitored for side effects.

Women requiring higher doses of the antithyroid medication to control hyperthyroidism should not breastfeed.

Thyroid Surgery

Surgery is the least-used option for treating Graves disease. Sometimes surgery may be used to treat

- pregnant women who cannot tolerate antithyroid medications

- people suspected of having thyroid cancer, though Graves disease does not cause cancer

- people for whom other forms of treatment are not successful

Before surgery, the healthcare provider may prescribe antithyroid medications to temporarily bring a patient's thyroid hormone levels into the normal range. This presurgical treatment prevents a condition called thyroid storm—a sudden, severe worsening of symptoms—that can occur when hyperthyroid patients have general anesthesia.

When surgery is used, many healthcare providers recommend the entire thyroid be removed to eliminate the chance that hyperthyroidism will return. If the entire thyroid is removed, lifelong thyroid hormone medication is necessary.

Although uncommon, certain problems can occur in thyroid surgery. The parathyroid glands can be damaged because they are located very close to the thyroid. These glands help control calcium and phosphorous levels in the body. Damage to the laryngeal nerve, also located close to the thyroid, can lead to voice changes or breathing problems.

But when surgery is performed by an experienced surgeon, less than 1 percent of patients have permanent complications.

Eye Care

The eye problems associated with Graves disease may not improve following thyroid treatment, so the two problems are often treated separately.

Eye drops can relieve dry, gritty, irritated eyes—the most common of the milder symptoms. If pain and swelling occur, healthcare providers may prescribe a steroid such as prednisone. Other medications that suppress the immune response may also provide relief.

Special lenses for glasses can help with light sensitivity and double vision. People with eye symptoms may be advised to sleep with their head elevated to reduce eyelid swelling. If the eyelids do not fully close, taping them shut at night can help prevent dry eyes.

In more severe cases, external radiation may be applied to the eyes to reduce inflammation. Like other types of radiation treatment, the benefits are not immediate; most people feel relief from symptoms 1 to 2 months after treatment.

Surgery may be used to improve bulging of the eyes and correct the vision changes caused by pressure on the optic nerve. A procedure called orbital decompression makes the eye socket bigger and gives the eye room to sink back to a more normal position. Eyelid surgery can return retracted eyelids to their normal position.

Can Treatment for Graves Disease Affect Pregnancy?

Treatment for Graves disease can sometimes affect pregnancy. After treatment with surgery or radioactive iodine, TSI antibodies can still be present in the blood, even when thyroid levels are normal. If a pregnant woman has received either of these treatments prior to becoming pregnant, the antibodies she produces may travel across the placenta to the baby's bloodstream and stimulate the fetal thyroid.

A pregnant woman who has been treated with surgery or radioactive iodine should inform her healthcare provider so her baby can be monitored for thyroid-related problems later in the pregnancy. Pregnant women may safely be treated with antithyroid medications.

Eating, Diet, and Nutrition

Experts recommend that people eat a balanced diet to obtain most nutrients.

Chapter 27

Thyroid Cancer

The thyroid is a gland at the base of the throat near the trachea (windpipe). It is shaped like a butterfly, with a right lobe and a left lobe. The isthmus, a thin piece of tissue, connects the two lobes. A healthy thyroid is a little larger than a quarter. It usually cannot be felt through the skin.

The thyroid uses iodine, a mineral found in some foods and in iodized salt, to help make several hormones. Thyroid hormones do the following:

- Control heart rate, body temperature, and how quickly food is changed into energy (metabolism).

- Control the amount of calcium in the blood.

Thyroid Nodules

Your doctor may find a lump (nodule) in your thyroid during a routine medical exam. A thyroid nodule is an abnormal growth of thyroid cells in the thyroid. Nodules may be solid or fluid-filled. When a thyroid nodule is found, an ultrasound of the thyroid and a fine-needle aspiration biopsy are often done to check for signs of cancer. Blood tests to check thyroid hormone levels and for antithyroid antibodies in the blood may also be done to check for other types of thyroid disease. Thyroid nodules usually don't cause symptoms or need treatment.

This chapter includes text excerpted from "Thyroid Cancer Treatment (PDQ®)—Patient Version," National Cancer Institute (NCI), August 17, 2016.

Sometimes the thyroid nodules become large enough that it is hard to swallow or breathe and more tests and treatment are needed. Only a small number of thyroid nodules are diagnosed as cancer.

Types

There are four main types of thyroid cancer:

1. Anaplastic thyroid cancer
2. Follicular thyroid cancer
3. Medullary thyroid cancer
4. Papillary thyroid cancer

Risks Factors

Anything that increases your risk of getting a disease is called a risk factor. Having a risk factor does not mean that you will get cancer; not having risk factors doesn't mean that you will not get cancer. Talk with your doctor if you think you may be at risk.

Risk factors for thyroid cancer include the following:

- Being between 25 and 65 years old

- Being female

- Being exposed to radiation to the head and neck as a child or being exposed to radiation from an atomic bomb. The cancer may occur as soon as 5 years after exposure.

- Having a history of goiter (enlarged thyroid).

- Having a family history of thyroid disease or thyroid cancer.

- Having certain genetic conditions such as familial medullary thyroid cancer (FMTC), multiple endocrine neoplasia type 2A syndrome, and multiple endocrine neoplasia type 2B syndrome.

- Being Asian

Causes

The genes in cells carry hereditary information from parent to child. A certain change in a gene that is passed from parent to child (inherited) may cause medullary thyroid cancer. A test has been developed that can find the changed gene before medullary thyroid cancer appears. The patient is tested first to see if he or she has the changed gene. If the patient has it, other family members may also be tested. Family members, including young children, who have the changed gene can decrease the chance of developing medullary thyroid cancer by having a thyroidectomy (surgery to remove the thyroid).

Signs and Symptoms

Thyroid cancer may not cause early signs or symptoms. It is sometimes found during a routine physical exam. Signs or symptoms may occur as the tumor gets bigger. Other conditions may cause the same signs or symptoms. Check with your doctor if you have any of the following:

- a lump (nodule) in the neck
- hoarseness
- trouble breathing
- trouble swallowing

Diagnosis

- Blood chemistry studies
- Blood hormone studies
- CT scan (CAT scan)
- Fine-needle aspiration biopsy of the thyroid
- Laryngoscopy
- Physical exam and history
- Surgical biopsy
- Ultrasound exam

Prognosis and Treatment

The prognosis (chance of recovery) and treatment options depend on the following:

- The age of the patient.
- The type of thyroid cancer.
- The stage of the cancer.

- The patient's general health.
- Whether the patient has multiple endocrine neoplasia type 2B (MEN 2B).
- Whether the cancer has just been diagnosed or has recurred (come back).

Stages of Thyroid Cancer

The process used to find out if cancer has spread within the thyroid or to other parts of the body is called staging. The information gathered from the staging process determines the stage of the disease. It is important to know the stage in order to plan treatment. The following tests and procedures may be used in the staging process:

- CT scan (CAT scan)
- Ultrasound exam
- Chest X-ray
- Sentinel lymph node biopsy

There Are Three Ways That Cancer Spreads in the Body

Cancer can spread through tissue, the lymph system, and the blood.

Cancer May Spread from Where It Began to Other Parts of the Body

When cancer spreads to another part of the body, it is called metastasis. Cancer cells break away from where they began (the primary tumor) and travel through the lymph system or blood.

- Lymph system. The cancer gets into the lymph system, travels through the lymph vessels, and forms a tumor (metastatic tumor) in another part of the body.
- Blood. The cancer gets into the blood, travels through the blood vessels, and forms a tumor (metastatic tumor) in another part of the body.

The metastatic tumor is the same type of cancer as the primary tumor. For example, if thyroid cancer spreads to the lung, the cancer cells in the lung are actually thyroid cancer cells. The disease is metastatic thyroid cancer, not lung cancer.

Stages are used to describe thyroid cancer according to the type of thyroid cancer and age of the patient:

Papillary and follicular thyroid cancer in patients younger than 45 years

- **Stage I:** In stage I papillary and follicular thyroid cancer, the tumor is any size and may have spread to nearby tissues and lymph nodes. Cancer has not spread to other parts of the body.

- **Stage II:** In stage II papillary and follicular thyroid cancer, the tumor is any size and cancer has spread from the thyroid to other parts of the body, such as the lungs or bone, and may have spread to lymph nodes.

Papillary and follicular thyroid cancer in patients 45 years and older

- **Stage I:** In stage I papillary and follicular thyroid cancer, cancer is found only in the thyroid and the tumor is 2 centimeters or smaller.

- **Stage II:** In stage II papillary and follicular thyroid cancer, cancer is only in the thyroid and the tumor is larger than 2 centimeters but not larger than 4 centimeters.

- **Stage III:** In stage III papillary and follicular thyroid cancer, either of the following is found:

  - the tumor is larger than 4 centimeters and only in the thyroid or the tumor is any size and cancer has spread to tissues just outside the thyroid, but not to lymph nodes; or

  - the tumor is any size and cancer may have spread to tissues just outside the thyroid and has spread to lymph nodes near the trachea or the larynx (voice box)

- **Stage IV:** Stage IV papillary and follicular thyroid cancer is divided into stages IVA, IVB, and IVC.

  - In stage IVA, either of the following is found:

    - the tumor is any size and cancer has spread outside the thyroid to tissues under the skin, the trachea, the esophagus, the larynx (voice box), and/or the recurrent laryngeal nerve (a nerve with 2 branches that go to the larynx); cancer may have spread to lymph nodes near the trachea or the larynx; or

- the tumor is any size and cancer may have spread to tissues just outside the thyroid. Cancer has spread to lymph nodes on one or both sides of the neck or between the lungs

- In stage IVB, cancer has spread to tissue in front of the spinal column or has surrounded the carotid artery or the blood vessels in the area between the lungs. Cancer may have spread to lymph nodes.

- In stage IVC, the tumor is any size and cancer has spread to other parts of the body, such as the lungs and bones, and may have spread to lymph nodes.

Medullary thyroid cancer for all ages

- **Stage 0:** Stage 0 medullary thyroid cancer is found only with a special screening test. No tumor can be found in the thyroid.

- **Stage I:** Stage I medullary thyroid cancer is found only in the thyroid and is 2 centimeters or smaller.

- **Stage II:** In stage II medullary thyroid cancer, either of the following is found:

  - the tumor is larger than 2 centimeters and only in the thyroid; or

  - the tumor is any size and has spread to tissues just outside the thyroid, but not to lymph nodes

- **Stage III:** In stage III medullary thyroid cancer, the tumor is any size, has spread to lymph nodes near the trachea and the larynx (voice box), and may have spread to tissues just outside the thyroid.

- **Stage IV:** Stage IV medullary thyroid cancer is divided into stages IVA, IVB, and IVC.

  - In stage IVA, either of the following is found:

    - the tumor is any size and cancer has spread outside the thyroid to tissues under the skin, the trachea, the esophagus, the larynx (voice box), and/or the recurrent laryngeal nerve (a nerve with 2 branches that go to the larynx); cancer may have spread to lymph nodes near the trachea or the larynx; or

    - the tumor is any size and cancer may have spread to tissues just outside the thyroid. Cancer has spread to lymph nodes on one or both sides of the neck or between the lungs

- In stage IVB, cancer has spread to tissue in front of the spinal column or has surrounded the carotid artery or the blood vessels in the area between the lungs. Cancer may have spread to lymph nodes.

- In stage IVC, the tumor is any size and cancer has spread to other parts of the body, such as the lungs and bones, and may have spread to lymph nodes.

Anaplastic Thyroid Cancer Is Considered Stage IV Thyroid Cancer
Anaplastic thyroid cancer grows quickly and has usually spread within the neck when it is found. Stage IV anaplastic thyroid cancer is divided into stages IVA, IVB, and IVC.

- In stage IVA, cancer is found in the thyroid and may have spread to lymph nodes.

- In stage IVB, cancer has spread to tissue just outside the thyroid and may have spread to lymph nodes.

- In stage IVC, cancer has spread to other parts of the body, such as the lungs and bones, and may have spread to lymph nodes.

Recurrent Thyroid Cancer

Recurrent thyroid cancer is cancer that has recurred (come back) after it has been treated. Thyroid cancer may come back in the thyroid or in other parts of the body.

Treatment Option Overview

Different types of treatment are available for patients with thyroid cancer. Some treatments are standard (the currently used treatment), and some are being tested in clinical trials. A treatment clinical trial is a research study meant to help improve current treatments or obtain information on new treatments for patients with cancer. When clinical trials show that a new treatment is better than the standard treatment, the new treatment may become the standard treatment. Patients may want to think about taking part in a clinical trial. Some clinical trials are open only to patients who have not started treatment.

Five Types of Standard Treatment Are Used

1. Surgery

   - Lobectomy

- Near-total thyroidectomy
- Total thyroidectomy
- Lymphadenectomy

2. Radiation Therapy, including Radioactive Iodine Therapy

- External radiation therapy
- Internal radiation therapy

3. Chemotherapy

4. Thyroid Hormone Therapy

5. Targeted Therapy

Patients May Want to Think about Taking Part in a Clinical Trial

For some patients, taking part in a clinical trial may be the best treatment choice. Clinical trials are part of the cancer research process. Clinical trials are done to find out if new cancer treatments are safe and effective or better than the standard treatment.

Many of today's standard treatments for cancer are based on earlier clinical trials. Patients who take part in a clinical trial may receive the standard treatment or be among the first to receive a new treatment.

Patients who take part in clinical trials also help improve the way cancer will be treated in the future. Even when clinical trials do not lead to effective new treatments, they often answer important questions and help move research forward.

Patients Can Enter Clinical Trials before, during, or after Starting Their Cancer Treatment

Some clinical trials only include patients who have not yet received treatment. Other trials test treatments for patients whose cancer has not gotten better. There are also clinical trials that test new ways to stop cancer from recurring (coming back) or reduce the side effects of cancer treatment.

Clinical trials are taking place in many parts of the country.

Follow-Up Tests May Be Needed

Some of the tests that were done to diagnose the cancer or to find out the stage of the cancer may be repeated. Some tests will be repeated in order to see how well the treatment is working. Decisions about whether to continue, change, or stop treatment may be based on the results of these tests.

Some of the tests will continue to be done from time to time after treatment has ended. The results of these tests can show if your condition has changed or if the cancer has recurred (come back). These tests are sometimes called follow-up tests or check-ups.

Chapter 28

Hypoparathyroidism

What Is Hypoparathyroidism?

Hypoparathyroidism is a rare condition in which the body doesn't make enough parathyroid hormone (PTH).

Parathyroid glands are four small endocrine glands located in the neck behind the thyroid gland that secrete PTH.

PTH regulates the amount of calcium and phosphorus that is stored in the bones and circulated in the blood. PTH has a direct effect on the body's calcium reservoir in the bones. It also signals the kidneys to either retain or secrete calcium and works with vitamin D to control how much calcium we absorb from our diet.

Decreased levels of PTH lead to low levels of calcium and high levels of phosphorus in the blood. This imbalance can lead to problems with bones, muscles, skin, and nerve endings.

What Are the Symptoms of Hypoparathyroidism?

The symptoms of hypoparathyroidism can include:

- calcium deposits (calcifications) may form in the brain or kidney

- cataracts on the eyes

- dry hair, brittle nails, and dry, coarse skin

This chapter includes text excerpted from "Hypoparathyroidism," *Eunice Kennedy Shriver* National Institute of Child Health and Human Development (NICHD), July 5, 2013.

- loss of memory

- malformations of the teeth, including weakened tooth enamel and misshapen roots of the teeth

- muscle cramps and spasms (called tetany) which cause pain in the face, hands, legs, and feet

- muscle weakness and generalized fatigue

- severe muscle spasms that may lead to convulsions

- tingling in the lips, fingers, and toes

In some cases, seizures during infancy or childhood may be the first sign of hypoparathyroidism.

How Many People Are Affected/at Risk for Hypoparathyroidism?

Hypoparathyroidism occurs in about 0.5 percent to 6.6 percent of people who have had their thyroid gland totally removed, but these rates vary significantly across hospitals. Rates at endocrine surgical centers that perform large numbers of thyroid surgeries have the lowest rates, between 0.9 percent and 1.6 percent.

What Causes Hypoparathyroidism?

The most common cause of hypoparathyroidism is injury to the parathyroid glands, such as during head and neck surgery. For example, thyroid surgery may lead to damage of the parathyroid glands or may damage the surrounding tissues.

In other cases, hypoparathyroidism is present at birth (called congenital), or it may be associated with an autoimmune disease that affects the parathyroid glands along with other glands such as the thyroid, ovaries, pancreas, or adrenal glands.

When hypoparathyroidism is present along with multiple other low hormone levels, it may be part of a rare congenital syndrome called autoimmune polyglandular failure type.

How Do Healthcare Providers Diagnose Hypoparathyroidism?

A healthcare provider will order a blood test to determine the levels of the following:

- calcium

- creatinine

- magnesium

- parathyroid hormone

- phosphorus

- 25-hydroxy vitamin D

Urine also may be tested to determine how much calcium is being removed (excreted) from the body.

How Is Hypoparathyroidism Treated?

The goal of treatment for hypoparathyroidism is to restore the body's calcium, magnesium, and phosphorus levels in the blood and urine to normal levels. This may be challenging, especially with conventional therapy.

The only therapies that are approved by the U.S. Food and Drug Administration (FDA) for hypoparathyroidism (from any cause) are synthetic forms of vitamin D and calcium and magnesium supplements.

Some individuals with hypoparathyroidism are encouraged to eat foods high in calcium such as dairy products, breakfast cereals, fortified orange juice, and green, leafy vegetables.

Hypoparathyroidism is one of the few hormone deficiency diseases that are not usually treated with the missing hormone. However, greater availability of various forms of parathyroid hormone (PTH) has led to several studies of investigational drugs for this condition.

What Are Possible Complications of Hypoparathyroidism and Its Treatments?

If congenital hypoparathyroidism is diagnosed and treated early, outcomes are usually good and the body grows normally.

If hypoparathyroidism is left untreated, complications can include blocked airway from severe muscle spasms, stunted growth, poorly formed or malformed teeth, development of cataracts, and calcium deposits in the brain.

In some cases, conventional treatments can lead to problems. Too much replacement of calcium and vitamin D can cause high blood calcium (a condition called hypercalcemia) and kidney problems, including reduced function and tissue damage.

Conventional therapy may also lead to kidney failure from a buildup of calcium in the kidney called nephrocalcinosis. This build up is not necessarily associated with hypercalcemia and may occur even when the blood calcium levels are kept in the normal range.

Chapter 29

Primary Hyperparathyroidism

What Is Primary Hyperparathyroidism?

Primary hyperparathyroidism is a disorder of the parathyroid glands, also called parathyroids. "Primary" means this disorder originates in the parathyroid glands. In primary hyperparathyroidism, one or more of the parathyroid glands are overactive. As a result, the gland releases too much parathyroid hormone (PTH). The disorder includes the problems that occur in the rest of the body as a result of too much PTH—for example, loss of calcium from bones.

In the United States, about 100,000 people develop primary hyperparathyroidism each year. The disorder is diagnosed most often in people between age 50 and 60, and women are affected about three times as often as men.

Secondary, or reactive, hyperparathyroidism can occur if a problem such as kidney failure causes the parathyroid glands to be overactive.

What Are the Parathyroid Glands?

The parathyroid glands are four pea-sized glands located on or near the thyroid gland in the neck. Occasionally, a person is born with one

This chapter includes text excerpted from "Primary Hyperparathyroidism," National Institute of Diabetes and Digestive and Kidney Diseases (NIDDK), August 2012. Reviewed October 2016.

or more of the parathyroid glands in another location. For example, a gland may be embedded in the thyroid, in the thymus—an immune system organ located in the chest—or elsewhere around this area. In most such cases, however, the parathyroid glands function normally.

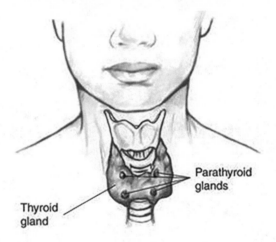

Figure 29.1. *Parathyroid Glands*

The parathyroid glands are part of the body's endocrine system. Endocrine glands produce, store, and release hormones, which travel in the bloodstream to target cells elsewhere in the body and direct the cells activity.

Though their names are similar, the thyroid and parathyroid glands are entirely different glands, each producing distinct hormones with specific functions. The parathyroid glands produce PTH, a hormone that helps maintain the correct balance of calcium in the body. PTH regulates the level of calcium in the blood, release of calcium from bone, absorption of calcium in the small intestine, and excretion of calcium in the urine.

When the level of calcium in the blood falls too low, normal parathyroid glands release just enough PTH to restore the blood calcium level.

What Are the Effects of High PTH Levels?

High PTH levels trigger the bones to release increased amounts of calcium into the blood, causing blood calcium levels to rise above normal. The loss of calcium from bones may weaken the bones. Also, the small intestine may absorb more calcium from food, adding to the excess calcium in the blood. In response to high blood calcium levels, the kidneys excrete more calcium in the urine, which can lead to kidney stones.

High blood calcium levels might contribute to other problems, such as heart disease, high blood pressure, and difficulty with concentration. However, more research is needed to better understand how primary hyperparathyroidism affects the cardiovascular system—the heart and blood vessels—and the central nervous system—the brain and spinal cord.

Why Is Calcium Important?

Calcium is essential for good health. Calcium plays an important role in bone and tooth development and, combined with phosphorus, strengthens bones and teeth. Calcium also helps muscles contract and nerves transmit signals.

What Causes Primary Hyperparathyroidism?

In about 80 percent of people with primary hyperparathyroidism, a benign, or noncancerous, tumor called an adenoma has formed in one of the parathyroid glands. The tumor causes the gland to become overactive. In most other cases, the excess hormone comes from two or more overactive parathyroid glands, a condition called multiple tumors or hyperplasia. Rarely, primary hyperparathyroidism is caused by cancer of a parathyroid gland.

In most cases, healthcare providers don't know why adenoma or multiple tumors occur in the parathyroid glands. Most people with primary hyperparathyroidism have no family history of the disorder, but some cases can be linked to an inherited problem. For example, familial multiple endocrine neoplasia type 1 is a rare, inherited syndrome that causes multiple tumors in the parathyroid glands as well as in the pancreas and the pituitary gland. Another rare genetic disorder, familial hypocalciuric hypercalcemia, causes a kind of hyperparathyroidism that is atypical, in part because it does not respond to standard parathyroid surgery.

What Are the Symptoms of Primary Hyperparathyroidism?

Most people with primary hyperparathyroidism have no symptoms. When symptoms appear, they are often mild and nonspecific, such as

- aches and pains in bones and joints
- fatigue and an increased need for sleep

- feelings of depression

- muscle weakness

  People with more severe disease may have

- confusion or impaired thinking and memory

- constipation

- increased thirst and urination

- loss of appetite

- nausea

- vomiting

These symptoms are mainly due to the high blood calcium levels that result from excessive PTH.

How Is Primary Hyperparathyroidism Diagnosed?

Healthcare providers diagnose primary hyperparathyroidism when a person has high blood calcium and PTH levels. High blood calcium is usually the first sign that leads healthcare providers to suspect parathyroid gland overactivity. Other diseases can cause high blood calcium levels, but only in primary hyperparathyroidism is the elevated calcium the result of too much PTH.

Routine blood tests that screen for a wide range of conditions, including high blood calcium levels, are helping healthcare providers diagnose primary hyperparathyroidism in people who have mild forms of the disorder and are symptom-free. For a blood test, blood is drawn at a healthcare provider's office or commercial facility and sent to a lab for analysis.

What Tests May Be Done to Check for Possible Complications?

Once the diagnosis of primary hyperparathyroidism is established, other tests may be done to assess complications:

- Bone mineral density test

- Ultrasound

- Computerized tomography (CT) scan

- Urine collection

- 25-hydroxy-vitamin D blood test

How Is Primary Hyperparathyroidism Treated?

- Surgery
    - Minimally invasive parathyroidectomy
    - Standard neck exploration
- Monitoring
- Medications

Eating, Diet, and Nutrition

Eating, diet, and nutrition have not been shown to play a role in causing or preventing primary hyperparathyroidism.

Vitamin D. Experts suggest correcting vitamin D deficiency in people with primary hyperparathyroidism to achieve a serum level of 25-hydroxy-vitamin D greater than 20 nanograms per deciliter (50 nanomoles per liter). Research is ongoing to determine optimal doses and regimens of vitamin D supplementation for people with primary hyperparathyroidism.

For the healthy public, the Institute of Medicine (IOM) guidelines for vitamin D intake are

- people ages 1 to 70 years may require 600 International Units (IUs)

- people age 71 and older may require as much as 800 IUs

The IOM also recommends that no more than 4,000 IUs of vitamin D be taken per day.

Calcium. People with primary hyperparathyroidism without symptoms who are being monitored do not need to restrict calcium in their diet. People with low calcium levels due to loss of all parathyroid tissue from surgery will need to take calcium supplements for the rest of their life.

Chapter 30

Parathyroid Cancer

About Parathyroid Cancer

The parathyroid glands are four pea-sized organs found in the neck near the thyroid gland. The parathyroid glands make parathyroid hormone (PTH or parathormone). PTH helps the body use and store calcium to keep the calcium in the blood at normal levels.

A parathyroid gland may become overactive and make too much PTH, a condition called hyperparathyroidism. Hyperparathyroidism can occur when a benign tumor (noncancer), called an adenoma, forms on one of the parathyroid glands, and causes it to grow and become overactive. Sometimes hyperparathyroidism can be caused by parathyroid cancer, but this is very rare.

The extra PTH causes:

• The calcium stored in the bones to move into the blood.

• The intestines to absorb more calcium from the food we eat.

This condition is called hypercalcemia (too much calcium in the blood).

The hypercalcemia caused by hyperparathyroidism is more serious and life-threatening than parathyroid cancer itself and treating hypercalcemia is as important as treating the cancer.

This chapter includes text excerpted from "Parathyroid Cancer Treatment (PDQ®)—Patient Version," National Cancer Institute (NCI), May 27, 2016.

Certain Factors Affect Prognosis (Chance of Recovery) and Treatment Options

The prognosis (chance of recovery) and treatment options depend on the following:

- Whether the calcium level in the blood can be controlled.
- The stage of the cancer.
- Whether the tumor and the capsule around the tumor can be completely removed by surgery.
- The patient's general health.

Risk Factors

Anything that increases the chance of getting a disease is called a risk factor. Risk factors for parathyroid cancer include the following rare disorders that are inherited (passed down from parent to child):

- Familial isolated hyperparathyroidism (FIHP).
- Multiple endocrine neoplasia type 1 (MEN1) syndrome.

Treatment with radiation therapy may increase the risk of developing a parathyroid adenoma.

Signs and Symptoms

Most parathyroid cancer signs and symptoms are caused by the hypercalcemia that develops. Signs and symptoms of hypercalcemia include the following:

- Being much more thirsty than usual
- Constipation
- Feeling very tired
- Loss of appetite
- Nausea and vomiting
- Trouble thinking clearly
- Urinating much more than usual
- Weakness
- Weight loss for no known reason

Other signs and symptoms of parathyroid cancer include the following:

- A broken bone.
- A lump in the neck.
- Change in voice such as hoarseness.
- Pain in the abdomen, side, or back that doesn't go away.
- Pain in the bones.
- Trouble swallowing

Other conditions may cause the same signs and symptoms as parathyroid cancer. Check with your doctor if you have any of these problems.

Diagnosis

Once blood tests are done and hyperparathyroidism is diagnosed, imaging tests may be done to help find which of the parathyroid glands is overactive. Sometimes the parathyroid glands are hard to find and imaging tests are done to find exactly where they are.

Parathyroid cancer may be hard to diagnose because the cells of a benign parathyroid adenoma and a malignant parathyroid cancer look alike. The patient's symptoms, blood levels of calcium and parathyroid hormone, and characteristics of the tumor are also used to make a diagnosis.

The following tests and procedures may be used:

- Angiogram
- Blood chemistry studies
- CT scan (CAT scan)
- Parathyroid hormone test
- Physical exam and history
- Sestamibi scan
- SPECT scan (single photon emission computed tomography scan)
- Ultrasound exam
- Venous sampling

Stages of Parathyroid Cancer

The process used to find out if cancer has spread to other parts of the body is called staging. The following imaging tests may be used to determine if cancer has spread to other parts of the body such as the lungs, liver, bone, heart, pancreas, or lymph nodes:

- CT scan (CAT scan)

- MRI (magnetic resonance imaging)

There Are Three Ways That Cancer Spreads in the Body

Cancer can spread through tissue, the lymph system, and the blood.

Cancer May Spread from Where It Began to Other Parts of the Body

When cancer spreads to another part of the body, it is called metastasis. Cancer cells break away from where they began (the primary tumor) and travel through the lymph system or blood.

- Lymph system. The cancer gets into the lymph system, travels through the lymph vessels, and forms a tumor (metastatic tumor) in another part of the body.

- Blood. The cancer gets into the blood, travels through the blood vessels, and forms a tumor (metastatic tumor) in another part of the body.

The metastatic tumor is the same type of cancer as the primary tumor. For example, if parathyroid cancer spreads to the lung, the cancer cells in the lung are actually parathyroid cancer cells. The disease is metastatic parathyroid cancer, not lung cancer.

There Is No Standard Staging Process for Parathyroid Cancer

Parathyroid cancer is described as either localized or metastatic:

- Localized parathyroid cancer is found in a parathyroid gland and may have spread to nearby tissues.

- Metastatic parathyroid cancer has spread to other parts of the body, such as the lungs, liver, bone, sac around the heart, pancreas, or lymph nodes.

Recurrent Parathyroid Cancer

Recurrent parathyroid cancer is cancer that has recurred (come back) after it has been treated. More than half of patients have a recurrence. The parathyroid cancer usually recurs between 2 and 5 years after the first surgery, but can recur up to 20 years later. It usually comes back in the tissues or lymph nodes of the neck. High blood calcium levels that appear after treatment may be the first sign of recurrence.

Treatment Option Overview

Different types of treatment are available for patients with parathyroid cancer. Some treatments are standard (the currently used treatment), and some are being tested in clinical trials. A treatment clinical trial is a research study meant to help improve current treatments or obtain information on new treatments for patients with cancer. When clinical trials show that a new treatment is better than the standard treatment, the new treatment may become the standard treatment. Patients may want to think about taking part in a clinical trial. Some clinical trials are open only to patients who have not started treatment.

Treatment Includes Control of Hypercalcemia (Too Much Calcium in the Blood) in Patients Who Have an Overactive Parathyroid Gland

In order to reduce the amount of parathyroid hormone that is being made and control the level of calcium in the blood, as much of the tumor as possible is removed in surgery. For patients who cannot have surgery, medication may be used.

Four Types of Standard Treatment Are Used

1. Surgery
   - En bloc resection
   - Tumor debulking
   - Metastasectomy
2. Radiation Therapy
   - External radiation therapy
   - Internal radiation therapy

3. Chemotherapy

4. Supportive Care

Patients May Want to Think about Taking Part in a Clinical Trial

For some patients, taking part in a clinical trial may be the best treatment choice. Clinical trials are part of the cancer research process. Clinical trials are done to find out if new cancer treatments are safe and effective or better than the standard treatment.

Many of today's standard treatments for cancer are based on earlier clinical trials. Patients who take part in a clinical trial may receive the standard treatment or be among the first to receive a new treatment.

Patients who take part in clinical trials also help improve the way cancer will be treated in the future. Even when clinical trials do not lead to effective new treatments, they often answer important questions and help move research forward.

Patients Can Enter Clinical Trials before, during, or after Starting Their Cancer Treatment

Some clinical trials only include patients who have not yet received treatment. Other trials test treatments for patients whose cancer has not gotten better. There are also clinical trials that test new ways to stop cancer from recurring (coming back) or reduce the side effects of cancer treatment.

Follow-Up Tests May Be Needed

Some of the tests that were done to diagnose the cancer or to find out the stage of the cancer may be repeated. Some tests will be repeated in order to see how well the treatment is working. Decisions about whether to continue, change, or stop treatment may be based on the results of these tests.

Some of the tests will continue to be done from time to time after treatment has ended. The results of these tests can show if your condition has changed or if the cancer has recurred (come back). These tests are sometimes called follow-up tests or check-ups.

Parathyroid cancer often recurs. Patients should have regular check-ups for the rest of their lives, to find and treat recurrences early.

Part Four

Adrenal Gland Disorders

Chapter 31

Addison Disease

Adrenal insufficiency is an endocrine, or hormonal, disorder that occurs when the adrenal glands do not produce enough of certain hormones. The adrenal glands are located just above the kidneys.

Adrenal insufficiency can be primary or secondary. Addison disease, the common term for primary adrenal insufficiency, occurs when the adrenal glands are damaged and cannot produce enough of the adrenal hormone cortisol. The adrenal hormone aldosterone may also be lacking. Addison disease affects 110 to 144 of every 1 million people in developed countries.

Secondary adrenal insufficiency occurs when the pituitary gland—a pea-sized gland at the base of the brain—fails to produce enough adrenocorticotropin (ACTH), a hormone that stimulates the adrenal glands to produce the hormone cortisol. If ACTH output is too low, cortisol production drops. Eventually, the adrenal glands can shrink due to lack of ACTH stimulation. Secondary adrenal insufficiency is much more common than Addison disease.

What Causes Addison Disease?

Autoimmune disorders cause most cases of Addison disease. Infections and medications may also cause the disease.

This chapter includes text excerpted from "Adrenal Insufficiency and Addison," National Institute of Diabetes and Digestive and Kidney Diseases (NIDDK), May 2014.

Autoimmune Disorders

Up to 80 percent of Addison disease cases are caused by an autoimmune disorder, which is when the body's immune system attacks the body's own cells and organs. In autoimmune Addison, which mainly occurs in middle-aged females, the immune system gradually destroys the adrenal cortex—the outer layer of the adrenal glands.

Primary adrenal insufficiency occurs when at least 90 percent of the adrenal cortex has been destroyed. As a result, both cortisol and aldosterone are often lacking. Sometimes only the adrenal glands are affected. Sometimes other endocrine glands are affected as well, as in polyendocrine deficiency syndrome.

Polyendocrine deficiency syndrome is classified into type 1 and type 2. Type 1 is inherited and occurs in children. In addition to adrenal insufficiency, these children may have

- Underactive parathyroid glands, which are four pea-sized glands located on or near the thyroid gland in the neck; they produce a hormone that helps maintain the correct balance of calcium in the body.

- Slow sexual development.

- Pernicious anemia, a severe type of anemia; anemia is a condition in which red blood cells are fewer than normal, which means less oxygen is carried to the body's cells. With most types of anemia, red blood cells are smaller than normal; however, in pernicious anemia, the cells are bigger than normal.

- Chronic fungal infections.

- Chronic hepatitis, a liver disease.

Researchers think type 2, which is sometimes called Schmidt syndrome, is also inherited. Type 2 usually affects young adults and may include

- An underactive thyroid gland, which produces hormones that regulate metabolism.

- Slow sexual development.

- Diabetes, in which a person has high blood glucose, also called high blood sugar or hyperglycemia.

- Vitiligo, a loss of pigment on areas of the skin.

Infections

Tuberculosis (TB), an infection that can destroy the adrenal glands, accounts for 10 to 15 percent of Addison disease cases in developed countries. When primary adrenal insufficiency was first identified by Dr. Thomas Addison in 1849, TB was the most common cause of the disease. As TB treatment improved, the incidence of Addison disease due to TB of the adrenal glands greatly decreased. However, recent reports show an increase in Addison disease from infections such as TB and cytomegalovirus. Cytomegalovirus is a common virus that does not cause symptoms in healthy people; however, it does affect babies in the womb and people who have a weakened immune system—mostly due to HIV/AIDS. Other bacterial infections, such as *Neisseria meningitidis,* which is a cause of meningitis, and fungal infections can also lead to Addison disease.

Other Causes

Less common causes of Addison disease are

- Cancer cells in the adrenal glands.

- Amyloidosis, a serious, though rare, group of diseases that occurs when abnormal proteins, called amyloids, build up in the blood and are deposited in tissues and organs.

- Surgical removal of the adrenal glands.

- Bleeding into the adrenal glands.

- Genetic defects including abnormal adrenal gland development, an inability of the adrenal glands to respond to acth, or a defect in adrenal hormone production.

- Medication-related causes, such as from anti-fungal medications and the anesthetic etomidate, which may be used when a person undergoes an emergency intubation—the placement of a flexible, plastic tube through the mouth and into the trachea, or windpipe, to assist with breathing.

What Other Tests Might a Healthcare Provider Perform after Diagnosis of Adrenal Insufficiency?

After Addison disease is diagnosed, healthcare providers may use the following tests to look at the adrenal glands, find out whether the disease is related to TB, or identify antibodies associated with autoimmune Addison disease.

- **Ultrasound of the abdomen.** Ultrasound uses a device, called a transducer, that bounces safe, painless sound waves off organs to create an image of their structure. A specially trained technician performs the procedure in a healthcare provider's office, an outpatient center, or a hospital, and a radiologist—a doctor who specializes in medical imaging—interprets the images; a patient does not need anesthesia. The images can show abnormalities in the adrenal glands, such as enlargement or small size, nodules, or signs of calcium deposits, which may indicate bleeding.

- **Tuberculin skin test.** A tuberculin skin test measures how a patient's immune system reacts to the bacteria that cause TB. A small needle is used to put some testing material, called tuberculin, under the skin. A nurse or lab technician performs the test in a healthcare provider's office; a patient does not need anesthesia. In 2 to 3 days, the patient returns to the healthcare provider, who will check to see if the patient had a reaction to the test. The test can show if adrenal insufficiency could be related to TB.

- To test whether a person has TB infection, which is when TB bacteria live in the body without making the person sick, a special TB blood test is used. To test whether a person has TB disease, which is when TB bacteria are actively attacking a person's lungs and making the person sick, other tests such as a chest X-ray and a sample of sputum—phlegm that is coughed up from deep in the lungs—may be needed.

- **Antibody blood tests.** A blood test involves drawing blood at a healthcare provider's office or a commercial facility and sending the sample to a lab for analysis. The blood test can detect antibodies—proteins made by the immune system to protect the body from foreign substances—associated with autoimmune Addison disease.

How Is Adrenal Insufficiency Treated?

Adrenal insufficiency is treated by replacing, or substituting, the hormones that the adrenal glands are not making. The dose of each medication is adjusted to meet the needs of the patient.

Cortisol is replaced with a corticosteroid, such as hydrocortisone, prednisone, or dexamethasone, taken orally one to three times each day, depending on which medication is chosen.

If aldosterone is also deficient, it is replaced with oral doses of a mineralocorticoid hormone, called fludrocortisone acetate (Florinef), taken once or twice daily. People with secondary adrenal insufficiency normally maintain aldosterone production, so they do not require aldosterone replacement therapy.

During adrenal crisis, low blood pressure, low blood glucose, low blood sodium, and high blood levels of potassium can be life threatening. Standard therapy involves immediate IV injections of corticosteroids and large volumes of IV saline solution with dextrose, a type of sugar. This treatment usually brings rapid improvement. When the patient can take liquids and medications by mouth, the amount of corticosteroids is decreased until a dose that maintains normal hormone levels is reached. If aldosterone is deficient, the person will need to regularly take oral doses of fludrocortisone acetate.

Researchers have found that using replacement therapy for dehydroepiandrosterone (DHEA) in adolescent girls who have secondary adrenal insufficiency and low levels of DHEA can improve pubic hair development and psychological stress. Further studies are needed before routine supplementation recommendations can be made.

Chapter 32

Primary Hyperaldosteronism (Conn Syndrome) and Familial Hyperaldosteronism

What Is Primary Hyperaldosteronism?

Primary hyperaldosteronism is a disorder caused by excess production of the hormone aldosterone by the adrenal glands. The main symptom of primary hyperaldosteronism is high blood pressure (hypertension), but other symptoms may include headaches, weakness, swelling (edema), and muscle spasms (tetany). The cause of primary hyperaldosteronism can vary. One cause may be an adenoma, or benign tumor, on the adrenal glands, which causes them to produce too much aldosterone. If primary hyperaldosteronism is caused by an adenoma, it is known as Conn's syndrome. The condition may also be caused by enlarged adrenal glands without adenomas (adrenal hyperplasia).

In some cases, primary hyperaldosteronism is inherited in an autosomal dominant manner, but in most cases the exact cause of the

This chapter contains text excerpted from the following sources: Text beginning with the heading "What Is Primary Hyperaldosteronism?" is excerpted from "Primary Hyperaldosteronism," Genetic and Rare Diseases Information Center (GARD), National Center for Advancing Translational Sciences (NCATS), July 26, 2016; Text beginning with the heading "What Is Familial Hyperaldosteronism?" is excerpted from "Familial Hyperaldosteronism," Genetics Home Reference (GHR), National Institutes of Health (NIH), September 20, 2016.

disease is unknown (idiopathic). A diagnosis is made by testing the blood for high levels of aldosterone. Treatment for Conn's syndrome includes surgical removal of the adenomas. Medication is used to treat primary hyperaldosteronism if it is caused by adrenal hyperplasia.

Related Diseases

The following diseases are related to Primary hyperaldosteronism.

• Familial hyperaldosteronism type 2

• Familial hyperaldosteronism type III

• Glucocorticoid-remediable aldosteronism

What Is Familial Hyperaldosteronism?

Familial hyperaldosteronism is a group of inherited conditions in which the adrenal glands, which are small glands located on top of each kidney, produce too much of the hormone aldosterone. Aldosterone helps control the amount of salt retained by the kidneys. Excess aldosterone causes the kidneys to retain more salt than normal, which in turn increases the body's fluid levels and blood pressure. People with familial hyperaldosteronism may develop severe high blood pressure (hypertension), often early in life. Without treatment, hypertension increases the risk of strokes, heart attacks, and kidney failure.

Familial hyperaldosteronism is categorized into three types, distinguished by their clinical features and genetic causes. In familial hyperaldosteronism type I, hypertension generally appears in childhood to early adulthood and can range from mild to severe. This type can be treated with steroid medications called glucocorticoids, so it is also known as glucocorticoid-remediable aldosteronism (GRA). In familial hyperaldosteronism type II, hypertension usually appears in early to middle adulthood and does not improve with glucocorticoid treatment. In most individuals with familial hyperaldosteronism type III, the adrenal glands are enlarged up to six times their normal size. These affected individuals have severe hypertension that starts in childhood. The hypertension is difficult to treat and often results in damage to organs such as the heart and kidneys. Rarely, individuals with type III have milder symptoms with treatable hypertension and no adrenal gland enlargement.

There are other forms of hyperaldosteronism that are not familial. These conditions are caused by various problems in the adrenal glands or kidneys. In some cases, a cause for the increase in aldosterone levels cannot be found.

Frequency

The prevalence of familial hyperaldosteronism is unknown. Familial hyperaldosteronism type II appears to be the most common variety. All types of familial hyperaldosteronism combined account for fewer than 1 out of 10 cases of hyperaldosteronism.

Genetic Changes

The various types of familial hyperaldosteronism have different genetic causes. Familial hyperaldosteronism type I is caused by the abnormal joining together (fusion) of two similar genes called *CYP11B1* and *CYP11B2*, which are located close together on chromosome 8. These genes provide instructions for making two enzymes that are found in the adrenal glands.

The *CYP11B1* gene provides instructions for making an enzyme called 11-beta-hydroxylase. This enzyme helps produce hormones called cortisol and corticosterone. The *CYP11B2* gene provides instructions for making another enzyme called aldosterone synthase, which helps produce aldosterone. When *CYP11B1* and *CYP11B2* are abnormally fused together, too much aldosterone synthase is produced. This overproduction causes the adrenal glands to make excess aldosterone, which leads to the signs and symptoms of familial hyperaldosteronism type I.

Familial hyperaldosteronism type III is caused by mutations in the *KCNJ5* gene. The *KCNJ5* gene provides instructions for making a protein that functions as a potassium channel, which means that it transports positively charged atoms (ions) of potassium into and out of cells. In the adrenal glands, the flow of ions through potassium channels produced from the *KCNJ5* gene is thought to help regulate the production of aldosterone. Mutations in the *KCNJ5* gene likely result in the production of potassium channels that are less selective, allowing other ions (predominantly sodium) to pass as well. The abnormal ion flow results in the activation of biochemical processes (pathways) that lead to increased aldosterone production, causing the hypertension associated with familial hyperaldosteronism type III.

The genetic cause of familial hyperaldosteronism type II is unknown.

Inheritance Pattern

This condition is inherited in an autosomal dominant pattern, which means one copy of the altered gene in each cell is sufficient to cause the disorder.

Other Names for This Condition

- Familial primary aldosteronism
- FH
- Hereditary aldosteronism
- Hyperaldosteronism, familial

Chapter 33

Cushing Syndrome

What Is Cushing Syndrome?

Cushing syndrome is a hormonal disorder caused by prolonged exposure of the body's tissues to high levels of the hormone cortisol. Sometimes called hypercortisolism, Cushing syndrome is relatively rare and most commonly affects adults aged 20 to 50. People who are obese and have type 2 diabetes, along with poorly controlled blood glucose-also called blood sugar-and high blood pressure, have an increased risk of developing the disorder.

What Are the Signs and Symptoms of Cushing Syndrome?

Signs and symptoms of Cushing syndrome vary, but most people with the disorder have upper body obesity, a rounded face, increased fat around the neck, and relatively slender arms and legs. Children tend to be obese with slowed growth rates.

Other signs appear in the skin, which becomes fragile and thin, bruises easily, and heals poorly. Purple or pink stretch marks may appear on the abdomen, thighs, buttocks, arms, and breasts. The bones are weakened, and routine activities such as bending, lifting, or rising from a chair may lead to backaches and rib or spinal column fractures.

This chapter includes text excerpted from "Cushing Syndrome," National Institute of Diabetes and Digestive and Kidney Diseases (NIDDK), August 2012. Reviewed October 2016.

Women with Cushing syndrome usually have excess hair growth on their face, neck, chest, abdomen, and thighs. Their menstrual periods may become irregular or stop. Men may have decreased fertility with diminished or absent desire for sex and, sometimes, erectile dysfunction.

Other common signs and symptoms include

- severe fatigue

- weak muscles

- high blood pressure

- high blood glucose

- increased thirst and urination

- irritability, anxiety, or depression

- a fatty hump between the shoulders

Sometimes other conditions have many of the same signs as Cushing syndrome, even though people with these disorders do not have abnormally elevated cortisol levels. For example, polycystic ovary syndrome can cause menstrual disturbances, weight gain beginning in adolescence, excess hair growth, and impaired insulin action and diabetes. Metabolic syndrome-a combination of problems that includes excess weight around the waist, high blood pressure, abnormal levels of cholesterol and triglycerides in the blood, and insulin resistance-also mimics the symptoms of Cushing syndrome.

What Causes Cushing Syndrome?

Cushing syndrome occurs when the body's tissues are exposed to high levels of cortisol for too long. Many people develop Cushing syndrome because they take glucocorticoids—steroid hormones that are chemically similar to naturally produced cortisol—such as prednisone for asthma, rheumatoid arthritis, lupus, and other inflammatory diseases. Glucocorticoids are also used to suppress the immune system after transplantation to keep the body from rejecting the new organ or tissue.

Other people develop Cushing syndrome because their bodies produce too much cortisol. Normally, the production of cortisol follows a precise chain of events. First, the hypothalamus, a part of the brain about the size of a small sugar cube, sends corticotropin-releasing hormone (CRH) to the pituitary gland. CRH causes the pituitary to

214

secrete adrenocorticotropin hormone (ACTH), which stimulates the adrenal glands. When the adrenals, which are located just above the kidneys, receive the ACTH, they respond by releasing cortisol into the bloodstream.

Cortisol performs vital tasks in the body including

- helping maintain blood pressure and cardiovascular function

- reducing the immune system's inflammatory response

- balancing the effects of insulin, which breaks down glucose for energy

- regulating the metabolism of proteins, carbohydrates, and fats

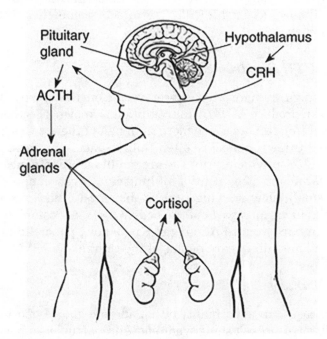

Figure 33.1. *Production of Cortisol*

The hypothalamus sends CRH to the pituitary, which responds by secreting ACTH. ACTH then causes the adrenals to release cortisol into the bloodstream.

One of cortisol's most important jobs is to help the body respond to stress. For this reason, women in their last 3 months of pregnancy and highly trained athletes normally have high levels of the hormone. People suffering from depression, alcoholism, malnutrition, or panic disorders also have increased cortisol levels.

When the amount of cortisol in the blood is adequate, the hypothalamus and pituitary release less CRH and ACTH. This process ensures the amount of cortisol released by the adrenal glands is precisely balanced to meet the body's daily needs. However, if something goes wrong with the adrenals or the regulating switches in the pituitary gland or hypothalamus, cortisol production can go awry.

Pituitary Adenomas

Pituitary adenomas cause 70 percent of Cushing syndrome cases, excluding those caused by glucocorticoid use. These benign, or noncancerous, tumors of the pituitary gland secrete extra ACTH. Most people with the disorder have a single adenoma. This form of the syndrome, known as Cushing disease, affects women five times more often than men.

Ectopic ACTH Syndrome

Some benign or, more often, cancerous tumors that arise outside the pituitary can produce ACTH. This condition is known as ectopic ACTH syndrome. Lung tumors cause more than half of these cases, and men are affected three times more often than women. The most common forms of ACTH-producing tumors are small cell lung cancer, which accounts for about 13 percent of all lung cancer cases, and carcinoid tumors—small, slow-growing tumors that arise from hormone-producing cells in various parts of the body. Other less common types of tumors that can produce ACTH are thymomas, pancreatic islet cell tumors, and medullary carcinomas of the thyroid.

Adrenal Tumors

In rare cases, an abnormality of the adrenal glands, most often an adrenal tumor, causes Cushing syndrome. Adrenal tumors are four to five times more common in women than men, and the average age of onset is about 40. Most of these cases involve noncancerous tumors of adrenal tissue called adrenal adenomas, which release excess cortisol into the blood.

Adrenocortical carcinomas—adrenal cancers—are the least common cause of Cushing syndrome. With adrenocortical carcinomas, cancer cells secrete excess levels of several adrenocortical hormones, including cortisol and adrenal androgens, a type of male hormone. Adrenocortical carcinomas usually cause very high hormone levels and rapid development of symptoms.

216

Familial Cushing Syndrome

Most cases of Cushing syndrome are not inherited. Rarely, however, Cushing syndrome results from an inherited tendency to develop tumors of one or more endocrine glands. Endocrine glands release hormones into the bloodstream. With primary pigmented micronodular adrenal disease, children or young adults develop small cortisol-producing tumors of the adrenal glands. With multiple endocrine neoplasia type 1 (MEN1), hormone-secreting tumors of the parathyroid glands, pancreas, and pituitary develop; Cushing syndrome in MEN1 may be due to pituitary, ectopic, or adrenal tumors.

How Is Cushing Syndrome Diagnosed?

Diagnosis is based on a review of a person's medical history, a physical examination, and laboratory tests. X-rays of the adrenal or pituitary glands can be useful in locating tumors.

Tests to Diagnose Cushing Syndrome

No single lab test is perfect and usually several are needed. The three most common tests used to diagnose Cushing syndrome are the 24-hour urinary free cortisol test, measurement of midnight plasma cortisol or late-night salivary cortisol, and the low-dose dexamethasone suppression test. Another test, the dexamethasone-corticotropin-releasing hormone test, may be needed to distinguish Cushing syndrome from other causes of excess cortisol.

- **24-hour urinary free cortisol level**. In this test, a person's urine is collected several times over a 24-hour period and tested for cortisol. Levels higher than 50 to 100 micrograms a day for an adult suggest Cushing syndrome. The normal upper limit varies in different laboratories, depending on which measurement technique is used.

- **Midnight plasma cortisol and late-night salivary cortisol measurements**. The midnight plasma cortisol test measures cortisol concentrations in the blood. Cortisol production is normally suppressed at night, but in Cushing syndrome, this suppression doesn't occur. If the cortisol level is more than 50 nanomoles per liter (nmol/L), Cushing syndrome is suspected. The test generally requires a 48-hour hospital stay to avoid falsely elevated cortisol levels due to stress.

- However, a late-night or bedtime saliva sample can be obtained at home, then tested to determine the cortisol level. Diagnostic ranges vary, depending on the measurement technique used.

- **Low-dose dexamethasone suppression test (LDDST).** In the LDDST, a person is given a low dose of dexamethasone, a synthetic glucocorticoid, by mouth every 6 hours for 2 days. Urine is collected before dexamethasone is administered and several times on each day of the test. A modified LDDST uses a onetime overnight dose.

Cortisol and other glucocorticoids signal the pituitary to release less ACTH, so the normal response after taking dexamethasone is a drop in blood and urine cortisol levels. If cortisol levels do not drop, Cushing syndrome is suspected.

The LDDST may not show a drop in cortisol levels in people with depression, alcoholism, high estrogen levels, acute illness, or stress, falsely indicating Cushing syndrome. On the other hand, drugs such as phenytoin and phenobarbital may cause cortisol levels to drop, falsely indicating that Cushing is not present in people who actually have the syndrome. For this reason, physicians usually advise their patients to stop taking these drugs at least 1 week before the test.

- **Dexamethasone-corticotropin-releasing hormone (CRH) test.** Some people have high cortisol levels but do not develop the progressive effects of Cushing syndrome, such as muscle weakness, fractures, and thinning of the skin. These people may have pseudo-Cushing syndrome, a condition sometimes found in people who have depression or anxiety disorders, drink excess alcohol, have poorly controlled diabetes, or are severely obese. Pseudo-Cushing does not have the same long-term effects on health as Cushing syndrome and does not require treatment directed at the endocrine glands.

The dexamethasone-CRH test rapidly distinguishes pseudo-Cushing from mild cases of Cushing. This test combines the LDDST and a CRH stimulation test. In the CRH stimulation test, an injection of CRH causes the pituitary to secrete ACTH. Pretreatment with dexamethasone prevents CRH from causing an increase in cortisol in people with pseudo-Cushing. Elevations of cortisol during this test suggest Cushing syndrome.

Tests to Find the Cause of Cushing Syndrome

Once Cushing syndrome has been diagnosed, other tests are used to find the exact location of the abnormality that leads to excess cortisol production. The choice of test depends, in part, on the preference of the endocrinologist or the center where the test is performed.

- **CRH stimulation test.** The CRH test, without pretreatment with dexamethasone, helps separate people with pituitary adenomas from those with ectopic ACTH syndrome or adrenal tumors. As a result of the CRH injection, people with pituitary adenomas usually experience a rise in blood levels of ACTH and cortisol because CRH acts directly on the pituitary. This response is rarely seen in people with ectopic ACTH syndrome and practically never in those with adrenal tumors.

- **High-dose dexamethasone suppression test (HDDST).** The HDDST is the same as the LDDST, except it uses higher doses of dexamethasone. This test helps separate people with excess production of ACTH due to pituitary adenomas from those with ectopic ACTH-producing tumors. High doses of dexamethasone usually suppress cortisol levels in people with pituitary adenomas but not in those with ectopic ACTH-producing tumors.

- **Radiologic imaging: direct visualization of the endocrine glands.** Imaging tests reveal the size and shape of the pituitary and adrenal glands and help determine if a tumor is present. The most common imaging tests are the computerized tomography (CT) scan and magnetic resonance imaging (MRI). A CT scan produces a series of X-ray pictures giving a cross-sectional image of a body part. MRI also produces images of internal organs but without exposing patients to ionizing radiation.

- Imaging procedures are used to find a tumor after a diagnosis has been made. Imaging is not used to make the diagnosis of Cushing syndrome because benign tumors are commonly found in the pituitary and adrenal glands. These tumors, sometimes called incidentalomas, do not produce hormones in quantities that are harmful. They are not removed unless blood tests show they are a cause of symptoms or they are unusually large. Conversely, pituitary tumors may not be detectable by imaging in almost half of people who ultimately need pituitary surgery for Cushing syndrome.

- **Petrosal sinus sampling**. This test is not always required, but in many cases, it is the best way to distinguish pituitary from ectopic causes of Cushing syndrome. Samples of blood are drawn from the petrosal sinuses-veins that drain the pituitary-by inserting tiny tubes through a vein in the upper thigh or groin region. A local anesthetic and mild sedation are given, and X-rays are taken to confirm the correct position of the tubes. Often CRH, the hormone that causes the pituitary to release ACTH, is given during this test to improve diagnostic accuracy.

Levels of ACTH in the petrosal sinuses are measured and compared with ACTH levels in a forearm vein. Higher levels of ACTH in the sinuses than in the forearm vein indicate a pituitary adenoma. Similar levels of ACTH in the petrosal sinuses and the forearm suggest ectopic ACTH syndrome.

How Is Cushing Syndrome Treated?

Treatment depends on the specific reason for excess cortisol and may include surgery, radiation, chemotherapy, or the use of cortisol-inhibiting drugs. If the cause is long-term use of glucocorticoid hormones to treat another disorder, the doctor will gradually reduce the dosage to the lowest dose adequate for control of that disorder. Once control is established, the daily dose of glucocorticoid hormones may be doubled and given on alternate days to lessen side effects. In some cases, noncorticosteroid drugs can be prescribed.

Pituitary Adenomas

Several therapies are available to treat the ACTH-secreting pituitary adenomas of Cushing disease. The most widely used treatment is surgical removal of the tumor, known as transsphenoidal adenomectomy. Using a special microscope and fine instruments, the surgeon approaches the pituitary gland through a nostril or an opening made below the upper lip. Because this procedure is extremely delicate, patients are often referred to centers specializing in this type of surgery. The success, or cure, rate of this procedure is more than 80 percent when performed by a surgeon with extensive experience. If surgery fails or only produces a temporary cure, surgery can be repeated, often with good results.

After curative pituitary surgery, the production of ACTH drops two levels below normal. This drop is natural and temporary, and patients are given a synthetic form of cortisol such as hydrocortisone or prednisone to compensate. Most people can stop this replacement therapy in less than 1 or 2 years, but some must be on it for life.

If transsphenoidal surgery fails or a patient is not a suitable candidate for surgery, radiation therapy is another possible treatment. Radiation to the pituitary gland is given over a 6-week period, with improvement occurring in 40 to 50 percent of adults and up to 85 percent of children. Another technique, called stereotactic radiosurgery or gamma knife radiation, can be given in a single high-dose treatment. It may take several months or years before people feel better from radiation treatment alone. Combining radiation with cortisol-inhibiting drugs can help speed recovery.

Drugs used alone or in combination to control the production of excess cortisol are ketoconazole, mitotane, aminoglutethimide, and metyrapone. Each drug has its own side effects that doctors consider when prescribing medical therapy for individual patients.

Ectopic ACTH Syndrome

To cure the overproduction of cortisol caused by ectopic ACTH syndrome, all of the cancerous tissue that is secreting ACTH must be eliminated. The choice of cancer treatment-surgery, radiation, chemotherapy, immunotherapy, or a combination of these treatments—depends on the type of cancer and how far it has spread. Because ACTH-secreting tumors may be small or widespread at the time of diagnosis, making them difficult to locate and treat directly, cortisol-inhibiting drugs are an important part of treatment. In some cases, if other treatments fail, surgical removal of the adrenal glands, called bilateral adrenalectomy, may replace drug therapy.

Adrenal Tumors

Surgery is the mainstay of treatment for benign and cancerous tumors of the adrenal glands. Primary pigmented micronodular adrenal disease and the inherited Carney complex-primary tumors of the heart that can lead to endocrine overactivity and Cushing syndrome-require surgical removal of the adrenal glands.

Chapter 34

Pheochromocytoma and Paraganglioma

About Pheochromocytoma and Paraganglioma

Paragangliomas form in nerve tissue in the adrenal glands and near certain blood vessels and nerves. Paragangliomas that form in the adrenal glands are called pheochromocytomas. Paragangliomas that form outside the adrenal glands are called extra-adrenal paragangliomas. In this chapter, extra-adrenal paragangliomas are called paragangliomas.

Pheochromocytomas and paragangliomas may be benign (not cancer) or malignant (cancer).

Pheochromocytoma Is a Rare Tumor That Forms in the Adrenal Medulla (the Center of the Adrenal Gland)

Pheochromocytoma forms in the adrenal glands. There are two adrenal glands, one on top of each kidney in the back of the upper abdomen. Each adrenal gland has two parts. The outer layer of the adrenal gland is the adrenal cortex. The center of the adrenal gland is the adrenal medulla.

This chapter includes text excerpted from "Pheochromocytoma and Paraganglioma Treatment (PDQ®)—Patient Version," National Cancer Institute (NCI), July 19, 2016.

Pheochromocytoma is a rare tumor of the adrenal medulla. Usually, pheochromocytoma affects one adrenal gland, but it may affect both adrenal glands. Sometimes there is more than one tumor in one adrenal gland.

The adrenal glands make important hormones called catecholamines. Adrenaline (epinephrine) and noradrenaline (norepinephrine) are two types of catecholamines that help control heart rate, blood pressure, blood sugar, and the way the body reacts to stress. Sometimes a pheochromocytoma will release extra adrenaline and noradrenaline into the blood and cause signs or symptoms of disease.

Paragangliomas Form outside the Adrenal Gland

Paragangliomas are rare tumors that form near the carotid artery, along nerve pathways in the head and neck, and in other parts of the body. Some paragangliomas make extra catecholamines called adrenaline and noradrenaline. The release of these extra catecholamines into the blood may cause signs or symptoms of disease.

Certain Inherited Disorders and Changes in Certain Genes Increase the Risk of Pheochromocytoma or Paraganglioma

Anything that increases your chance of getting a disease is called a risk factor. Having a risk factor doesn't mean that you will get cancer; not having risk factors doesn't mean that you will not get cancer. Talk to your doctor if you think you may be at risk.

The following inherited syndromes or gene changes increase the risk of pheochromocytoma or paraganglioma:

- Multiple endocrine neoplasia 2 syndrome, types A and B (MEN2A and MEN2B).

- Von Hippel-Lindau (VHL) syndrome.

- Neurofibromatosis type 1 (NF1).

- Hereditary paraganglioma syndrome.

- Carney-Stratakis dyad (paraganglioma and gastrointestinal stromal tumor [GIST]).

- Carney triad (paraganglioma, GIST, and pulmonary chondroma).

Signs and Symptoms of Pheochromocytoma and Paraganglioma Include High Blood Pressure and Headache

Some tumors do not make extra adrenaline or noradrenaline and do not cause signs and symptoms. These tumors are sometimes found when a lump forms in the neck or when a test or procedure is done for another reason. Signs and symptoms of pheochromocytoma and paraganglioma occur when too much adrenaline or noradrenaline is released into the blood. These and other signs and symptoms may be caused by pheochromocytoma and paraganglioma or by other conditions. Check with your doctor if you have any of the following:

- high blood pressure

- headache

- heavy sweating for no known reason

- a strong, fast, or irregular heartbeat

- being shaky

- being extremely pale

The most common sign is high blood pressure. It may be hard to control. Very high blood pressure can cause serious health problems such as irregular heartbeat, heart attack, stroke, or death.

Signs and Symptoms of Pheochromocytoma and Paraganglioma May Occur at Any Time or Be Brought on by Certain Events

Signs and symptoms of pheochromocytoma and paraganglioma may occur when one of the following events happens:

- hard physical activity

- a physical injury or having a lot of emotional stress

- childbirth

- going under anesthesia

- surgery, including procedures to remove the tumor

- eating foods high in tyramine (such as red wine, chocolate, and cheese)

Tests That Examine the Blood and Urine Are Used to Detect (Find) and Diagnose Pheochromocytoma and Paraganglioma

- physical exam and history

- twenty-four-hour urine test

- blood catecholamine studies

- CT scan (CAT scan)

- MRI (magnetic resonance imaging)

Genetic Counseling Is Part of the Treatment Plan for Patients with Pheochromocytoma or Paraganglioma

All patients who are diagnosed with pheochromocytoma or paraganglioma should have genetic counseling to find out their risk for having an inherited syndrome and other related cancers.

Genetic testing may be recommended by a genetic counselor for patients who:

- Have a personal or family history of traits linked with inherited pheochromocytoma or paraganglioma syndrome.

- Have tumors in both adrenal glands.

- Have more than one tumor in one adrenal gland.

- Have signs or symptoms of extra catecholamines being released into the blood or malignant (cancerous) paraganglioma.

- Are diagnosed before age 40.

Genetic testing is sometimes recommended for patients with pheochromocytoma who:

- Are aged 40 to 50 years.

- Have a tumor in one adrenal gland.

- Do not have a personal or family history of an inherited syndrome.

When certain gene changes are found during genetic testing, the testing is usually offered to family members who are at risk but do not have signs or symptoms.

Genetic testing is not recommended for patients older than 50 years.

Certain Factors Affect Prognosis (Chance of Recovery) and Treatment Options

The prognosis (chance of recovery) and treatment options depend on the following:

- Whether the tumor is benign or malignant.

- Whether the tumor is in one area only or has spread to other places in the body.

- Whether there are signs or symptoms caused by a higher-than-normal amount of catecholamines.

- Whether the tumor has just been diagnosed or has recurred (come back).

Stages of Pheochromocytoma and Paraganglioma

The extent or spread of cancer is usually described as stage. It is important to know whether the cancer has spread in order to plan treatment. The following tests and procedures may be used to determine if the tumor has spread to other parts of the body:

- **CT scan (CAT scan)**: A procedure that makes a series of detailed pictures of areas inside the body, such as the neck, chest, abdomen, and pelvis, taken from different angles. The pictures are made by a computer linked to an X-ray machine. A dye may be injected into a vein or swallowed to help the organs or tissues show up more clearly. The abdomen and pelvis are imaged to detect tumors that release catecholamine. This procedure is also called computed tomography, computerized tomography, or computerized axial tomography.

- **MRI (magnetic resonance imaging)**: A procedure that uses a magnet, radio waves, and a computer to make a series of detailed pictures of areas inside the body such as the neck, chest, abdomen, and pelvis. This procedure is also called nuclear magnetic resonance imaging (NMRI).

- **MIBG scan**: A procedure used to find neuroendocrine tumors, such as pheochromocytoma and paraganglioma. A very small amount of a substance called radioactive MIBG is injected into a vein and travels through the bloodstream. Neuroendocrine tumor cells take up the radioactive MIBG and are detected by as canner. Scans may be taken over 1–3 days. An iodine solution

227

may be given before or during the test to keep the thyroid gland from absorbing too much of the MIBG.

- **Octreotide scan**: A type of radionuclide scan used to find certain tumors, including tumors that release catecholamine. A very small amount of radioactive octreotide (a hormone that attaches to certain tumors) is injected into a vein and travels through the bloodstream. The radioactive octreotide attaches to the tumor and a special camera that detects radioactivity is used to show where the tumors are in the body.

- **FDG-PET scan (fluorodeoxyglucose-positron emission tomography scan)**: A procedure to find malignant tumor cells in the body. A small amount of FDG, a type of radioactive glucose (sugar), is injected into a vein. The PET scanner rotates around the body and makes a picture of where glucose is being used in the body. Malignant tumor cells show up brighter in the picture because they are more active and take up more glucose than normal cells do.

There Are Three Ways That Cancer Spreads in the Body

Cancer can spread through tissue, the lymph system, and the blood:

- Tissue. The cancer spreads from where it began by growing into nearby areas.

- Lymph system. The cancer spreads from where it began by getting into the lymph system. The cancer travels through the lymph vessels to other parts of the body.

- Blood. The cancer spreads from where it began by getting into the blood. The cancer travels through the blood vessels to other parts of the body.

Cancer May Spread from Where It Began to Other Parts of the Body

When cancer spreads to another part of the body, it is called metastasis. Cancer cells break away from where they began (the primary tumor) and travel through the lymph system or blood.

- Lymph system. The cancer gets into the lymph system, travels through the lymph vessels, and forms a tumor (metastatic tumor) in another part of the body.

228

- Blood. The cancer gets into the blood, travels through the blood vessels, and forms a tumor (metastatic tumor) in another part of the body.

The metastatic tumor is the same type of cancer as the primary tumor. For example, if pheochromocytoma spreads to the bone, the cancer cells in the bone are actually pheochromocytoma cells. The disease is metastatic pheochromocytoma, not bone cancer.

There Is No Standard Staging System for Pheochromocytoma and Paraganglioma

Pheochromocytoma and Paraganglioma Are Described as Localized, Regional, or Metastatic

Localized Pheochromocytoma and Paraganglioma

The tumor is found in one or both adrenal glands (pheochromocytoma) or in one area only (paraganglioma).

Regional Pheochromocytoma and Paraganglioma

Cancer has spread to lymph nodes or other tissues near where the tumor began.

Metastatic Pheochromocytoma and Paraganglioma

The cancer has spread to other parts of the body, such as the liver, lungs, bone, or distant lymph nodes.

Recurrent Pheochromocytoma and Paraganglioma

Recurrent pheochromocytoma or paraganglioma is cancer that has recurred (come back) after it has been treated. The cancer may come back in the same place or in another part of the body.

Treatment Option Overview

Different types of treatments are available for patients with pheochromocytoma or paraganglioma. Some treatments are standard (the currently used treatment), and some are being tested in clinical trials. A treatment clinical trial is a research study meant to help improve current treatments or obtain information on new treatments for patients with cancer. When clinical trials show that a new treatment is better than the standard treatment, the new treatment may become the standard treatment. Patients may want to think about taking part in a clinical trial. Some clinical trials are open only to patients who have not started treatment.

Patients with Pheochromocytoma and Paraganglioma That Cause Signs or Symptoms Are Treated with Drug Therapy

Drug therapy begins when pheochromocytoma or paraganglioma is diagnosed. This may include:

- Drugs that keep the blood pressure normal. For example, one type of drug called alpha blockers stops noradrenaline from making small blood vessels more narrow. Keeping the blood vessels open and relaxed improves blood flow and lowers blood pressure.

- Drugs that keep the heart rate normal. For example, one type of drug called beta blockers stops the effect of too much noradrenaline and slows the heart rate.

- Drugs that block the effect of extra hormones made by the adrenal gland.

Drug therapy is often given for one to three weeks before surgery.

Six Types of Standard Treatment Are Used

Surgery

Surgery to remove pheochromocytoma is usually an adrenalectomy (removal of one or both adrenal glands). During this surgery, the tissues and lymph nodes inside the abdomen will be checked and if the tumor has spread, these tissues may also be removed. Drugs may be given before, during, and after surgery to keep blood pressure and heart rate normal.

After surgery to remove the tumor, catecholamine levels in the blood or urine are checked. Normal catecholamine levels are a sign that all the pheochromocytoma cells were removed.

If both adrenal glands are removed, life-long hormone therapy to replace hormones made by the adrenal glands is needed.

Radiation Therapy

Radiation therapy is a cancer treatment that uses high-energy X-rays or other types of radiation to kill cancer cells or keep them from growing.

There are two types of radiation therapy:

- External radiation therapy uses a machine outside the body to send radiation toward the cancer.

- Internal radiation therapy uses a radioactive substance sealed in needles, seeds, wires, or catheters that are placed directly into or near the cancer.

The way the radiation therapy is given depends on the type of cancer being treated and whether it is localized, regional, metastatic, or recurrent. External radiation therapy and 131I-MIBG therapy are used to treat pheochromocytoma.

Pheochromocytoma is sometimes treated with 131I-MIBG, which carries radiation directly to tumor cells. 131I-MIBG is a radioactive substance that collects in certain kinds of tumor cells, killing them with the radiation that is given off. The 131I-MIBG is given by infusion. Not all pheochromocytomas take up 131I-MIBG, so a test is done first to check for this before treatment begins.

Chemotherapy

Chemotherapy is a cancer treatment that uses drugs to stop the growth of cancer cells, either by killing the cells or by stopping them from dividing. When chemotherapy is taken by mouth or injected into a vein or muscle, the drugs enter the bloodstream and can reach cancer cells throughout the body (systemic chemotherapy). When chemotherapy is placed directly into the cerebrospinal fluid, an organ, or a body cavity such as the abdomen, the drugs mainly affect cancer cells in those areas (regional chemotherapy). Combination chemotherapy is treatment using more than one anticancer drug. The way the chemotherapy is given depends on the type of cancer being treated and whether it is localized, regional, metastatic, or recurrent.

Ablation Therapy

Ablation is a treatment to remove or destroy a body part or tissue or its function. Ablation therapies used to help kill cancer cells include:

- Radiofrequency ablation: A procedure that uses radio waves to heat and destroy abnormal cells. The radio waves travel through electrodes (small devices that carry electricity). Radiofrequency ablation may be used to treat cancer and other conditions.

- Cryoablation: A procedure in which tissue is frozen to destroy abnormal cells. Liquid nitrogen or liquid carbon dioxide is used to freeze the tissue.

Embolization Therapy

Embolization therapy is a treatment to block the artery leading to the adrenal gland. Blocking the flow of blood to the adrenal glands helps kill cancer cells growing there.

Targeted Therapy

Targeted therapy is a treatment that uses drugs or other substances to identify and attack specific cancer cells without harming normal cells. Targeted therapies are used to treat metastatic and recurrent pheochromocytoma.

Sunitinib (a type of tyrosine kinase inhibitor) is a new treatment being studied for metastatic pheochromocytoma. Tyrosine kinase inhibitor therapy is a type of targeted therapy that blocks signals needed for tumors to grow.

Follow-Up Tests Will Be Needed

Some of the tests that were done to diagnose the cancer or to find out the extent of the cancer may be repeated. Some tests will be repeated in order to see how well the treatment is working. Decisions about whether to continue, change, or stop treatment will be based on the results of these tests.

Some of the tests will continue to be done from time to time after treatment has ended. The results of these tests can show if your condition has changed or if the cancer has recurred (come back). These tests are sometimes called follow-up tests.

For patients with pheochromocytoma or paraganglioma that causes symptoms, catecholamine levels in the blood and urine will be checked on a regular basis. Catecholamine levels that are higher than normal can be a sign that the cancer has come back.

For patients with paraganglioma that does not cause symptoms, follow-up tests such as CT, MRI, or MIBG scan should be done every year.

For patients with inherited pheochromocytoma, catecholamine levels in the blood and urine will be checked on a regular basis. Other screening tests will be done to check for other tumors that are linked to the inherited syndrome.

Talk to your doctor about which tests should be done and how often. Patients with pheochromocytoma or paraganglioma need lifelong follow-up.

Pheochromocytoma during Pregnancy

Although it is rarely diagnosed during pregnancy, pheochromocytoma can be very serious for the mother and the newborn. Women who have an increased risk of pheochromocytoma should have prenatal testing. Pregnant women with pheochromocytoma should be treated by a team of doctors who are experts in this type of care.

Signs of pheochromocytoma in pregnancy may include any of the following:

* High blood pressure during the first 3 months of pregnancy.

* Sudden periods of high blood pressure.

* High blood pressure that is very hard to treat.

The diagnosis of pheochromocytoma in pregnant women includes testing for catecholamine levels in blood and urine.

Treatment of Pregnant Women with Pheochromocytoma May Include Surgery

Treatment of pheochromocytoma during pregnancy may include the following:

* Surgery to completely remove the cancer during the second trimester (the fourth through the sixth month of pregnancy).

* Surgery to completely remove the cancer combined with delivery of the fetus by cesarean section.

Chapter 35

Adrenal Gland Cancer

There are two adrenal glands. The adrenal glands are small and shaped like a triangle. One adrenal gland sits on top of each kidney. Each adrenal gland has two parts. The outer layer of the adrenal gland is the adrenal cortex. The center of the adrenal gland is the adrenal medulla.

The adrenal cortex makes important hormones that:

• Balance the water and salt in the body.

• Help keep blood pressure normal.

• Help control the body's use of protein, fat, and carbohydrates.

• Cause the body to have masculine or feminine characteristics.

Adrenocortical carcinoma is also called cancer of the adrenal cortex. A tumor of the adrenal cortex may be functioning (makes more hormones than normal) or nonfunctioning (does not make more hormones than normal). Most adrenocortical tumors are functioning. The hormones made by functioning tumors may cause certain signs or symptoms of disease.

The adrenal medulla makes hormones that help the body react to stress. Cancer that forms in the adrenal medulla is called pheochromocytoma and is not discussed in this chapter.

Adrenocortical carcinoma and pheochromocytoma can occur in both adults and children. Treatment for children, however, is different than treatment for adults.

This chapter includes text excerpted from "Adrenocortical Carcinoma Treatment (PDQ®)—Patient Version," National Cancer Institute (NCI), May 27, 2016.

Having Certain Genetic Conditions Increases the Risk of Adrenocortical Carcinoma

Anything that increases your risk of getting a disease is called a risk factor. Having a risk factor does not mean that you will get cancer; not having risk factors doesn't mean that you will not get cancer. Talk with your doctor if you think you may be at risk.

Risk factors for adrenocortical carcinoma include having the following hereditary diseases:

- Li-Fraumeni syndrome
- Beckwith-Wiedemann syndrome
- Carney complex

Symptoms of Adrenocortical Carcinoma Include Pain in the Abdomen

These and other signs and symptoms may be caused by adrenocortical carcinoma:

- A feeling of fullness in the abdomen
- A lump in the abdomen
- Pain the abdomen or back

A nonfunctioning adrenocortical tumor may not cause signs or symptoms in the early stages.

A functioning adrenocortical tumor makes too much of one of the following hormones:

- Cortisol
- Aldosterone
- Testosterone
- Estrogen

Too much cortisol may cause:

- Weight gain in the face, neck, and trunk of the body and thin arms and legs.
- Growth of fine hair on the face, upper back, or arms.
- A round, red, full face.
- A lump of fat on the back of the neck.

- A deepening of the voice and swelling of the sex organs or breasts in both males and females.

- Muscle weakness

- High blood sugar

- High blood pressure

Too much aldosterone may cause:

- High blood pressure

- Muscle weakness or cramps

- Frequent urination

- Feeling thirsty

Too much testosterone (in women) may cause:

- Growth of fine hair on the face, upper back, or arms

- Acne

- Balding

- A deepening of the voice

- No menstrual periods

Men who make too much testosterone do not usually have signs or symptoms.

Too much estrogen (in women) may cause:

- Irregular menstrual periods in women who have not gone through menopause.

- Vaginal bleeding in women who have gone through menopause.

- Weight gain

Too much estrogen (in men) may cause:

- Growth of breast tissue

- Lower sex drive

- Impotence

These and other signs and symptoms may be caused by adrenocortical carcinoma or by other conditions. Check with your doctor if you have any of these problems.

Imaging Studies and Tests That Examine the Blood and Urine Are Used to Detect (Find) and Diagnose Adrenocortical Carcinoma

The tests and procedures used to diagnose adrenocortical carcinoma depend on the patient's signs and symptoms. The following tests and procedures may be used:

- Adrenal angiography

- Adrenal venography

- Biopsy

- Blood chemistry study

- CT scan (CAT scan)

- High-dose dexamethasone suppression test

- Low-dose dexamethasone suppression test

- MIBG scan

- MRI (magnetic resonance imaging)

- PET scan (positron emission tomography scan)

- Physical exam and history

- Twenty-four-hour urine test

Stages of Adrenocortical Carcinoma

The process used to find out if cancer has spread within the adrenal gland or to other parts of the body is called staging. The information gathered from the staging process determines the stage of the disease. It is important to know the stage in order to plan treatment. The following tests and procedures may be used in the staging process:

- **CT scan (CAT scan):** A procedure that makes a series of detailed pictures of areas inside the body, such as the abdomen or chest, taken from different angles. The pictures are made by a computer linked to an X-ray machine. A dye may be injected into a vein or swallowed to help the organs or tissues show up more clearly. This procedure is also called computed tomography, computerized tomography, or computerized axial tomography.

- **MRI (magnetic resonance imaging) with gadolinium**: A procedure that uses a magnet, radio waves, and a computer to make a series of detailed pictures of areas inside the body. A substance called gadolinium may be injected into a vein. The gadolinium collects around the cancer cells so they show up brighter in the picture. This procedure is also called nuclear magnetic resonance imaging (NMRI).

- **PET scan (positron emission tomography scan)**: A procedure to find malignant tumor cells in the body. A small amount of radioactive glucose (sugar) is injected into a vein. The PET scanner rotates around the body and makes a picture of where glucose is being used in the body. Malignant tumor cells show up brighter in the picture because they are more active and take up more glucose than normal cells do.

- **Ultrasound exam**: A procedure in which high-energy sound waves (ultrasound) are bounced off internal tissues or organs, such as the vena cava, and make echoes. The echoes form a picture of body tissues called a sonogram.

- **Adrenalectomy**: A procedure to remove the affected adrenal gland. A tissue sample is viewed under a microscope by a pathologist to check for signs of cancer.

There Are Three Ways That Cancer Spreads in the Body

Cancer can spread through tissue, the lymph system, and the blood:

- Tissue. The cancer spreads from where it began by growing into nearby areas.

- Lymph system. The cancer spreads from where it began by getting into the lymph system. The cancer travels through the lymph vessels to other parts of the body.

- Blood. The cancer spreads from where it began by getting into the blood. The cancer travels through the blood vessels to other parts of the body.

Cancer May Spread from Where It Began to Other Parts of the Body

When cancer spreads to another part of the body, it is called metastasis. Cancer cells break away from where they began (the primary tumor) and travel through the lymph system or blood.

- Lymph system. The cancer gets into the lymph system, travels through the lymph vessels, and forms a tumor (metastatic tumor) in another part of the body.

- Blood. The cancer gets into the blood, travels through the blood vessels, and forms a tumor (metastatic tumor) in another part of the body.

The metastatic tumor is the same type of cancer as the primary tumor. For example, if adrenocortical carcinoma spreads to the lung, the cancer cells in the lung are actually adrenocortical carcinoma cells. The disease is metastatic adrenocortical carcinoma, not lung cancer.

The Following Stages Are Used for Adrenocortical Carcinoma

Stage I

In stage I, the tumor is 5 centimeters or smaller and is found in the adrenal gland only.

Stage II

In stage II, the tumor is larger than 5 centimeters and is found in the adrenal gland only.

Stage III

In stage III, the tumor can be any size and has spread:

- to fat or lymph nodes near the adrenal gland; or
- to nearby tissues, but not to the organs near the adrenal gland

Stage IV

In stage IV, the tumor can be any size and has spread:

- to nearby tissues and to fat and lymph nodes near the adrenal gland; or
- to organs near the adrenal gland and may have spread to nearby lymph nodes; or
- to other parts of the body, such as the liver or lung

Recurrent Adrenocortical Carcinoma

Recurrent adrenocortical carcinoma is cancer that has recurred (come back) after it has been treated. The cancer may come back in the adrenal cortex or in other parts of the body.

Treatment Option Overview

Different types of treatments are available for patients with adrenocortical carcinoma. Some treatments are standard (the currently used treatment), and some are being tested in clinical trials. A treatment clinical trial is a research study meant to help improve current treatments or obtain information on new treatments for patients with cancer. When clinical trials show that a new treatment is better than the standard treatment, the new treatment may become the standard treatment. Patients may want to think about taking part in a clinical trial. Some clinical trials are open only to patients who have not started treatment.

Five Types of Standard Treatment Are Used

1. Surgery

2. Radiation Therapy

   - External radiation therapy

   - Internal radiation therapy

3. Chemotherapy

4. Biologic Therapy

5. Targeted Therapy

Follow-Up Tests May Be Needed

Some of the tests that were done to diagnose the cancer or to find out the stage of the cancer may be repeated. Some tests will be repeated in order to see how well the treatment is working. Decisions about whether to continue, change, or stop treatment may be based on the results of these tests.

Some of the tests will continue to be done from time to time after treatment has ended. The results of these tests can show if your condition has changed or if the cancer has recurred (come back). These tests are sometimes called follow-up tests or check-ups.

Treatment Options for Recurrent Adrenocortical Carcinoma

Treatment of recurrent adrenocortical carcinoma may include the following as palliative therapy to relieve symptoms and improve the quality of life:

- surgery

- radiation therapy

- a clinical trial of chemotherapy or biologic therapy

Chapter 36

X-Linked Adrenal Hypoplasia Congenita (AHC)

X-linked adrenal hypoplasia congenita is an inherited disorder that mainly affects males. It involves many hormone-producing (endocrine) tissues in the body, particularly a pair of small glands on top of each kidney called the adrenal glands. These glands produce a variety of hormones that regulate many essential functions in the body. Congenital adrenal hypoplasia is characterized by adrenal insufficiency, which may be life threatening, and hypogonadotropic hypogonadism. Congenital adrenal hypoplasia is caused by mutations in the NR0B1 gene. It is inherited in an X-linked recessive pattern.

Symptoms

X-linked adrenal hypoplasia congenita is a disorder that mainly affects males. One of the main signs of this disorder is adrenal insufficiency, which occurs when the adrenal glands do not produce enough hormones. Adrenal insufficiency typically begins in infancy or childhood and can cause vomiting, difficulty with feeding, dehydration, extremely low blood sugar (hypoglycemia), and shock. If untreated, these complications may be life-threatening.

Affected males may also have a shortage of male sex hormones, which leads to underdeveloped reproductive tissues, undescended

This chapter includes text excerpted from "X-Linked Adrenal Hypoplasia Congenita," Genetic and Rare Diseases Information Center (GARD), National Center for Advancing Translational Sciences (NCATS), September 1, 2016.

testicles, delayed puberty, and an inability to father children. Together, these characteristics are known as hypogonadotropic hypogonadism.

The onset and severity of these signs and symptoms can vary, even among affected members of the same family.

- Absence of pubertal development
- Adrenal hypoplasia
- Cryptorchidism
- Dehydration
- Delayed puberty
- Failure to thrive
- Hyperpigmentation of the skin
- Hypocortisolemia
- Hypogonadotrophic hypogonadism
- Hyponatremia
- Low gonadotropins (secondary hypogonadism)
- Muscular dystrophy
- Renal salt wasting
- X-linked recessive inheritance

Causes

X-linked adrenal hypoplasia congenita is caused by mutations in the *NR0B1* gene. The *NR0B1* gene provides instructions to make a protein called DAX1. This protein plays an important role in the development and function of several hormone-producing tissues including the adrenal glands, two hormone-secreting glands in the brain (the hypothalamus and pituitary), and the gonads (ovaries in females and testes in males). The hormones produced by these glands control many important body functions.

Some *NR0B1* mutations result in the production of an inactive version of the DAX1 protein, while other mutations delete the entire gene. The resulting shortage of DAX1 disrupts the normal development and function of hormone-producing tissues in the body. The signs and symptoms of adrenal insufficiency and hypogonadotropic hypogonadism occur when endocrine glands do not produce the right amounts of certain hormones.

Inheritance

X-linked adrenal hypoplasia congenita is inherited in an X-linked recessive pattern. A condition is considered X-linked if the mutated gene that causes the disorder is located on the X chromosome, one of the two sex chromosomes. In males (who have only one X chromosome), one altered copy of the gene in each cell is sufficient to cause the condition. In females (who have two X chromosomes), a mutation must be present in both copies of the gene to cause the disorder. Males are affected by X-linked recessive disorders much more frequently than females. A characteristic of X-linked inheritance is that fathers cannot pass X-linked traits to their sons.

In X-linked recessive inheritance, a female with one mutated copy of the gene in each cell is called a carrier. She can pass on the altered gene, but usually does not experience signs and symptoms of the disorder. In rare cases, however, females who carry a *NR0B1* mutation may experience adrenal insufficiency or signs of hypogonadotropic hypogonadism such as underdeveloped reproductive tissues, delayed puberty, and an absence of menstruation.

Chapter 37

Congenital Adrenal Hyperplasia (CAH)

What Is Congenital Adrenal Hyperplasia (CAH)?

CAH refers to a group of genetic disorders that affect the adrenal glands. These glands sit on top of the kidneys and release hormones the body needs to function. CAH is caused by three disturbances:

- **Too little cortisol**. The adrenal glands of infants born with CAH cannot make enough of the hormone cortisol. This hormone affects energy levels, blood sugar levels, blood pressure, and the body's response to stress, illness, and injury.

- **Too little aldosterone**. In about 75 percent of cases, infants born with CAH cannot make enough of the hormone aldosterone, which helps the body maintain the proper level of sodium (salt) and water and helps maintain blood pressure.

- **Too much androgens**. In certain cases, infants born with CAH produce too much of male hormones, androgens. Proper levels of these hormones are needed for normal growth and development in both boys and girls.

This chapter includes text excerpted from "Congenital Adrenal Hyperplasia (CAH)," *Eunice Kennedy Shriver* National Institute of Child Health and Human Development (NICHD), July 9, 2013.

CAH can also cause imbalances in the hormone adrenaline, which affects blood sugar levels, blood pressure, and the body's response to stress.

The hormone imbalances in most cases of CAH (about 95 percent) are caused by too little of a substance called 21-hydroxylase. The adrenal glands need 21-hydroxylase to make proper amounts of hormones. This type of CAH is sometimes referred to as 21-hydroxylase deficiency. In CAH due to 21-hydroxylase deficiency, the adrenal glands cannot make enough cortisol or aldosterone. In addition, the glands make too much androgen. People with 21-hydroxylase deficiency also may not produce enough adrenaline.

About 5 percent of cases of CAH are caused by deficiency in a substance similar to 21-hydroxylase, called 11-hydroxylase. This type of CAH is sometimes referred to as 11-hydroxylase deficiency. In CAH due to 11-hydroxylase deficiency, the adrenal glands make too little cortisol and too many androgens. This type of CAH does not result in aldosterone deficiency.

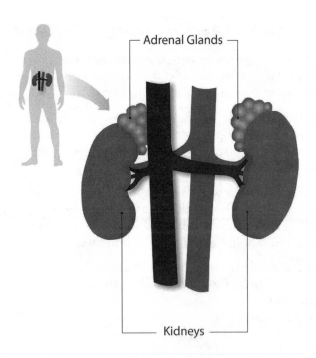

Figure 37.1. *Position of the Adrenal Glands and Kidneys in the Human Body*

Other very rare types of CAH include 3-betahydroxy-steroid dehydrogenase deficiency, lipoid CAH, and 17-hydroxylase deficiency. They are not discussed here.

CAH can be categorized as classic or nonclassic types based on severity:

- **Classic CAH** is more severe than the nonclassic form. It can be life threatening in newborns if it is not diagnosed. Classic CAH can be caused by either 21-hydroxylase or 11-hydroxylase deficiency.

- **Nonclassic CAH** is sometimes called late-onset CAH. It is a milder form of the disorder that usually is diagnosed in late childhood or early adolescence. Sometimes, people have nonclassic CAH and never know it. This form of CAH is almost always caused by 21-hydroxylase deficiency.

What Causes CAH?

CAH is caused by changes (mutations) in one of several genes. These changes lead to deficiencies in 21-hydroxylase or, less commonly, 11-hydroxylase. Both of these are chemicals called enzymes. The adrenal glands need these enzymes to make proper amounts of the hormones: cortisol, aldosterone, androgens, and adrenaline.

How Is CAH Inherited?

The genes for CAH are passed down from parents to their children. In general, people have two copies of every gene in their bodies. They receive one copy from each parent. For an infant to have CAH, both copies must have an error that affects an adrenal-gland enzyme.

CAH is an example of an autosomal recessive disorder:

- Autosomal means the gene is not on the X chromosome or Y chromosome.

- Recessive means that both copies of the gene must have the error for the disease or disorder to occur.

If both parents have CAH, all of their children will also have it. If each parent carries one affected gene and one normal gene (called a "carrier"), there is a one-in-four chance of their child having CAH.

Autosomal recessive

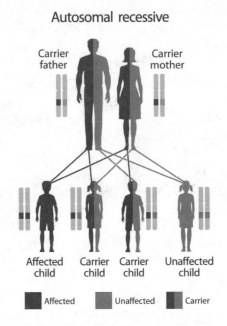

Figure 37.2. *Inheritance of an Autosomal Recessive Disorder from Carrier Parents*

How Many People Are Affected by or at Risk for CAH?

Classic CAH occurs in about one of every 15,000 births worldwide. Nonclassic CAH is among the most common genetic disorders. It occurs in about one of every 1,000 people, but could occur in as many as 1 in 20 people in some communities. It is more common in Ashkenazi Jews, Hispanics, Italians, and Yugoslavians.

What Are the Symptoms of CAH?

Classic CAH

Symptoms of classic CAH due to 21-hydroxylase deficiency (95 percent of classic CAH cases) can be grouped into two types according to their severity: **salt wasting** and **simple virilizing** (also called **nonsalt wasting**).

Symptoms of classic CAH due to 11-hydroxylase deficiency (5 percent of classic CAH cases) are similar to those of simple virilizing CAH. About two-thirds of people with classic 11-hydroxylase deficiency also have high blood pressure (hypertension).

Salt-wasting CAH:

Salt-wasting CAH is the severe form of classic 21-hydroxylase deficiency. In this type of CAH, the adrenal glands make too little aldosterone, causing the body to be unable to retain enough sodium (salt). Too much sodium is lost in urine (thus the name, "salt-wasting"). If undiagnosed, symptoms of classic salt-wasting CAH appear within days or weeks of birth and, in some cases, death occurs.

Symptoms may include:

- dehydration

- poor feeding

- diarrhea

- vomiting

- heart rhythm problems (arrhythmias)

- low blood pressure

- very low blood sodium levels

- low blood glucose

- too much acid in the blood, called metabolic acidosis

- weight loss

- shock, a condition where not enough blood gets to the brain and other organs. Shock in infants with salt-wasting is called adrenal crisis. Signs include confusion, irritability, rapid heart rate, and/or coma.

Even when carefully treated, children with salt-wasting CAH are still at risk for adrenal crises when they become ill or are under physical stress. The body needs more than the usual amount of adrenal hormones during illness, injury, or physical stress. This means a child with CAH must be given more medication during these times to prevent an adrenal crisis.

Salt-wasting CAH also involves symptoms caused by low cortisol and high androgens. These symptoms may include:

- In female newborns, external genitalia can be ambiguous, i.e., not typical female appearing, with normal internal reproductive organs (ovaries, uterus, and fallopian tubes)

- Enlarged genitalia in male newborns

- Development of certain qualities called virilization in boys or girls before the normal age of puberty, sometimes as early as age 2 or 3. This is a condition characterized by:

  - rapid growth

  - appearance of pubic and armpit hair

  - deep voice

  - failure to menstruate, or abnormal or irregular menstrual periods (females)

  - well-developed muscles

  - enlarged penis (males)

  - unusually tall height as children, but being shorter than normal as adults

  - possible difficulties getting pregnant (females)

  - excess facial hair (females)

  - early beard (males)

  - severe acne

  - benign testicular tumors and infertility (males)

Simple virilizing (non-salt wasting) CAH:

Simple virilizing CAH is the moderate form of classic 21-hydroxylase deficiency. This type of CAH involves less severe aldosterone deficiency. Therefore, there are no severe or life-threatening sodium-deficiency symptoms in newborns. Like salt-wasting CAH, simple virilizing CAH involves too little cortisol and too much androgen. Female newborns have ambiguous genitalia and young children display virilization.

Nonclassic CAH

Almost all cases of nonclassic CAH are caused by a mild 21-hydroxylase deficiency. Most symptoms of nonclassic CAH are related to increased androgens. Symptoms can show up in childhood, adolescence, or early adulthood.

Symptoms of nonclassic CAH can include:

- rapid growth in childhood and early teens but shorter height than both parents

- early signs of puberty

- acne

- irregular menstrual periods (females)

- fertility problems (in about 10 percent to 15 percent of women)

- excess facial or body hair in women

- male-pattern baldness (hair loss near the temples)

- enlarged penis (males)

- small testicles (males)

Some people have nonclassic CAH and never know it because the symptoms are so mild.

How Do Healthcare Providers Diagnose CAH?

During Pregnancy

If a woman already has a child with CAH and becomes pregnant with the same partner, her fetus has a one in four chance of having CAH. For this reason, prenatal testing can be done for some forms of CAH. A healthcare provider checks for the disorder by using techniques called amniocentesis or chorionic villus sampling.

- **Amniocentesis**. This involves inserting a needle into the womb, through the abdomen, to withdraw a small amount of fluid from the sac that surrounds the fetus. The procedure is usually done between the 15th and 20th week of pregnancy.

- **Chorionic villus sampling**. This is similar to amniocentesis. A healthcare provider inserts a needle into the womb, either through the abdomen or the cervix, and extracts a small piece of tissue from the chorionic villi (the tissue that will later become the placenta). This procedure is usually done between the 10th and 12th week of pregnancy.

After a healthcare provider takes a sample using one of these techniques, he or she will perform a genetic test on the sample. This test will reveal whether the fetus has a gene change that causes CAH.

Parents may also choose to wait until birth to have the newborn tested. Talking to their healthcare providers may help parents identify the option that is right for them.

At Birth

All U.S. states have neonatal screening for CAH. Infants who test positive need to have follow-up testing done to confirm the diagnosis. If, for some reason, the neonatal screening is negative but there is high suspicion for CAH (such as ambiguous genitalia), further evaluation is also indicated.

Later in Life

Newborns do not show symptoms of nonclassic CAH, and the test done on newborns does not detect nonclassic CAH. Nonclassic CAH is diagnosed in childhood or adulthood, when symptoms appear. To diagnose nonclassic CAH, a healthcare provider may:

- Ask whether family members have CAH.

- Do a physical exam.

- Take blood and urine to measure hormone levels.

- Do a genetic test to determine if the patient has the gene change that causes CAH.

An X-ray can help to diagnose CAH in children. Because some children with CAH grow too quickly, their bones will be more developed than normal for their age.

What Are the Treatments for CAH?

Treatments for CAH include medication and surgery as well as psychological support.

Medication

Classic CAH

- Newborns with classic CAH should start treatment very soon after birth to reduce the effects of CAH. Classic CAH is treated with steroids that replace the low hormones.

- Infants and children usually take a form of cortisol called hydrocortisone.

- Adults take hydrocortisone, prednisone, or dexamethasone, which also replace cortisol.

- Patients with classic CAH also take another medicine, fludrocortisone, to replace aldosterone.

- Eating salty foods or taking salt pills may also help salt-wasters retain salt.

The body needs more cortisol when it is under physical stress. Adults and children with classic CAH need close medical attention and may need to take more of their medication during these times. They may also need more medication if they:

- have an illness with a high fever

- undergo surgery

- sustain a major injury

People who have classic CAH need to wear a medical alert identification bracelet or necklace. To alert medical professionals in case of an emergency, the bracelet or necklace should read: "adrenal insufficiency, requires hydrocortisone." Adults or parents also need to learn how to give an injection of hydrocortisone if there is an emergency.

Patients with classic CAH need to take medication daily for their entire lives. If a patient stops taking his or her medication, symptoms will return.

The body makes different amounts of cortisol at different times in life, so sometimes a patient's dose of medication may be too high or too low. Taking too much medication to replace cortisol can cause symptoms of Cushing syndrome. These include:

- weight gain
- slowed growth
- stretch marks on the skin
- rounded face
- high blood pressure
- bone loss
- high blood sugar

It is important to alert the healthcare provider if these symptoms appear so that he or she can adjust the medication dose.

Nonclassic CAH

People with nonclassic CAH may not need treatment if they do not have symptoms. Individuals with symptoms are given low doses of the same cortisol replacing medication taken by people with classic CAH.

Symptoms of nonclassic CAH that signal that the patient may need treatment are:

- early puberty

- excess body hair

- irregular menstrual periods (females)

- infertility

It may be possible for patients with nonclassic CAH to stop medication as adults if their symptoms go away.

Surgery

Classic CAH

Girls who are born with ambiguous external genitalia usually have surgery. For example, surgery is necessary if changes to the genitals have affected urine flow. Surgery to make the genitals look more female also can be done.

The Endocrine Society, which supports hormonal research and clinical practice, recommends that this feminizing surgery be considered during infancy. If it is done, the group recommends choosing an experienced surgeon who practices in a center that sees many CAH cases.

The Congenital Adrenal Hyperplasia Research, Education and Support (CARES) Foundation strongly recommends delaying surgery until:

- The child is medically stable,

- Parents are fully informed of the risks and benefits, and

- A surgeon with expertise in this type of procedure is found.

Parents should also find a psychologist, social worker, or other mental health professional to support them in their decision making. It is important to find an experienced mental health provider whose expertise includes working with children who have CAH and their special needs.

Nonclassic CAH

- CAH Girls with nonclassic CAH have normal genitals, so they do not need surgery.

If My Children Have CAH Can They Go to Day Care and School?

Yes, children with CAH can attend day care and school. Before enrolling children in day care, parents should explain that the child has adrenal insufficiency, which might require the administration of emergency medication. Parents should discuss the day care provider's policy on giving medications to children. They should also provide a set of written instructions, as well as a list of emergency contact names and numbers.

Before a child starts school, parents should consider meeting with the teacher, principal, and school nurse to explain the child's condition. Parents can also discuss precautions to take if the child becomes ill.

I Have CAH and Want to Start a Family. What Should I Be Thinking About?

Anyone with CAH, or from a family in which CAH has been diagnosed, should consider genetic counseling. Genetic counselors discuss all options for having a child. They explain the risks and benefits of each option.

The genes for CAH are passed down from parents to their children. In general, people have two copies of every gene in their bodies. They receive one copy from each parent. For an infant to have CAH, both copies must have an error that affects an adrenal-gland enzyme.

CAH is an example of an autosomal recessive disorder:

- Autosomal means the gene is not on the X chromosome or Y chromosome.

- Recessive means that both copies of the gene must have the error for the disease or disorder to occur.

If both parents have CAH, all of their children also will have it. If each parent carries one affected gene and one normal gene, there is a one in four chance of a child having CAH.

For Women

Women with CAH can get pregnant. In some of the women, high levels of androgens disrupt the regular release of the egg from the ovary, a process known as ovulation. Some women also have irregular menstrual cycles. These problems can make it more difficult to get pregnant. These women often can be helped with medicines. Women with CAH who want to become pregnant can meet with a reproductive endocrinologist. This is a healthcare provider who specializes in fertility issues.

Women with CAH who become pregnant should continue taking their medications.

For Men

Men with CAH can father children. The main challenges for these men are low testosterone (a hormone important for male fertility and sexual function), and growths in the testicles called adrenal rest tissue. These problems can cause reduced sperm production. These issues tend to occur when hormone imbalances are not well controlled with medicines. Men who wish to father children should take all medicines as directed. A healthcare provider may recommend that males with CAH who have gone through puberty get an ultrasound of the testicles. The ultrasound provides a picture of the inside of the testicle and can help a healthcare provider detect abnormal growths. Future ultrasounds can be compared with the original to quickly identify any problems.

Chapter 38

Managing Adrenal Insufficiency

What Are the Adrenal Glands?

Your body has two adrenal glands. Each gland is located above a kidney. The adrenal glands secrete many hormones needed for the body's normal functioning. Two of these hormones are cortisol and aldosterone. Cortisol helps the body use sugar and protein for energy and enables the body to recover from infections and stresses (for example: surgery and illness). Aldosterone maintains the right amount of sodium (salt), potassium, and water in the body.

What Is Adrenal Insufficiency (AI)?

People with adrenal insufficiency (AI) do not have enough of the hormones cortisol and aldosterone. Without the right levels of these hormones, your body cannot maintain essential life functions. AI may be permanent or temporary.

When AI is permanent, medication must be taken daily for an entire lifetime. Causes of permanent AI include the following:

- Addison Disease

- Congenital adrenal hyperplasia (CAH) discovered in childhood

This chapter includes text excerpted from "Managing Adrenal Insufficiency," National Institutes of Health (NIH), May 14, 2016.

- Complete surgical removal of the pituitary gland
- Surgical removal of the adrenals

Temporary AI is caused by some medications, infections, and/or surgeries. Causes of temporary AI include the following:

- Transsphenoidal surgery for Cushing disease that removes a tumor from the pituitary gland.
- Removal of a tumor causing the adrenal glands to make too much cortisol.
- Medical treatment for Cushing syndrome with drugs that lower cortisol levels.
- Medical treatment with steroids for prolonged periods of time.

What Are the Signs and Symptoms of AI?

When your essential life functions are not being maintained because of a lack of adrenal hormones, you will not feel well. Your symptoms can include:

- unusual tiredness and weakness
- dizziness when standing up
- nausea, vomiting, and diarrhea
- loss of appetite
- upset stomach
- joint aches and pains

Other symptoms you may experience over time include:

- weight loss
- darkened skin
- craving for salt

If any of these symptoms appear and you know that you have a risk for developing AI, call your healthcare provider immediately.

What Medication Is Used to Treat AI?

To keep your AI under control, you must take medication daily to replace missing hormones. This medication is in pill form and must be taken in the amounts and at the times prescribed by your healthcare provider. This medication is often referred to as your replacement dose. Many medications can replace cortisol; they are called glucocorticoids. At National Institutes of Health (NIH), hydrocortisone, dexamethasone, or prednisone are usually recommended. If you miss a dose, follow the instructions of your healthcare provider.

If you are missing the hormone aldosterone, your body cannot maintain the right levels of sodium (salt) and fluids. To replace aldosterone, you will be given a drug called fludrocortisone (Florinef). Adults usually take tablets of fludrocortisone (Florinef). Children with AI who have trouble swallowing pills can take fludrocortisone (Florinef) tablets dissolved in water or crushed. Occasionally, you will be given salt tablets. If you miss a dose of fludrocortisone (Florinef), take it as soon as possible.

What Are the Side Effects of These Drugs?

Replacement doses of hydrocortisone rarely cause side effects. Sometimes, an upset stomach may occur. If this happens, take your medication with meals. If you notice anything else out of the ordinary, call your healthcare provider. If the dose is too high, patients can gain weight or develop signs of Cushing syndrome.

What Do I Do When I Do Not Feel Well?

There may be times when you do not feel well. When you are sick, be sure to take the right amount of medication at the right time of day. If you feel sick for more than three days, contact your healthcare provider. There may be times when you will need to take more than your normal replacement dose of hydrocortisone. Normally functioning adrenal glands produce more hydrocortisone when the body is under the physical stress of fever (over 100 degrees Fahrenheit), infection, surgery, trauma with loss of consciousness, vomiting, or diarrhea. It is important to drink plenty of sugar and salt-containing fluids when you are sick to prevent dehydration or low blood sugar.

If you are sick with a fever (over 100 degrees Fahrenheit), infection, vomiting, or diarrhea, you should call your healthcare provider right away. Your healthcare provider may give you written instructions for sick days ("sick day rules"). Generally, this means doubling your usual hydrocortisone dose for 1 to 3 days. It is important to discuss the decision to increase the dose with your healthcare provider. It is important you increase your hormone dose only for physical stresses.

You should not increase it for mental stress (such as a bad day at work, anxiety, or loneliness).

What If I Am So Ill That I Cannot Take My Medication?

If you are too ill to take your pills, or you cannot keep them down (for example vomiting), you must take a glucocorticoid medicine by injection. You or someone who lives with you will need to learn how to give you this injection.

The injection will take the place of both hydrocortisone and Florinef pills. If you find it necessary to give yourself an injectable medication, call your healthcare provider, or go to the nearest hospital emergency room immediately after giving the injection.

You should have the injectable medication with you at all times, make sure to check the expiration date periodically. If used, you should replace as soon as possible.

How Much Medicine Should I Take Once I Feel Better?

As soon as your illness is over and the symptoms are gone (for example, fever, vomiting, and diarrhea), you can usually return to taking your usual amount of medication. You should discuss this with your healthcare provider.

How Do I Give Myself an Injection?

Injectable glucocorticoid is given intramuscularly, which means it is injected into a large muscle. When giving yourself an injection, the easiest and best place to do it is in the thigh on the same side as your dominant hand (for example, the right thigh if you are right-handed). Adults should always carry injectable medication with them. If you have a child with AI, you or the child's caregiver must always carry the child's medication. If the child is in school, the school nurse must know about your child's condition and be able to give an injection of glucocorticoid.

What Else Do I Need to Know about AI?

You can control AI by taking an active role in your care. Taking care of yourself involves:

1. learning about your disease

2. taking your medication every day

3. recognizing illness and taking special care of yourself

4. getting regular medical check-ups

5. wearing a Medic-Alert bracelet at all times

    - This will be given to you before you leave the Clinical Center. If you are ordering medical alert identification we advise writing on it "adrenal insufficiency, requires cortef."

Inform your healthcare providers of the diagnosis of AI before any surgical procedure to determine whether "stress dosing" is needed. You may want to check in with your local Emergency Medical System to find out about policy/procedures for managing AI in your area.

Chapter 39

Laparoscopic Adrenal Gland Removal

Adrenal glands are triangular-shaped organs located at the top of each kidney. They are classified as endocrine glands because they produce hormones, such aldosterone, cortisol, epinephrine, and norepinephrine, as well as a small amount of estrogen and androgen. These hormones control many bodily functions, including metabolism, blood chemistry, immune system regulation, blood pressure, electrolytes, glucose usage and the ability to react quickly in times of stress (the "fight or flight" response).

When the adrenal glands produce more or less of these hormones than the body needs, a variety of illnesses can develop. For example, overproduction of aldosterone can result in hyperaldosteronism, which causes low blood pressure and low potassium levels, whereas too little aldosterone may have the opposite effect, hypoaldosteronism. Similarly, if the adrenal glands produce too much cortisol, Cushing's syndrome could be the result, while underproduction is associated with Addison's disease. And either under- or overproduction of some hormones can lead to several types of tumors, some benign and some cancerous.

Disorders of the adrenal glands can be treated in a number of ways, including medication and hormone replacement, but when removal becomes necessary, there are at least five ways the surgery, called

"Laparoscopic Adrenal Gland Removal," © 2017 Omnigraphics. Reviewed October 2016.

adrenalectomy, may be performed. Four of them come under the heading of the "open" approach, in which a six-to-twelve-inch incision is made in the abdomen, flank, or back to give the surgeon access to the adrenal gland and surrounding area. The alternative is laparoscopic surgery, a procedure in which three to five holes of just one-quarter to one-half inch are required.

Laparoscopic Adrenalectomy Procedure

Removal of the adrenal gland may be recommended for patients with functioning adrenal-gland disorders, in which the organ is producing excess hormones, or non-functioning disorders, a condition in which the gland does not produce any hormones. Either may be caused by a benign or malignant tumor.

Preparation for surgery

- When an adrenal tumor is suspected, the doctor will typically order urine and blood tests to determine the level of various hormones in the body.

- A computerized tomography (CT) scan or magnetic resonance imaging (MRI) might then be used to confirm the presence of the tumor and pinpoint its location.

- Depending on the patient's age and condition, a chest X-ray and an electrocardiogram (EKG) might be administered.

- Prior to the operation, some patients may need to take medication to control the symptoms of the adrenal disorder. Others might need to discontinue certain drugs.

- The surgeon will review the procedure in detail, explaining the benefits and potential risks of the operation, and ask the patient to sign a consent form.

- The patient will be advised not to eat or drink after midnight on the day of the surgery.

How laparoscopic adrenalectomy is performed

- The procedure will take place in a hospital with the patient under general anesthesia, so he or she is asleep during the surgery.

- The patient will be positioned on his or her back or side, depending on how the adrenal gland will be removed.

- One or more IV lines will be inserted in order to administer fluids during the procedure.

- The surgeon will make three to five small incisions and insert tubes into them through which various instruments will be introduced.

- One such instrument, called a laparoscope, connects to a camera that is attached to a television screen and gives the surgeon a magnified view of the internal organs.

- Other instruments, such as forceps and scissors, inserted through the rest of the tubes allow the doctor to separate the adrenal gland from the kidney.

- Once the gland is detached it is placed in a small bag, also introduced through a tube, which makes it easier to remove from the body.

- Finally, the instruments and tubes are withdrawn, the surgeon closes the incisions, and dressings are applied.

After surgery

- When the adrenalectomy is completed, the patient is moved to a recovery room where he or she will rest for several hours and be monitored closely by hospital staff.

- Assuming no complications, the patient will then be moved to a regular hospital room for one to three days.

- Although laparoscopic surgery is much less invasive than an open procedure, some discomfort at the incision sites is to be expected, so during their hospital stay patient are usually given pain medication.

- No special home care is generally required. Patients can engage in light activities almost immediately, resume showering as long as the incision sites are kept dry, and change dressings as needed.

- The doctor may prescribe pain pills and will let the patient know when he or she can begin taking regular medicines again.

- Within about a week, most patients are able to resume normal activities, including work, climbing stairs, driving, and light lifting.

- The surgeon will schedule a follow-up visit about two weeks after the surgery to be sure that recovery is proceeding satisfactorily and discuss any of the patient's concerns.

Advantages of Laparoscopic Adrenal Gland Removal

In some cases, such as when a tumor is very large, open surgery must be used, but laparoscopic adrenalectomy is now commonly performed whenever possible. Some of the advantages of this technique include:

- less time in surgery
- smaller incisions
- shorter hospital stays
- less post-operative pain
- fewer complications
- faster recovery time
- less scarring
- very high success rate

Risks and Complications

Although laparoscopic adrenal gland removal is considerably less invasive and generally safer than open surgery, any surgical procedure carries risks, and post-operative complications, though rare and usually not serious, can occur. Some of these include:

- excessive bleeding during surgery
- injury to other internal organs during the procedure
- adverse reaction to general anesthesia
- high blood pressure
- excessive post-operative pain
- infection at the wound site
- drainage and bleeding from the wound
- swelling and redness
- nausea

- dizziness

- fluid retention

- sudden weight gain

Life after Adrenal Gland Removal

The long-term effects of adrenalectomy vary from individual to individual, but one major determining factor is whether one or both glands have been removed. In general, a single adrenal gland can produce enough hormones to meet the body's needs. A lot depends on the type of tumor or disorder that necessitated the surgery in the first place, but most patients are able to function normally with one adrenal gland without the need for hormone replacement. The doctor will monitor the function of the remaining organ to be sure it is working properly and recommend medication if necessary.

If both adrenal glands have been removed, or if the remaining gland is not functioning properly, the patient may need to take steroids, such as hydrocortisone or fludrocortisone to replace the hormones that had been produced by these organs. These substances may be necessary to support life, so it's critical that their use be continued unless instructed otherwise by a doctor. It is also wise for the patient to inform all of his or her healthcare providers of the operation and get a medical alert bracelet stating that an adrenalectomy has been performed and that in an emergency special life-saving medication may be required.

References

1. "Adrenal Gland Removal," DoveMed.com, October 18, 2015.

2. "Adrenal Gland Removal," George Washington University Medical Faculty Associates, n.d.

3. "Laparoscopic Adrenal Gland Removal," Society of American Gastrointestinal and Endoscopic Surgeons, n.d.

4. Norman, James MD, FACS, FACE. "Surgical Approaches to the Adrenal Gland," EndocrineWeb.com, April 18, 2016.

Part Five

Pancreatic and Diabetic Disorders

Chapter 40

Pancreatitis

What Is Pancreatitis?

Pancreatitis is inflammation of the pancreas. The pancreas is a large gland behind the stomach and close to the duodenum—the first part of the small intestine. The pancreas secretes digestive juices, or enzymes, into the duodenum through a tube called the pancreatic duct. Pancreatic enzymes join with bile—a liquid produced in the liver and stored in the gallbladder—to digest food. The pancreas also releases the hormones insulin and glucagon into the bloodstream. These hormones help the body regulate the glucose it takes from food for energy.

Normally, digestive enzymes secreted by the pancreas do not become active until they reach the small intestine. But when the pancreas is inflamed, the enzymes inside it attack and damage the tissues that produce them.

Pancreatitis can be acute or chronic. Either form is serious and can lead to complications. In severe cases, bleeding, infection, and permanent tissue damage may occur.

Both forms of pancreatitis occur more often in men than women.

What Is Acute Pancreatitis?

Acute pancreatitis is inflammation of the pancreas that occurs suddenly and usually resolves in a few days with treatment. Acute

This chapter includes text excerpted from "Pancreatitis," National Institute of Diabetes and Digestive and Kidney Diseases (NIDDK), August 2012. Reviewed October 2016.

pancreatitis can be a life-threatening illness with severe complications. Each year, about 210,000 people in the United States are admitted to the hospital with acute pancreatitis. The most common cause of acute pancreatitis is the presence of gallstones—small, pebble-like substances made of hardened bile—that cause inflammation in the pancreas as they pass through the common bile duct. Chronic, heavy alcohol use is also a common cause. Acute pancreatitis can occur within hours or as long as 2 days after consuming alcohol. Other causes of acute pancreatitis include abdominal trauma, medications, infections, tumors, and genetic abnormalities of the pancreas.

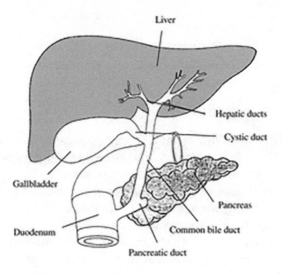

Figure 40.1. *Pancreas*

The gallbladder and the ducts that carry bile and other digestive enzymes from the liver, gallbladder, and pancreas to the small intestine are called the biliary system.

Symptoms

Acute pancreatitis usually begins with gradual or sudden pain in the upper abdomen that sometimes extends through the back. The pain may be mild at first and feel worse after eating. But the pain is often severe and may become constant and last for several days. A person with acute pancreatitis usually looks and feels very ill and needs immediate medical attention. Other symptoms may include

- a swollen and tender abdomen

- nausea and vomiting

274

- fever

- a rapid pulse

Severe acute pancreatitis may cause dehydration and low blood pressure. The heart, lungs, or kidneys can fail. If bleeding occurs in the pancreas, shock and even death may follow.

Diagnosis

While asking about a person's medical history and conducting a thorough physical examination, the doctor will order a blood test to assist in the diagnosis. During acute pancreatitis, the blood contains at least three times the normal amount of amylase and lipase, digestive enzymes formed in the pancreas. Changes may also occur in other body chemicals such as glucose, calcium, magnesium, sodium, potassium, and bicarbonate. After the person's condition improves, the levels usually return to normal.

Diagnosing acute pancreatitis is often difficult because of the deep location of the pancreas. The doctor will likely order one or more of the following tests:

- **Abdominal ultrasound.** Sound waves are sent toward the pancreas through a handheld device that a technician glides over the abdomen. The sound waves bounce off the pancreas, gallbladder, liver, and other organs, and their echoes make electrical impulses that create a picture—called a sonogram—on a video monitor. If gallstones are causing inflammation, the sound waves will also bounce off them, showing their location.

- **Computerized tomography (CT) scan.** The CT scan is a non-invasive X-ray that produces three-dimensional pictures of parts of the body. The person lies on a table that slides into a donut-shaped machine. The test may show gallstones and the extent of damage to the pancreas.

- **Endoscopic ultrasound (EUS).** After spraying a solution to numb the patient's throat, the doctor inserts an endoscope—a thin, flexible, lighted tube—down the throat, through the stomach, and into the small intestine. The doctor turns on an ultrasound attachment to the scope that produces sound waves to create visual images of the pancreas and bile ducts.

- **Magnetic resonance cholangiopancreatography (MRCP).** MRCP uses magnetic resonance imaging, a noninvasive test

275

that produces cross-section images of parts of the body. After being lightly sedated, the patient lies in a cylinder-like tube for the test. The technician injects dye into the patient's veins that helps show the pancreas, gallbladder, and pancreatic and bile ducts.

Treatment

Treatment for acute pancreatitis requires a few days' stay in the hospital for intravenous (IV) fluids, antibiotics, and medication to relieve pain. The person cannot eat or drink so the pancreas can rest. If vomiting occurs, a tube may be placed through the nose and into the stomach to remove fluid and air.

Unless complications arise, acute pancreatitis usually resolves in a few days. In severe cases, the person may require nasogastric feeding—a special liquid given in a long, thin tube inserted through the nose and throat and into the stomach—for several weeks while the pancreas heals.

Before leaving the hospital, the person will be advised not to smoke, drink alcoholic beverages, or eat fatty meals. In some cases, the cause of the pancreatitis is clear, but in others, more tests are needed after the person is discharged and the pancreas is healed.

Therapeutic Endoscopic Retrograde Cholangiopancreatography (ERCP) for Acute and Chronic Pancreatitis

ERCP is a specialized technique used to view the pancreas, gallbladder, and bile ducts and treat complications of acute and chronic pancreatitis—gallstones, narrowing or blockage of the pancreatic duct or bile ducts, leaks in the bile ducts, and pseudocysts—accumulations of fluid and tissue debris.

Soon after a person is admitted to the hospital with suspected narrowing of the pancreatic duct or bile ducts, a physician with specialized training performs ERCP.

After lightly sedating the patient and giving medication to numb the throat, the doctor inserts an endoscope—a long, flexible, lighted tube with a camera—through the mouth, throat, and stomach into the small intestine. The endoscope is connected to a computer and screen. The doctor guides the endoscope and injects a special dye into the pancreatic or bile ducts that helps the pancreas, gallbladder, and bile ducts appear on the screen while X-rays are taken.

The following procedures can be performed using ERCP:

Sphincterotomy. Using a small wire on the endoscope, the doctor finds the muscle that surrounds the pancreatic duct or bile ducts and makes a tiny cut to enlarge the duct opening. When a pseudocyst is present, the duct is drained.

Gallstone removal. The endoscope is used to remove pancreatic or bile duct stones with a tiny basket. Gallstone removal is sometimes performed along with a sphincterotomy.

Stent placement. Using the endoscope, the doctor places a tiny piece of plastic or metal that looks like a straw in a narrowed pancreatic or bile duct to keep it open.

Balloon dilatation. Some endoscopes have a small balloon that the doctor uses to dilate, or stretch, a narrowed pancreatic or bile duct. A temporary stent may be placed for a few months to keep the duct open.

People who undergo therapeutic ERCP are at slight risk for complications, including severe pancreatitis, infection, bowel perforation, or bleeding. Complications of ERCP are more common in people with acute or recurrent pancreatitis. A patient who experiences fever, trouble swallowing, or increased throat, chest, or abdominal pain after the procedure should notify a doctor immediately.

Complications

Gallstones that cause acute pancreatitis require surgical removal of the stones and the gallbladder. If the pancreatitis is mild, gallbladder removal—called cholecystectomy—may proceed while the person is in the hospital. If the pancreatitis is severe, gallstones may be removed using therapeutic endoscopic retrograde cholangiopancreatography (ERCP)—a specialized technique used to view the pancreas, gallbladder, and bile ducts and treat complications of acute and chronic pancreatitis. Cholecystectomy is delayed for a month or more to allow for full recovery.

If an infection develops, ERCP or surgery may be needed to drain the infected area, also called an abscess. Exploratory surgery may also be necessary to find the source of any bleeding, to rule out conditions that resemble pancreatitis, or to remove severely damaged pancreatic tissue.

Pseudocysts—accumulations of fluid and tissue debris—that may develop in the pancreas can be drained using ERCP or EUS.

If pseudocysts are left untreated, enzymes and toxins can enter the bloodstream and affect the heart, lungs, kidneys, or other organs.

Acute pancreatitis sometimes causes kidney failure. People with kidney failure need blood-cleansing treatments called dialysis or a kidney transplant.

In rare cases, acute pancreatitis can cause breathing problems. Hypoxia, a condition that occurs when body cells and tissues do not get enough oxygen, can develop. Doctors treat hypoxia by giving oxygen to the patient. Some people still experience lung failure—even with oxygen—and require a respirator for a while to help them breathe.

What Is Chronic Pancreatitis?

Chronic pancreatitis is inflammation of the pancreas that does not heal or improve—it gets worse over time and leads to permanent damage. Chronic pancreatitis, like acute pancreatitis, occurs when digestive enzymes attack the pancreas and nearby tissues, causing episodes of pain. Chronic pancreatitis often develops in people who are between the ages of 30 and 40.

The most common cause of chronic pancreatitis is many years of heavy alcohol use. The chronic form of pancreatitis can be triggered by one acute attack that damages the pancreatic duct. The damaged duct causes the pancreas to become inflamed. Scar tissue develops and the pancreas is slowly destroyed.

Other causes of chronic pancreatitis are

- hereditary disorders of the pancreas

- cystic fibrosis—the most common inherited disorder leading to chronic pancreatitis

- hypercalcemia—high levels of calcium in the blood

- hyperlipidemia or hypertriglyceridemia—high levels of blood fats

- some medicines

- certain autoimmune conditions

- unknown causes

Hereditary pancreatitis can present in a person younger than age 30, but it might not be diagnosed for several years. Episodes of abdominal pain and diarrhea lasting several days come and go over time and can progress to chronic pancreatitis. A diagnosis of hereditary pancreatitis is likely if the person has two or more family members with pancreatitis in more than one generation.

Symptoms

Most people with chronic pancreatitis experience upper abdominal pain, although some people have no pain at all. The pain may spread to the back, feel worse when eating or drinking, and become constant and disabling. In some cases, abdominal pain goes away as the condition worsens, most likely because the pancreas is no longer making digestive enzymes. Other symptoms include

- nausea
- vomiting
- weight loss
- diarrhea
- oily stools

People with chronic pancreatitis often lose weight, even when their appetite and eating habits are normal. The weight loss occurs because the body does not secrete enough pancreatic enzymes to digest food, so nutrients are not absorbed normally. Poor digestion leads to malnutrition due to excretion of fat in the stool.

Diagnosis

Chronic pancreatitis is often confused with acute pancreatitis because the symptoms are similar. As with acute pancreatitis, the doctor will conduct a thorough medical history and physical examination. Blood tests may help the doctor know if the pancreas is still making enough digestive enzymes, but sometimes these enzymes appear normal even though the person has chronic pancreatitis.

In more advanced stages of pancreatitis, when malabsorption and diabetes can occur, the doctor may order blood, urine, and stool tests to help diagnose chronic pancreatitis and monitor its progression.

After ordering X-rays of the abdomen, the doctor will conduct one or more of the tests used to diagnose acute pancreatitis—abdominal ultrasound, CT scan, EUS, and MRCP.

Treatment

Treatment for chronic pancreatitis may require hospitalization for pain management, IV hydration, and nutritional support. Nasogastric feedings may be necessary for several weeks if the person continues to lose weight.

When a normal diet is resumed, the doctor may prescribe synthetic pancreatic enzymes if the pancreas does not secrete enough of its own. The enzymes should be taken with every meal to help the person digest food and regain some weight. The next step is to plan a nutritious diet that is low in fat and includes small, frequent meals. A dietitian can assist in developing a meal plan. Drinking plenty of fluids and limiting caffeinated beverages is also important.

People with chronic pancreatitis are strongly advised not to smoke or consume alcoholic beverages, even if the pancreatitis is mild or in the early stages.

Complications

People with chronic pancreatitis who continue to consume large amounts of alcohol may develop sudden bouts of severe abdominal pain.

As with acute pancreatitis, ERCP is used to identify and treat complications associated with chronic pancreatitis such as gallstones, pseudocysts, and narrowing or obstruction of the ducts. Chronic pancreatitis also can lead to calcification of the pancreas, which means the pancreatic tissue hardens from deposits of insoluble calcium salts. Surgery may be necessary to remove part of the pancreas.

In cases involving persistent pain, surgery or other procedures are sometimes recommended to block the nerves in the abdominal area that cause pain.

When pancreatic tissue is destroyed in chronic pancreatitis and the insulin-producing cells of the pancreas, called beta cells, have been damaged, diabetes may develop. People with a family history of diabetes are more likely to develop the disease. If diabetes occurs, insulin or other medicines are needed to keep blood glucose at normal levels. A healthcare provider works with the patient to develop a regimen of medication, diet, and frequent blood glucose monitoring.

How Common Is Pancreatitis in Children?

Chronic pancreatitis in children is rare. Trauma to the pancreas and hereditary pancreatitis are two known causes of childhood pancreatitis. Children with cystic fibrosis—a progressive and incurable lung disease—may be at risk of developing pancreatitis. But more often the cause of pancreatitis in children is unknown.

Chapter 41

Insulin Resistance and Prediabetes

What Is Insulin?

Insulin is a hormone made in the pancreas, an organ located behind the stomach. The pancreas contains clusters of cells called islets. Beta cells within the islets make insulin and release it into the blood.

Insulin plays a major role in metabolism—the way the body uses digested food for energy. The digestive tract breaks down carbohydrates—sugars and starches found in many foods—into glucose. Glucose is a form of sugar that enters the bloodstream. With the help of insulin, cells throughout the body absorb glucose and use it for energy.

Insulin's Role in Blood Glucose Control

When blood glucose levels rise after a meal, the pancreas releases insulin into the blood. Insulin and glucose then travel in the blood to cells throughout the body.

- Insulin helps muscle, fat, and liver cells absorb glucose from the bloodstream, lowering blood glucose levels.

This chapter includes text excerpted from "Insulin Resistance and Prediabetes," National Institute of Diabetes and Digestive and Kidney Diseases (NIDDK), June 13, 2014.

- Insulin stimulates the liver and muscle tissue to store excess glucose. The stored form of glucose is called glycogen.

- Insulin also lowers blood glucose levels by reducing glucose production in the liver.

In a healthy person, these functions allow blood glucose and insulin levels to remain in the normal range.

What Is Insulin Resistance?

Insulin resistance is a condition in which the body produces insulin but does not use it effectively. When people have insulin resistance, glucose builds up in the blood instead of being absorbed by the cells, leading to type 2 diabetes or prediabetes.

Most people with insulin resistance don't know they have it for many years—until they develop type 2 diabetes, a serious, lifelong disease. The good news is that if people learn they have insulin resistance early on, they can often prevent or delay diabetes by making changes to their lifestyle.

Insulin resistance can lead to a variety of serious health disorders.

What Happens with Insulin Resistance?

In insulin resistance, muscle, fat, and liver cells do not respond properly to insulin and thus cannot easily absorb glucose from the bloodstream. As a result, the body needs higher levels of insulin to help glucose enter cells.

The beta cells in the pancreas try to keep up with this increased demand for insulin by producing more. As long as the beta cells are able to produce enough insulin to overcome the insulin resistance, blood glucose levels stay in the healthy range.

Over time, insulin resistance can lead to type 2 diabetes and prediabetes because the beta cells fail to keep up with the body's increased need for insulin. Without enough insulin, excess glucose builds up in the bloodstream, leading to diabetes, prediabetes, and other serious health disorders.

What Causes Insulin Resistance?

Although the exact causes of insulin resistance are not completely understood, scientists think the major contributors to insulin resistance are excess weight and physical inactivity.

Excess Weight

Some experts believe obesity, especially excess fat around the waist, is a primary cause of insulin resistance. Scientists used to think that fat tissue functioned solely as energy storage. However, studies have shown that belly fat produces hormones and other substances that can cause serious health problems such as insulin resistance, high blood pressure, imbalanced cholesterol, and cardiovascular disease (CVD).

Belly fat plays a part in developing chronic, or long-lasting, inflammation in the body. Chronic inflammation can damage the body over time, without any signs or symptoms. Scientists have found that complex interactions in fat tissue draw immune cells to the area and trigger low-level chronic inflammation. This inflammation can contribute to the development of insulin resistance, type 2 diabetes, and CVD. Studies show that losing the weight can reduce insulin resistance and prevent or delay type 2 diabetes.

Physical Inactivity

Many studies have shown that physical inactivity is associated with insulin resistance, often leading to type 2 diabetes. In the body, more glucose is used by muscle than other tissues. Normally, active muscles burn their stored glucose for energy and refill their reserves with glucose taken from the bloodstream, keeping blood glucose levels in balance.

Studies show that after exercising, muscles become more sensitive to insulin, reversing insulin resistance and lowering blood glucose levels. Exercise also helps muscles absorb more glucose without the need for insulin. The more muscle a body has, the more glucose it can burn to control blood glucose levels.

Other Causes

Other causes of insulin resistance may include ethnicity; certain diseases; hormones; steroid use; some medications; older age; sleep problems, especially sleep apnea; and cigarette smoking.

Does Sleep Matter?

Yes. Studies show that untreated sleep problems, especially sleep apnea, can increase the risk of obesity, insulin resistance, and type 2 diabetes. Night shift workers may also be at increased risk for these problems. Sleep apnea is a common disorder in which a person's breathing is interrupted during sleep. People may often move out of deep sleep and into light sleep when their breathing pauses or becomes shallow. This results in poor sleep quality that causes problem sleepiness, or excessive tiredness, during the day.

Many people aren't aware of their symptoms and aren't diagnosed. People who think they might have sleep problems should talk with their healthcare provider.

What Is Prediabetes?

Prediabetes is a condition in which blood glucose or A1C levels—which reflect average blood glucose levels—are higher than normal but not high enough for a diagnosis of diabetes. Prediabetes is becoming more common in the United States. The U.S. Department of Health and Human Services (HHS) estimates that at least 86 million U.S. adults ages 20 or older had prediabetes in 2012. People with prediabetes are at increased risk of developing type 2 diabetes and CVD, which can lead to heart attack or stroke.

How Does Insulin Resistance Relate to Type 2 Diabetes and Prediabetes?

Insulin resistance increases the risk of developing type 2 diabetes and prediabetes. Prediabetes usually occurs in people who already have insulin resistance. Although insulin resistance alone does not cause type 2 diabetes, it often sets the stage for the disease by placing a high demand on the insulin-producing beta cells. In prediabetes, the beta cells can no longer produce enough insulin to overcome insulin resistance, causing blood glucose levels to rise above the normal range.

Once a person has prediabetes, continued loss of beta cell function usually leads to type 2 diabetes. People with type 2 diabetes have high blood glucose. Over time, high blood glucose damages nerves and blood vessels, leading to complications such as heart disease, stroke, blindness, kidney failure, and lower-limb amputations.

Studies have shown that most people with prediabetes develop type 2 diabetes within 10 years, unless they change their lifestyle. Lifestyle changes include losing 5 to 7 percent of their body weight—10 to 14 pounds for people who weigh 200 pounds—by making changes in their diet and level of physical activity.

What Are the Symptoms of Insulin Resistance and Prediabetes?

Insulin resistance and prediabetes usually have no symptoms. People may have one or both conditions for several years without knowing they have them. Even without symptoms, healthcare providers can identify people at high risk by their physical characteristics, also known as risk factors.

People with a severe form of insulin resistance may have dark patches of skin, usually on the back of the neck. Sometimes people have a dark ring around their neck. Dark patches may also appear on elbows, knees, knuckles, and armpits. This condition is called acanthosis nigricans.

Who Should Be Tested for Prediabetes?

The American Diabetes Association (ADA) recommends that testing to detect prediabetes be considered in adults who are overweight or obese and have one or more additional risk factors for diabetes. The section "Body Mass Index (BMI)" explains how to determine if a person is overweight or obese. However, not everyone who is overweight will get type 2 diabetes. People without these risk factors should begin testing at age 45.

Risk factors for prediabetes—in addition to being overweight or obese or being age 45 or older—include the following:

- being physically inactive

- having a parent or sibling with diabetes

- having a family background that is African American, Alaska Native, American Indian, Asian American,

- Hispanic/Latino, or Pacific Islander American

- giving birth to a baby weighing more than 9 pounds

- being diagnosed with gestational diabetes—diabetes that develops only during pregnancy

- having high blood pressure—140/90 mmHg or above—or being treated for high blood pressure

- HDL cholesterol level below 35 mg/dL or a triglyceride level above 250 mg/dL

- having polycystic ovary syndrome (PCOS)

- having prediabetes, impaired fasting glucose (IFG), or impaired glucose tolerance (IGT) on an earlier testing

- having other conditions associated with insulin resistance, such as obesity or acanthosis nigricans

- having CVD

If test results are normal, testing should be repeated at least every 3 years. Testing is important for early diagnosis. Catching prediabetes early gives people time to change their lifestyle and prevent type 2 diabetes and CVD. Healthcare providers may recommend more frequent testing depending on initial results and risk status.

In addition to weight, the location of excess fat on the body can be important. A waist measurement of 40 inches or more for men and 35 inches or more for women is linked to insulin resistance and increases a person's risk for type 2 diabetes. This is true even if a person's BMI falls within the normal range.

Body Mass Index (BMI)

Body mass index is a measurement of body weight relative to height. Adults ages 20 or older can follow the steps below using the BMI chart to find out whether they are normal weight, overweight, or obese:

- People should find their height in the left-hand column.

- They should move across the row to the number closest to their weight.

- Then, they should check the number at the top of that column.

The number at the top of the column is the BMI. The words above the BMI number indicate whether that person is normal weight, overweight, or obese. People who are overweight or obese should consider talking with a healthcare provider or registered dietitian about ways to lose weight to reduce the risk of diabetes.

The BMI chart has certain limitations. The chart may overestimate body fat in athletes and others who have a muscular build and underestimate body fat in older adults and others who have lost muscle. BMI for children and teens must be determined based on age and sex in addition to height and weight.

How Are Insulin Resistance and Prediabetes Diagnosed?

Healthcare providers use blood tests to determine whether a person has prediabetes, but they do not usually test specifically for insulin resistance. Insulin resistance can be assessed by measuring the level of insulin in the blood.

However, the test that most accurately measures insulin resistance, called the euglycemic clamp, is too costly and complicated to be used in most healthcare providers' offices. The clamp is a research tool used by scientists to learn more about glucose metabolism. Research has shown that if blood tests indicate prediabetes, insulin resistance most likely is present.

Blood Tests for Prediabetes

All blood tests involve drawing blood at a healthcare provider's office or commercial facility and sending the sample to a lab for analysis. Lab analysis of blood is needed to ensure test results are accurate. Glucose measuring devices used in a healthcare provider's office, such as finger-stick devices, are not accurate enough for diagnosis but may be used as a quick indicator of high blood glucose.

Prediabetes can be detected with one of the following blood tests:

- the A1C test

- the fasting plasma glucose (FPG) test

- the oral glucose tolerance test (OGTT)

A1C test. Sometimes called hemoglobin A1c, HbA1c, or glycohemoglobin test, this test reflects average blood glucose levels over the past 3 months. This test is the most reliable test for prediabetes, but it is not as sensitive as the other tests. In some individuals, it may miss prediabetes that could be caught by glucose tests.

Although some healthcare providers can quickly measure A1C in their office, that type of measurement—called a point-of-care test—is not considered reliable for diagnosis. For diagnosis of prediabetes, the A1C test should be analyzed in a laboratory using a method that is certified by the NGSP.

The A1C test can be unreliable for diagnosing prediabetes in people with certain conditions that are known to interfere with the results. Interference should be suspected when A1C results seem very different from the results of a blood glucose test. People of African,

Mediterranean, or Southeast Asian descent, or people with family members with sickle cell anemia or a thalassemia, are particularly at risk of interference. People in these groups may have a less common type of hemoglobin, known as a hemoglobin variant, that can interfere with some A1C tests.

An A1C of 5.7 to 6.4 percent indicates prediabetes.

Fasting plasma glucose test. This test measures blood glucose in people who have not eaten anything for at least 8 hours. This test is most reliable when done in the morning. Prediabetes found with this test is called IFG.

Fasting glucose levels of 100 to 125 mg/dL indicate prediabetes.

OGTT. This test measures blood glucose after people have not eaten for at least 8 hours and 2 hours after they drink a sweet liquid provided by a healthcare provider or laboratory. Prediabetes found with this test is called IGT.

A blood glucose level between 140 and 199 mg/dL indicates prediabetes.

The following table lists the blood test levels for a diagnosis of prediabetes.

	A1C (percent)	Fasting Plasma Glucose (mg/dL)	Oral Glucose Tolerance Test (mg/dL)
Diabetes	6.5 or above	126 or above	200 or above
Prediabetes	5.7 to 6.4	100 to 125	140 to 199
Normal	About 5	99 or below	139 or below

Definitions: mg = milligram, dL = deciliter
For all three tests, within the prediabetes range, the higher the test result, the greater the risk of diabetes.

Figure 41.1. *Blood Test Levels for Diagnosis of Diabetes and Prediabetes*

Understanding Test Results

A blood test indicating prediabetes means that insulin resistance has progressed to the point where the beta cells in the pancreas can no longer compensate and a person's blood glucose levels are rising toward type 2 diabetes. The higher the test results, the greater the risk of type 2 diabetes.

Test numbers. For example, people with an A1C below 5.7 percent may still be at risk for diabetes if they have a family history of type 2 diabetes or have gained excess weight around the waist. People with an A1C above 6.0 percent should be considered at very high risk of developing diabetes. A level of 6.5 percent or above means a person has diabetes.

Follow up. People whose test results indicate they have prediabetes may be retested in 1 year and should consider making lifestyle changes to reduce their risk of developing type 2 diabetes.

Varying results. Although all these tests can be used to test for prediabetes, in some people one test will indicate a diagnosis of prediabetes or diabetes when another test does not. People with differing test results may be in an early stage of the disease, where blood glucose levels have not risen high enough to show on every test.

Healthcare providers repeat laboratory tests to confirm test results. Diabetes develops over time, so even with variations in test results, healthcare providers can tell when overall blood glucose levels are becoming too high.

Can Insulin Resistance and Prediabetes Be Reversed?

Yes. Physical activity and weight loss help the body respond better to insulin. The Diabetes Prevention Program (DPP) was a federally funded study of 3,234 people at high risk for diabetes.

The DPP and other large studies proved that people with prediabetes can often prevent or delay diabetes if they lose a modest amount of weight by cutting fat and calorie intake and increasing physical activity—for example, walking 30 minutes a day, 5 days a week.

People at High Risk for Diabetes

DPP study participants were overweight and had prediabetes. Many had family members with type 2 diabetes. Prediabetes, obesity, and a family history of diabetes are strong risk factors for type 2 diabetes. About half of the DPP participants were from minority groups with high rates of diabetes, including African Americans, Alaska Natives, American Indians, Asian Americans, Hispanics/Latinos, and Pacific Islander Americans.

DPP participants also included others at high risk for developing type 2 diabetes, such as women with a history of gestational diabetes and people ages 60 and older.

Approaches to Preventing Diabetes

The DPP tested three approaches to preventing diabetes:

- **Making lifestyle changes.** People in the lifestyle change group exercised, usually by walking 5 days a week for about 30 minutes a day, and lowered their intake of fat and calories.

- **Taking the diabetes medication metformin.** Those who took metformin also received information about physical activity and diet.

- **Receiving education about diabetes.** The third group only received information about physical activity and diet and took a placebo—a pill without medication in it.

People in the lifestyle change group showed the best outcomes. However people who took metformin also benefited. The results showed that by losing an average of 15 pounds in the first year of the study, people in the lifestyle change group reduced their risk of developing type 2 diabetes by 58 percent over 3 years.

Lifestyle change was even more effective in those ages 60 and older. People in this group reduced their risk by 71 percent.

People in the metformin group also benefited, reducing their risk by 31 percent.

Lasting Results

The Diabetes Prevention Program Outcomes Study (DPPOS) has shown that the benefits of weight loss and metformin last for at least 10 years. The DPPOS has continued to follow most DPP participants since the DPP ended in 2001. The DPPOS showed that 10 years after enrolling in the DPP

- people in the lifestyle change group reduced their risk for developing diabetes by 34 percent

- those in the lifestyle change group ages 60 or older had even greater benefit, reducing their risk of developing diabetes by 49 percent

- participants in the lifestyle change group also had fewer heart and blood vessel disease risk factors, including lower blood pressure and triglyceride levels, even though they took fewer medications to control their heart disease risk

- those in the metformin group reduced their risk of developing diabetes by 18 percent

Even though controlling weight with lifestyle changes is challenging, it produces long-term health rewards by lowering the risk for type 2 diabetes, lowering blood glucose levels, and reducing other heart disease risk factors.

What Steps Can Help Reverse Insulin Resistance and Prediabetes?

By losing weight and being more physically active, people can reverse insulin resistance and prediabetes, thus preventing or delaying type 2 diabetes. People can decrease their risk by

- eating a healthy diet and reaching and maintaining a healthy weight

- increasing physical activity

- not smoking

- taking medication

Chapter 42

Diabetes

What Is Diabetes?

Diabetes is a disease in which blood glucose levels are above normal. Most of the food we eat is turned into glucose, or sugar, for our bodies to use for energy. The pancreas, an organ that lies near the stomach, makes a hormone called insulin to help glucose get into the cells of our bodies. When you have diabetes, your body either doesn't make enough insulin or can't use its own insulin as well as it should. This causes sugar to build up in your blood.

Diabetes can cause serious health complications including heart disease, blindness, kidney failure, and lower-extremity amputations. Diabetes is the seventh leading cause of death in the United States.

What Are the Symptoms of Diabetes?

People who think they might have diabetes must visit a physician for diagnosis. They might have SOME or NONE of the following symptoms:

- frequent urination

- excessive thirst

- unexplained weight loss

This chapter includes text excerpted from "Basics about Diabetes," Centers for Disease Control and Prevention (CDC), March 31, 2015.

- extreme hunger
- sudden vision changes
- tingling or numbness in hands or feet
- feeling very tired much of the time
- very dry skin
- sores that are slow to heal
- more infections than usual

Nausea, vomiting, or stomach pains may accompany some of these symptoms in the abrupt onset of insulin-dependent diabetes, now called type 1 diabetes.

What Are the Types of Diabetes?

Type 1 diabetes, which was previously called insulin-dependent diabetes mellitus (IDDM) or juvenile-onset diabetes, may account for about 5 percent of all diagnosed cases of diabetes. **Type 2 diabetes**, which was previously called non-insulin-dependent diabetes mellitus (NIDDM) or adult-onset diabetes, may account for about 90 percent to 95 percent of all diagnosed cases of diabetes. **Gestational diabetes** is a type of diabetes that only pregnant women get. If not treated, it can cause problems for mothers and babies. Gestational diabetes develops in 2 percent to 10 percent of all pregnancies but usually disappears when a pregnancy is over. **Other specific types of diabetes** resulting from specific genetic syndromes, surgery, drugs, malnutrition, infections, and other illnesses may account for 1 percent to 5 percent of all diagnosed cases of diabetes.

What Are the Risk Factors for Diabetes?

Risk factors for type 2 diabetes include older age, obesity, family history of diabetes, prior history of gestational diabetes, impaired glucose tolerance, physical inactivity, and race/ethnicity. African Americans, Hispanic/Latino Americans, American Indians, and some Asian Americans and Pacific Islanders are at particularly high risk for type 2 diabetes.

Risk factors are less well defined for type 1 diabetes than for type 2 diabetes, but autoimmune, genetic, and environmental factors are involved in developing this type of diabetes.

Gestational diabetes occurs more frequently in African Americans, Hispanic/Latino Americans, American Indians, and people with a family history of diabetes than in other groups. Obesity is also associated with higher risk. Women who have had gestational diabetes have a 35 percent to 60 percent chance of developing diabetes in the next 10–20 years.

Other specific types of diabetes, which may account for 1 percent to 5 percent of all diagnosed cases, result from specific genetic syndromes, surgery, drugs, malnutrition, infections, and other illnesses.

What Is the Treatment for Diabetes?

Healthy eating, physical activity, and insulin injections are the basic therapies for type 1 diabetes. The amount of insulin taken must be balanced with food intake and daily activities. Blood glucose levels must be closely monitored through frequent blood glucose testing.

Healthy eating, physical activity, and blood glucose testing are the basic therapies for type 2 diabetes. In addition, many people with type 2 diabetes require oral medication, insulin, or both to control their blood glucose levels.

People with diabetes must take responsibility for their day-to-day care, and keep blood glucose levels from going too low or too high.

People with diabetes should see a healthcare provider who will monitor their diabetes control and help them learn to manage their diabetes. In addition, people with diabetes may see endocrinologists, who may specialize in diabetes care; ophthalmologists for eye examinations; podiatrists for routine foot care; and dietitians and diabetes educators who teach the skills needed for daily diabetes management.

What Causes Type 1 Diabetes?

The causes of type 1 diabetes appear to be much different than those for type 2 diabetes, though the exact mechanisms for developing both diseases are unknown. The appearance of type 1 diabetes is suspected to follow exposure to an "environmental trigger," such as an unidentified virus, stimulating an immune attack against the beta cells of the pancreas (that produce insulin) in some genetically predisposed people.

Can Diabetes Be Prevented?

Researchers are making progress in identifying the exact genetics and "triggers" that predispose some individuals to develop type 1 diabetes, but prevention remains elusive.

A number of studies have shown that regular physical activity can significantly reduce the risk of developing type 2 diabetes. Type 2 diabetes is associated with obesity.

Is There a Cure for Diabetes?

In response to the growing health burden of diabetes, the diabetes community has three choices: prevent diabetes; cure diabetes; and improve the quality of care of people with diabetes to prevent devastating complications. All three approaches are actively being pursued by the U.S. Department of Health and Human Services (HHS).

Both the National Institutes of Health (NIH) and the Centers for Disease Control and Prevention (CDC) are involved in prevention activities. The NIH is involved in research to cure both type 1 and type 2 diabetes, especially type 1. CDC focuses most of its programs on making sure that the proven science to prevent complications is put into daily practice for people with diabetes. The basic idea is that if all the important research and science are not applied meaningfully in the daily lives of people with diabetes, then the research is, in essence, wasted.

Several approaches to "cure" diabetes are currently under investigation:

- Pancreas transplantation

- Islet cell transplantation (islet cells produce insulin)

- Artificial pancreas development

- Genetic manipulation (fat or muscle cells that don't normally make insulin have a human insulin gene inserted—then these "pseudo" islet cells are transplanted into people with type 1 diabetes).

Each of these approaches still has a lot of challenges, such as preventing immune rejection; finding an adequate number of insulin cells; keeping cells alive; and others. But progress is being made in all areas.

Chapter 43

Hypoglycemia

What Is Hypoglycemia?

Hypoglycemia, also called low blood glucose or low blood sugar, occurs when the level of glucose in your blood drops below normal. For many people with diabetes, that means a level of 70 milligrams per deciliter (mg/dL) or less. Your numbers might be different, so check with your healthcare provider to find out what level is too low for you.

What Are the Symptoms of Hypoglycemia?

Symptoms of hypoglycemia tend to come on quickly and can vary from person to person. You may have one or more mild-to-moderate symptoms listed in the table below. Sometimes people don't feel any symptoms.

Severe hypoglycemia is when your blood glucose level becomes so low that you're unable to treat yourself and need help from another person. Severe hypoglycemia is dangerous and needs to be treated right away. This condition is more common in people with type 1 diabetes.

This chapter includes text excerpted from "Low Blood Glucose (Hypoglycemia)," National Institute of Diabetes and Digestive and Kidney Diseases (NIDDK), August 30, 2016.

Table 43.1. Hypoglycemia Symptoms

Mild-to-Moderate		Severe
• shaky or jittery • sweaty • hungry • headachy • blurred vision • sleepy or tired • dizzy or lightheaded • confused or disoriented • pale	• uncoordinated • irritable or nervous • argumentative or combative • changed behavior or personality • trouble concentrating • weak • fast or irregular heart beat	• unable to eat or drink • seizures or convulsions (jerky movements) • unconsciousness

Some symptoms of hypoglycemia during sleep are

• crying out or having nightmares

• sweating enough to make your pajamas or sheets damp

• feeling tired, irritable, or confused after waking up

What Causes Hypoglycemia in Diabetes?

Hypoglycemia can be a side effect of insulin or other types of diabetes medicines that help your body make more insulin. Two types of diabetes pills can cause hypoglycemia: sulfonylureas and meglitinides. Ask your healthcare team if your diabetes medicine can cause hypoglycemia.

Although other diabetes medicines don't cause hypoglycemia by themselves, they can increase the chances of hypoglycemia if you also take insulin, a sulfonylurea, or a meglitinide.

What Other Factors Contribute to Hypoglycemia in Diabetes?

If you take insulin or diabetes medicines that increase the amount of insulin your body makes—but don't match your medications with your food or physical activity—you could develop hypoglycemia. The following factors can make hypoglycemia more likely:

Not Eating Enough Carbohydrates (Carbs)

When you eat foods containing carbohydrates, your digestive system breaks down the sugars and starches into glucose. Glucose then enters your bloodstream and raises your blood glucose level. If you don't eat enough carbohydrates to match your medication, your blood glucose could drop too low.

Skipping or Delaying a Meal

If you skip or delay a meal, your blood glucose could drop too low. Hypoglycemia also can occur when you are asleep and haven't eaten for several hours.

Increasing Physical Activity

Increasing your physical activity level beyond your normal routine can lower your blood glucose level for up to 24 hours after the activity.

Drinking Too Much Alcohol without Enough Food

Alcohol makes it harder for your body to keep your blood glucose level steady, especially if you haven't eaten in a while. The effects of alcohol can also keep you from feeling the symptoms of hypoglycemia, which may lead to severe hypoglycemia.

Being Sick

When you're sick, you may not be able to eat as much or keep food down, which can cause low blood glucose.

How Can I Prevent Hypoglycemia If I Have Diabetes?

If you are taking insulin, a sulfonylurea, or a meglitinide, using your diabetes management plan and working with your healthcare team to adjust your plan as needed can help you prevent hypoglycemia. The following actions can also help prevent hypoglycemia:

Check Blood Glucose Levels

Knowing your blood glucose level can help you decide how much medicine to take, what food to eat, and how physically active to be. To find out your blood glucose level, check yourself with a blood glucose meter as often as your doctor advises.

Hypoglycemia unawareness. Sometimes people with diabetes don't feel or recognize the symptoms of hypoglycemia, a problem called hypoglycemia unawareness. If you have had hypoglycemia without feeling any symptoms, you may need to check your blood glucose more often so you know when you need to treat your hypoglycemia or take steps to prevent it. Be sure to check your blood glucose before you drive.

If you have hypoglycemia unawareness or have hypoglycemia often, ask your healthcare provider about a continuous glucose monitor (CGM). A CGM checks your blood glucose level at regular times throughout the day and night. CGMs can tell you if your blood glucose is falling quickly and sound an alarm if your blood glucose falls too low. CGM alarms can wake you up if you have hypoglycemia during sleep.

Eat Regular Meals and Snacks

Your meal plan is key to preventing hypoglycemia. Eat regular meals and snacks with the correct amount of carbohydrates to help keep your blood glucose level from going too low. Also, if you drink alcoholic beverages, it's best to eat some food at the same time.

Be Physically Active Safely

Physical activity can lower your blood glucose during the activity and for hours afterward. To help prevent hypoglycemia, you may need to check your blood glucose before, during, and after physical activity and adjust your medicine or carbohydrate intake. For example, you might eat a snack before being physically active or decrease your insulin dose as directed by your healthcare provider to keep your blood glucose from dropping too low.

Work with Your Healthcare Team

Tell your healthcare team if you have had hypoglycemia. Your healthcare team may adjust your diabetes medicines or other aspects of your management plan. Learn about balancing your medicines, eating plan, and physical activity to prevent hypoglycemia. Ask if you should have a glucagon emergency kit to carry with you at all times.

How Do I Treat Hypoglycemia?

If you begin to feel one or more hypoglycemia symptoms, check your blood glucose. If your blood glucose level is below your target or less than 70, eat or drink 15 grams of carbohydrates right away. Examples include

- four glucose tablets or one tube of glucose gel

- 1/2 cup (4 ounces) of fruit juice—not low-calorie or reduced sugar*
- 1/2 can (4 to 6 ounces) of soda—not low-calorie or reduced sugar
- 1 tablespoon of sugar, honey, or corn syrup
- 2 tablespoons of raisins

Wait 15 minutes and check your blood glucose again. If your glucose level is still low, eat or drink another 15 grams of glucose or carbohydrates. Check your blood glucose again after another 15 minutes. Repeat these steps until your glucose level is back to normal.

If your next meal is more than 1 hour away, have a snack to keep your blood glucose level in your target range. Try crackers or a piece of fruit.

* People who have kidney disease shouldn't drink orange juice for their 15 grams of carbohydrates because it contains a lot of potassium. Apple, grape, or cranberry juice are good options.

Treating Hypoglycemia If You Take Acarbose or Miglitol

If you take acarbose or miglitol along with diabetes medicines that can cause hypoglycemia, you will need to take glucose tablets or glucose gel if your blood glucose level is too low. Eating or drinking other sources of carbohydrates won't raise your blood glucose level quickly enough.

What If I Have Severe Hypoglycemia and Can't Treat Myself?

Someone will need to give you a glucagon injection if you have severe hypoglycemia. An injection of glucagon will quickly raise your blood glucose level. Talk with your healthcare provider about when and how to use a glucagon emergency kit. If you have an emergency kit, check the date on the package to make sure it hasn't expired.

If you are likely to have severe hypoglycemia, teach your family, friends, and coworkers when and how to give you a glucagon injection. Also, tell your family, friends, and coworkers to call 911 right away after giving you a glucagon injection or if you don't have a glucagon emergency kit with you.

If you have hypoglycemia often or have had severe hypoglycemia, you should wear a medical alert bracelet or pendant. A medical alert ID tells other people that you have diabetes and need care right away. Getting prompt care can help prevent the serious problems that hypoglycemia can cause.

301

Chapter 44

Cancer of the Pancreas

About Pancreatic Cancer

The pancreas is a gland about 6 inches long that is shaped like a thin pear lying on its side. The wider end of the pancreas is called the head, the middle section is called the body, and the narrow end is called the tail. The pancreas lies between the stomach and the spine. The pancreas has two main jobs in the body:

- To make juices that help digest (break down) food.

- To make hormones, such as insulin and glucagon, that help control blood sugar levels. Both of these hormones help the body use and store the energy it gets from food.

The digestive juices are made by exocrine pancreas cells and the hormones are made by endocrine pancreas cells. About 95 percent of pancreatic cancers begin in exocrine cells.

Smoking and Health History Can Affect the Risk of Pancreatic Cancer

Anything that increases your risk of getting a disease is called a risk factor. Having a risk factor does not mean that you will get cancer; not having risk factors doesn't mean that you will not get cancer. Talk with your doctor if you think you may be at risk.

This chapter includes text excerpted from "Pancreatic Cancer Treatment (PDQ®)—Patient Version," National Cancer Institute (NCI), June 30, 2016.

Risk factors for pancreatic cancer include the following:

- Smoking
- Being very overweight
- Having a personal history of diabetes or chronic pancreatitis.
- Having a family history of pancreatic cancer or pancreatitis.
- Having certain hereditary conditions, such as:
- Multiple endocrine neoplasia type 1 (MEN1) syndrome
- Hereditary nonpolyposis colon cancer (HNPCC; Lynch syndrome)
- von Hippel-Lindau syndrome
- Peutz-Jeghers syndrome
- Hereditary breast and ovarian cancer syndrome.
- Familial atypical multiple mole melanoma (FAMMM) syndrome

Signs and Symptoms of Pancreatic Cancer Include Jaundice, Pain, and Weight Loss

Pancreatic cancer may not cause early signs or symptoms. Signs and symptoms may be caused by pancreatic cancer or by other conditions. Check with your doctor if you have any of the following:

- Dark urine
- Feeling very tired
- Jaundice (yellowing of the skin and whites of the eyes)
- Light-colored stools
- Loss of appetite
- Pain in the upper or middle abdomen and back
- Weight loss for no known reason

Pancreatic Cancer Is Difficult to Detect (Find) and Diagnose Early

Pancreatic cancer is difficult to detect and diagnose for the following reasons:

- There aren't any noticeable signs or symptoms in the early stages of pancreatic cancer.

- The signs and symptoms of pancreatic cancer, when present, are like the signs and symptoms of many other illnesses.

- The pancreas is hidden behind other organs such as the stomach, small intestine, liver, gallbladder, spleen, and bile ducts.

Tests That Examine the Pancreas Are Used to Detect (Find), Diagnose, and Stage Pancreatic Cancer

Pancreatic cancer is usually diagnosed with tests and procedures that make pictures of the pancreas and the area around it. The process used to find out if cancer cells have spread within and around the pancreas is called staging. Tests and procedures to detect, diagnose, and stage pancreatic cancer are usually done at the same time. In order to plan treatment, it is important to know the stage of the disease and whether or not the pancreatic cancer can be removed by surgery.

The following tests and procedures may be used:

- Abdominal ultrasound

- Biopsy

- Blood chemistry studies

- CT scan (CAT scan)

- Endoscopic retrograde cholangiopancreatography (ERCP)

- Endoscopic ultrasound (EUS)

- Laparoscopy

- MRI (magnetic resonance imaging)

- Percutaneous transhepatic cholangiography (PTC)

- PET scan (positron emission tomography scan)

- Physical exam and history

- Tumor marker test

Certain Factors Affect Prognosis (Chance of Recovery) and Treatment Options

The prognosis (chance of recovery) and treatment options depend on the following:

- Whether or not the tumor can be removed by surgery.

- The stage of the cancer (the size of the tumor and whether the cancer has spread outside the pancreas to nearby tissues or lymph nodes or to other places in the body).

- The patient's general health.

- Whether the cancer has just been diagnosed or has recurred (come back).

Pancreatic cancer can be controlled only if it is found before it has spread, when it can be completely removed by surgery. If the cancer has spread, palliative treatment can improve the patient's quality of life by controlling the symptoms and complications of this disease.

Stages of Pancreatic Cancer

The process used to find out if cancer has spread within the pancreas or to other parts of the body is called staging. The information gathered from the staging process determines the stage of the disease. It is important to know the stage of the disease in order to plan treatment. The results of some of the tests used to diagnose pancreatic cancer are often also used to stage the disease.

There Are Three Ways That Cancer Spreads in the Body

Cancer can spread through tissue, the lymph system, and the blood:

- Tissue. The cancer spreads from where it began by growing into nearby areas.

- Lymph system. The cancer spreads from where it began by getting into the lymph system. The cancer travels through the lymph vessels to other parts of the body.

- Blood. The cancer spreads from where it began by getting into the blood. The cancer travels through the blood vessels to other parts of the body.

Cancer May Spread from Where It Began to Other Parts of the Body

When cancer spreads to another part of the body, it is called metastasis. Cancer cells break away from where they began (the primary tumor) and travel through the lymph system or blood.

- Lymph system. The cancer gets into the lymph system, travels through the lymph vessels, and forms a tumor (metastatic tumor) in another part of the body.

- Blood. The cancer gets into the blood, travels through the blood vessels, and forms a tumor (metastatic tumor) in another part of the body.

The metastatic tumor is the same type of cancer as the primary tumor. For example, if pancreatic cancer spreads to the liver, the cancer cells in the liver are actually pancreatic cancer cells. The disease is metastatic pancreatic cancer, not liver cancer.

The Following Stages Are Used for Pancreatic Cancer

Stage 0 (Carcinoma in Situ)

In stage 0, abnormal cells are found in the lining of the pancreas. These abnormal cells may become cancer and spread into nearby normal tissue. Stage 0 is also called carcinoma in situ.

In stage I, cancer has formed and is found in the pancreas only. Stage I is divided into stage IA and stage IB, based on the size of the tumor.

- Stage IA: The tumor is 2 centimeters or smaller.

- Stage IB: The tumor is larger than 2 centimeters.

Stage II

In stage II, cancer may have spread to nearby tissue and organs, and may have spread to lymph nodes near the pancreas. Stage II is divided into stage IIA and stage IIB, based on where the cancer has spread.

- Stage IIA: Cancer has spread to nearby tissue and organs but has not spread to nearby lymph nodes.

- Stage IIB: Cancer has spread to nearby lymph nodes and may have spread to nearby tissue and organs.

Stage III

In stage III, cancer has spread to the major blood vessels near the pancreas and may have spread to nearby lymph nodes.

Stage IV

In stage IV, cancer may be of any size and has spread to distant organs, such as the liver, lung, and peritoneal cavity. It may have also spread to organs and tissues near the pancreas or to lymph nodes.

Recurrent Pancreatic Cancer

Recurrent pancreatic cancer is cancer that has recurred (come back) after it has been treated. The cancer may come back in the pancreas or in other parts of the body.

Treatment Option Overview

Different types of treatment are available for patients with pancreatic cancer. Some treatments are standard (the currently used treatment), and some are being tested in clinical trials. A treatment clinical trial is a research study meant to help improve current treatments or obtain information on new treatments for patients with cancer. When clinical trials show that a new treatment is better than the standard treatment, the new treatment may become the standard treatment. Patients may want to think about taking part in a clinical trial. Some clinical trials are open only to patients who have not started treatment.

Five Types of Standard Treatment Are Used

Surgery

One of the following types of surgery may be used to take out the tumor:

- Whipple procedure: A surgical procedure in which the head of the pancreas, the gallbladder, part of the stomach, part of the small intestine, and the bile duct are removed. Enough of the pancreas is left to produce digestive juices and insulin.

- Total pancreatectomy: This operation removes the whole pancreas, part of the stomach, part of the small intestine, the common bile duct, the gallbladder, the spleen, and nearby lymph nodes.

- Distal pancreatectomy: The body and the tail of the pancreas and usually the spleen are removed.

If the cancer has spread and cannot be removed, the following types of palliative surgery may be done to relieve symptoms and improve quality of life:

- Surgical biliary bypass: If cancer is blocking the small intestine and bile is building up in the gallbladder, a biliary bypass may be done. During this operation, the doctor will cut the gallbladder or bile duct and sew it to the small intestine to create a new pathway around the blocked area.

- Endoscopic stent placement: If the tumor is blocking the bile duct, surgery may be done to put in a stent (a thin tube) to drain bile that has built up in the area. The doctor may place the stent through a catheter that drains to the outside of the body or the stent may go around the blocked area and drain the bile into the small intestine.

- Gastric bypass: If the tumor is blocking the flow of food from the stomach, the stomach may be sewn directly to the small intestine so the patient can continue to eat normally.

Radiation Therapy

Radiation therapy is a cancer treatment that uses high-energy X-rays or other types of radiation to kill cancer cells or keep them from growing. There are two types of radiation therapy:

- External radiation therapy uses a machine outside the body to send radiation toward the cancer.

- Internal radiation therapy uses a radioactive substance sealed in needles, seeds, wires, or catheters that are placed directly into or near the cancer.

The way the radiation therapy is given depends on the type and stage of the cancer being treated. External radiation therapy is used to treat pancreatic cancer.

Chemotherapy

Chemotherapy is a cancer treatment that uses drugs to stop the growth of cancer cells, either by killing the cells or by stopping them from dividing. When chemotherapy is taken by mouth or injected into a vein or muscle, the drugs enter the bloodstream and can reach cancer cells throughout the body (systemic chemotherapy). When chemotherapy is placed directly into the cerebrospinal fluid, an organ, or a body cavity such as the abdomen, the drugs mainly affect cancer cells in those areas (regional chemotherapy). Combination chemotherapy is treatment using more than one anticancer drug. The way the chemotherapy is given depends on the type and stage of the cancer being treated.

Chemoradiation Therapy

Chemoradiation therapy combines chemotherapy and radiation therapy to increase the effects of both.

Targeted Therapy

Targeted therapy is a type of treatment that uses drugs or other substances to identify and attack specific cancer cells without harming normal cells. Tyrosine kinase inhibitors (TKIs) are targeted therapy drugs that block signals needed for tumors to grow. Erlotinib is a type of TKI used to treat pancreatic cancer.

There Are Treatments for Pain Caused by Pancreatic Cancer

Pain can occur when the tumor presses on nerves or other organs near the pancreas. When pain medicine is not enough, there are treatments that act on nerves in the abdomen to relieve the pain. The doctor may inject medicine into the area around affected nerves or may cut the nerves to block the feeling of pain. Radiation therapy with or without chemotherapy can also help relieve pain by shrinking the tumor.

Patients with Pancreatic Cancer Have Special Nutritional Needs

Surgery to remove the pancreas may affect its ability to make pancreatic enzymes that help to digest food. As a result, patients may have problems digesting food and absorbing nutrients into the body. To prevent malnutrition, the doctor may prescribe medicines that replace these enzymes.

New Types of Treatment Are Being Tested in Clinical Trials

Biologic Therapy

Biologic therapy is a treatment that uses the patient's immune system to fight cancer. Substances made by the body or made in a laboratory are used to boost, direct, or restore the body's natural defenses against cancer. This type of cancer treatment is also called biotherapy or immunotherapy.

Patients May Want to Think about Taking Part in a Clinical Trial

For some patients, taking part in a clinical trial may be the best treatment choice. Clinical trials are part of the cancer research process. Clinical trials are done to find out if new cancer treatments are safe and effective or better than the standard treatment.

Many of today's standard treatments for cancer are based on earlier clinical trials. Patients who take part in a clinical trial may receive the standard treatment or be among the first to receive a new treatment.

Patients who take part in clinical trials also help improve the way cancer will be treated in the future. Even when clinical trials do not lead to effective new treatments, they often answer important questions and help move research forward.

Patients Can Enter Clinical Trials before, during, or after Starting Their Cancer Treatment

Some clinical trials only include patients who have not yet received treatment. Other trials test treatments for patients whose cancer has not gotten better. There are also clinical trials that test new ways to stop cancer from recurring (coming back) or reduce the side effects of cancer treatment.

Follow-Up Tests May Be Needed

Some of the tests that were done to diagnose the cancer or to find out the stage of the cancer may be repeated. Some tests will be repeated in order to see how well the treatment is working. Decisions about whether to continue, change, or stop treatment may be based on the results of these tests.

Some of the tests will continue to be done from time to time after treatment has ended. The results of these tests can show if your condition has changed or if the cancer has recurred (come back). These tests are sometimes called follow-up tests or check-ups.

Treatment Options for Recurrent Pancreatic Cancer

Treatment of recurrent pancreatic cancer may include the following:

- Palliative surgery or stent placement to bypass blocked areas in ducts or the small intestine.

- Palliative radiation therapy to shrink the tumor.

- Other palliative medical care to reduce symptoms, such as nerve blocks to relieve pain.

- Chemotherapy

- Clinical trials of chemotherapy, new anticancer therapies, or biologic therapy.

Chapter 45

Islet Cell Tumors

About Pancreatic Neuroendocrine Tumors (Islet Cell Tumors)

The pancreas is a gland about 6 inches long that is shaped like a thin pear lying on its side. The wider end of the pancreas is called the head, the middle section is called the body, and the narrow end is called the tail. The pancreas lies behind the stomach and in front of the spine. There are two kinds of cells in the pancreas:

- **Endocrine pancreas cells** make several kinds of hormones (chemicals that control the actions of certain cells or organs in the body), such as insulin to control blood sugar. They cluster together in many small groups (islets) throughout the pancreas. Endocrine pancreas cells are also called islet cells or islets of Langerhans. Tumors that form in islet cells are called islet cell tumors, pancreatic endocrine tumors, or pancreatic neuroendocrine tumors (pancreatic NETs).

- **Exocrine pancreas cells** make enzymes that are released into the small intestine to help the body digest food. Most of the pancreas is made of ducts with small sacs at the end of the ducts, which are lined with exocrine cells.

This chapter includes text excerpted from "Pancreatic Neuroendocrine Tumors (Islet Cell Tumors) Treatment (PDQ®)—Patient Version," National Cancer Institute (NCI), July 30, 2015.

Pancreatic neuroendocrine tumors (NETs) may be benign (not cancer) or malignant (cancer). When pancreatic NETs are malignant, they are called pancreatic endocrine cancer or islet cell carcinoma.

Pancreatic NETs are much less common than pancreatic exocrine tumors and have a better prognosis.

Pancreatic NETs May or May Not Cause Signs or Symptoms

Pancreatic NETs may be functional or nonfunctional:

• Functional tumors make extra amounts of hormones, such as gastrin, insulin, and glucagon, that cause signs and symptoms.

• Nonfunctional tumors do not make extra amounts of hormones. Signs and symptoms are caused by the tumor as it spreads and grows. Most nonfunctional tumors are malignant (cancer).

Most pancreatic NETs are functional tumors.

There Are Different Kinds of Functional Pancreatic NETs

Pancreatic NETs make different kinds of hormones such as gastrin, insulin, and glucagon. Functional pancreatic NETs include the following:

• **Gastrinoma:** A tumor that forms in cells that make gastrin. Gastrin is a hormone that causes the stomach to release an acid that helps digest food. Both gastrin and stomach acid are increased by gastrinomas. When increased stomach acid, stomach ulcers, and diarrhea are caused by a tumor that makes gastrin, it is called Zollinger-Ellison syndrome. A gastrinoma usually forms in the head of the pancreas and sometimes forms in the small intestine. Most gastrinomas are malignant (cancer).

• **Insulinoma:** A tumor that forms in cells that make insulin. Insulin is a hormone that controls the amount of glucose (sugar) in the blood. It moves glucose into the cells, where it can be used by the body for energy. Insulinomas are usually slow-growing tumors that rarely spread. An insulinoma forms in the head, body, or tail of the pancreas. Insulinomas are usually benign (not cancer).

• **Glucagonoma:** A tumor that forms in cells that make glucagon. Glucagon is a hormone that increases the amount of glucose in the blood. It causes the liver to break down glycogen. Too much

glucagon causes hyperglycemia (high blood sugar). A glucagonoma usually forms in the tail of the pancreas. Most gluca-
gonomas are malignant (cancer).

- **Other types of tumors**: There are other rare types of functional pancreatic NETs that make hormones, including hormones that control the balance of sugar, salt, and water in the
  body. These tumors include:

  - VIPomas, which make vasoactive intestinal peptide. VIPoma
    may also be called Verner-Morrison syndrome.

  - Somatostatinomas, which make somatostatin.

These other types of tumors are grouped together because they are
treated in much the same way.

Having Certain Syndromes Can Increase the Risk of Pancreatic NETs

Anything that increases your risk of getting a disease is called a
risk factor. Having a risk factor does not mean that you will get cancer;
not having risk factors doesn't mean that you will not get cancer. Talk
with your doctor if you think you may be at risk.

Multiple endocrine neoplasia type 1 (MEN1) syndrome is a risk
factor for pancreatic NETs.

Different Types of Pancreatic NETs Have Different Signs and Symptoms

Signs or symptoms can be caused by the growth of the tumor and/
or by hormones the tumor makes or by other conditions. Some tumors
may not cause signs or symptoms. Check with your doctor if you have
any of these problems.

Signs and Symptoms of a Non-Functional Pancreatic NET

A non-functional pancreatic NET may grow for a long time without
causing signs or symptoms. It may grow large or spread to other parts
of the body before it causes signs or symptoms, such as:

- diarrhea

- indigestion

- a lump in the abdomen

- pain in the abdomen or back

- yellowing of the skin and whites of the eyes

Signs and Symptoms of a Functional Pancreatic NET

The signs and symptoms of a functional pancreatic NET depend on the type of hormone being made.

Too much gastrin may cause:

- Stomach ulcers that keep coming back.

- Pain in the abdomen, which may spread to the back. The pain may come and go and it may go away after taking an antacid.

- The flow of stomach contents back into the esophagus (gastro-esophageal reflux).

- Diarrhea

Too much insulin may cause:

- Low blood sugar. This can cause blurred vision, headache, and feeling lightheaded, tired, weak, shaky, nervous, irritable, sweaty, confused, or hungry.

- Fast heartbeat.

Too much glucagon may cause:

- Skin rash on the face, stomach, or legs.

- High blood sugar. This can cause headaches, frequent urination, dry skin and mouth, or feeling hungry, thirsty, tired, or weak.

- Blood clots. Blood clots in the lung can cause shortness of breath, cough, or pain in the chest. Blood clots in the arm or leg can cause pain, swelling, warmth, or redness of the arm or leg.

- Diarrhea

- Weight loss for no known reason.

- Sore tongue or sores at the corners of the mouth.

Too much vasoactive intestinal peptide (VIP) may cause:

- Very large amounts of watery diarrhea.

- Dehydration. This can cause feeling thirsty, making less urine, dry skin and mouth, headaches, dizziness, or feeling tired.

- Low potassium level in the blood. This can cause muscle weakness, aching, or cramps, numbness and tingling, frequent urination, fast heartbeat, and feeling confused or thirsty.

- Cramps or pain in the abdomen.

- Weight loss for no known reason.

Too much somatostatin may cause:

- High blood sugar. This can cause headaches, frequent urination, dry skin and mouth, or feeling hungry, thirsty, tired, or weak.

- Diarrhea

- Steatorrhea (very foul-smelling stool that floats).

- Gallstones

- Yellowing of the skin and whites of the eyes.

- Weight loss for no known reason.

Lab Tests and Imaging Tests Are Used to Detect (Find) and Diagnose Pancreatic NETs

The following tests and procedures may be used:

- Abdominal CT scan (CAT scan)

- Angiogram

- Biopsy

- Blood chemistry studies

- Bone scan

- Chromogranin A test

- Endoscopic retrograde cholangiopancreatography (ERCP)

- Endoscopic ultrasound (EUS)

- Intraoperative ultrasound

- Laparotomy

- MRI (magnetic resonance imaging)

- Physical exam and history

- Somatostatin receptor scintigrapy

Other Kinds of Lab Tests Are Used to Check for the Specific Type of Pancreatic NETs

The following tests and procedures may be used:

Gastrinoma

- **Fasting serum gastrin test**: A test in which a blood sample is checked to measure the amount of gastrin in the blood. This test is done after the patient has had nothing to eat or drink for at least 8 hours. Conditions other than gastrinoma can cause an increase in the amount of gastrin in the blood.

- **Basal acid output test**: A test to measure the amount of acid made by the stomach. The test is done after the patient has had nothing to eat or drink for at least 8 hours. A tube is inserted through the nose or throat, into the stomach. The stomach contents are removed and four samples of gastric acid are removed through the tube. These samples are used to find out the amount of gastric acid made during the test and the pH level of the gastric secretions.

- **Secretin stimulation test**: If the basal acid output test result is not normal, a secretin stimulation test may be done. The tube is moved into the small intestine and samples are taken from the small intestine after a drug called secretin is injected. Secretin causes the small intestine to make acid. When there is a gastrinoma, the secretin causes an increase in how much gastric acid is made and the level of gastrin in the blood.

- **Somatostatin receptor scintigraphy**: A type of radionuclide scan that may be used to find small pancreatic NETs. A small amount of radioactive octreotide (a hormone that attaches to tumors) is injected into a vein and travels through the blood. The radioactive octreotide attaches to the tumor and a special camera that detects radioactivity is used to show where the tumors are in the body. This procedure is also called octreotide scan and SRS.

Insulinoma

- **Fasting serum glucose and insulin test**: A test in which a blood sample is checked to measure the amounts of glucose (sugar) and insulin in the blood. The test is done after the patient has had nothing to eat or drink for at least 24 hours.

Glucagonoma

- **Fasting serum glucagon test**: A test in which a blood sample is checked to measure the amount of glucagon in the blood. The test is done after the patient has had nothing to eat or drink for at least 8 hours.

Other Tumor Types

- VIPoma

  - **Serum VIP (vasoactive intestinal peptide) test**: A test in which a blood sample is checked to measure the amount of VIP.

  - **Blood chemistry studies**: A procedure in which a blood sample is checked to measure the amounts of certain substances released into the blood by organs and tissues in the body. An unusual (higher or lower than normal) amount of a substance can be a sign of disease. In VIPoma, there is a lower than normal amount of potassium.

  - **Stool analysis**: A stool sample is checked for a higher than normal sodium (salt) and potassium levels.

- Somatostatinoma

  - **Fasting serum somatostatin test**: A test in which a blood sample is checked to measure the amount of somatostatin in the blood. The test is done after the patient has had nothing to eat or drink for at least 8 hours.

  - **Somatostatin receptor scintigraphy**: A type of radionuclide scan that may be used to find small pancreatic NETs. A small amount of radioactive octreotide (a hormone that attaches to tumors) is injected into a vein and travels through the blood. The radioactive octreotide attaches to the tumor and a special camera that detects radioactivity is used to show where the tumors are in the body. This procedure is also called octreotide scan and SRS.

Certain Factors Affect Prognosis (Chance of Recovery) and Treatment Options

Pancreatic NETs can often be cured. The prognosis (chance of recovery) and treatment options depend on the following:

- The type of cancer cell.

- Where the tumor is found in the pancreas.

- Whether the tumor has spread to more than one place in the pancreas or to other parts of the body.

- Whether the patient has MEN1 syndrome.

- The patient's age and general health.

- Whether the cancer has just been diagnosed or has recurred (come back).

Stages of Pancreatic Neuroendocrine Tumors

The process used to find out if cancer has spread within the pancreas or to other parts of the body is called staging. The results of the tests and procedures used to diagnose pancreatic neuroendocrine tumors (NETs) are also used to find out whether the cancer has spread.

Although there is a standard staging system for pancreatic NETs, it is not used to plan treatment. Treatment of pancreatic NETs is based on the following:

- Whether the cancer is found in one place in the pancreas.

- Whether the cancer is found in several places in the pancreas.

- Whether the cancer has spread to lymph nodes near the pancreas or to other parts of the body such as the liver, lung, peritoneum, or bone.

There Are Three Ways That Cancer Spreads in the Body

Cancer can spread through tissue, the lymph system, and the blood:

- Tissue. The cancer spreads from where it began by growing into nearby areas.

- Lymph system. The cancer spreads from where it began by getting into the lymph system. The cancer travels through the lymph vessels to other parts of the body.

- Blood. The cancer spreads from where it began by getting into the blood. The cancer travels through the blood vessels to other parts of the body.

Cancer May Spread from Where It Began to Other Parts of the Body

When cancer spreads to another part of the body, it is called metastasis. Cancer cells break away from where they began (the primary tumor) and travel through the lymph system or blood.

- Lymph system. The cancer gets into the lymph system, travels through the lymph vessels, and forms a tumor (metastatic tumor) in another part of the body.

- Blood. The cancer gets into the blood, travels through the blood vessels, and forms a tumor (metastatic tumor) in another part of the body.

The metastatic tumor is the same type of tumor as the primary tumor. For example, if a pancreatic neuroendocrine tumor spreads to the liver, the tumor cells in the liver are actually neuroendocrine tumor cells. The disease is metastatic pancreatic neuroendocrine tumor, not liver cancer.

Recurrent Pancreatic Neuroendocrine Tumors

Recurrent pancreatic neuroendocrine tumors (NETs) are tumors that have recurred (come back) after being treated. The tumors may come back in the pancreas or in other parts of the body.

Treatment Option Overview

Different types of treatments are available for patients with pancreatic neuroendocrine tumors (NETs). Some treatments are standard (the currently used treatment), and some are being tested in clinical trials. A treatment clinical trial is a research study meant to help improve current treatments or obtain information on new treatments for patients with cancer. When clinical trials show that a new treatment is better than the standard treatment, the new treatment may become the standard treatment. Patients may want to think about taking part in a clinical trial. Some clinical trials are open only to patients who have not started treatment.

Six Types of Standard Treatment Are Used

1. Surgery
   - Cryosurgical ablation

- Distal pancreatectomy

- Enucleation

- Liver resection

- Pancreatoduodenectomy

- Parietal cell vagotomy

- Radiofrequency ablation

- Total gastrectomy

2. Chemotherapy

- Regional chemotherapy

- Systemic chemotherapy

3. Hormone Therapy

4. Hepatic Arterial Occlusion or Chemoembolization

5. Targeted Therapy

6. Supportive Care

Follow-Up Tests May Be Needed

Some of the tests that were done to diagnose the cancer or to find out the stage of the cancer may be repeated. Some tests will be repeated in order to see how well the treatment is working. Decisions about whether to continue, change, or stop treatment may be based on the results of these tests.

Some of the tests will continue to be done from time to time after treatment has ended. The results of these tests can show if your condition has changed or if the cancer has recurred (come back). These tests are sometimes called follow-up tests or check-ups.

Chapter 46

Zollinger-Ellison Syndrome

What Is Zollinger-Ellison Syndrome?

Zollinger-Ellison syndrome is a rare disorder that occurs when one or more tumors form in the pancreas and duodenum. The tumors, called gastrinomas, release large amounts of gastrin that cause the stomach to produce large amounts of acid. Normally, the body releases small amounts of gastrin after eating, which triggers the stomach to make gastric acid that helps break down food and liquid in the stomach. The extra acid causes peptic ulcers to form in the duodenum and elsewhere in the upper intestine.

The tumors seen with Zollinger-Ellison syndrome are sometimes cancerous and may spread to other areas of the body.

What Are the Stomach, Duodenum, and Pancreas?

The stomach, duodenum, and pancreas are digestive organs that break down food and liquid.

- The stomach stores swallowed food and liquid. The muscle action of the lower part of the stomach mixes the food and liquid with digestive juice. Partially digested food and liquid slowly move into the duodenum and are further broken down.

This chapter includes text excerpted from "Zollinger-Ellison Syndrome," National Institute of Diabetes and Digestive and Kidney Diseases (NIDDK), December 2013.

- The duodenum is the first part of the small intestine—the tube-shaped organ between the stomach and the large intestine—where digestion of the food and liquid continues.

- The pancreas is an organ that makes the hormone insulin and enzymes for digestion. A hormone is a natural chemical produced in one part of the body and released into the blood to trigger or regulate particular functions of the body. Insulin helps cells throughout the body remove glucose, also called sugar, from blood and use it for energy. The pancreas is located behind the stomach and close to the duodenum.

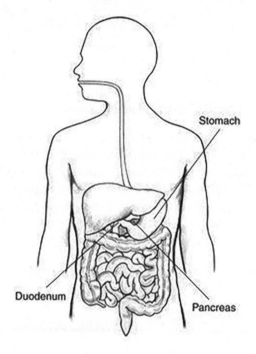

Figure 46.1. *Digestive Organs*

The stomach, duodenum, and pancreas are digestive organs that break down food and liquid.

What Causes Zollinger-Ellison Syndrome?

Experts do not know the exact cause of Zollinger-Ellison syndrome. About 25 to 30 percent of gastrinomas are caused by an inherited genetic disorder called multiple endocrine neoplasia type 1 (MEN1). MEN1 causes hormone-releasing tumors in the endocrine glands and the duodenum. Symptoms of MEN1 include increased hormone levels in the blood, kidney stones, diabetes, muscle weakness, weakened bones, and fractures.

How Common Is Zollinger-Ellison Syndrome?

Zollinger-Ellison syndrome is rare and only occurs in about one in every 1 million people. Although anyone can get Zollinger-Ellison syndrome, the disease is more common among men 30 to 50 years old. A child who has a parent with MEN1 is also at increased risk for Zollinger-Ellison syndrome.

What Are the Signs and Symptoms of Zollinger-Ellison Syndrome?

Zollinger-Ellison syndrome signs and symptoms are similar to those of peptic ulcers. A dull or burning pain felt anywhere between the navel and midchest is the most common symptom of a peptic ulcer. This discomfort usually

- occurs when the stomach is empty—between meals or during the night—and may be briefly relieved by eating food
- lasts for minutes to hours
- comes and goes for several days, weeks, or months

Other symptoms include

- Bloating
- Burping
- Diarrhea
- Nausea
- Poor appetite
- Vomiting
- Weight loss

Some people with Zollinger-Ellison syndrome have only diarrhea, with no other symptoms. Others develop gastroesophageal reflux (GER), which occurs when stomach contents flow back up into the esophagus—a muscular tube that carries food and liquids to the stomach. In addition to nausea and vomiting, reflux symptoms include a painful, burning feeling in the midchest.

Seek Help for Emergency Symptoms

A person who has any of the following emergency symptoms should call or see a healthcare provider right away:

- Chest pain

- Sharp, sudden, persistent, and severe stomach pain

- Red blood in stool or black stools

- Red blood in vomit or vomit that looks like coffee grounds

These symptoms could be signs of a serious problem, such as

- Internal bleeding—when gastric acid or a peptic ulcer breaks a blood vessel

- Perforation—when a peptic ulcer forms a hole in the duodenal wall

- Obstruction—when a peptic ulcer blocks the path of food trying to leave the stomach

How Is Zollinger-Ellison Syndrome Diagnosed?

A healthcare provider diagnoses Zollinger-Ellison syndrome based on the following:

- Blood tests

- Imaging tests to look for gastrinomas

- Measurement of stomach acid

- Medical history

- Physical exam

- Signs and symptoms

- Upper gastrointestinal (GI) endoscopy

Medical History

Taking a medical and family history is one of the first things a healthcare provider may do to help diagnose Zollinger-Ellison syndrome. The healthcare provider may ask about family cases of MEN1 in particular.

Physical Exam

A physical exam may help diagnose Zollinger-Ellison syndrome. During a physical exam, a healthcare provider usually

- examines a person's body
- uses a stethoscope to listen to bodily sounds
- taps on specific areas of the person's body

Signs and Symptoms

A healthcare provider may suspect Zollinger-Ellison syndrome if

- diarrhea accompanies peptic ulcer symptoms or if peptic ulcer treatment fails.

- a person has peptic ulcers without the use of nonsteroidal anti-inflammatory drugs (NSAIDs) such as aspirin and ibuprofen or a bacterial *Helicobacter pylori (H. pylori)* infection. NSAID use and *H. pylori* infection may cause peptic ulcers.

- a person has severe ulcers that bleed or cause holes in the duodenum or stomach.

- a healthcare provider diagnoses a person or the person's family member with MEN1 or a person has symptoms of MEN1.

Blood Tests

The healthcare provider may use blood tests to check for an elevated gastrin level. A technician or nurse draws a blood sample during an office visit or at a commercial facility and sends the sample to a lab for analysis. A healthcare provider will ask the person to fast for several hours prior to the test and may ask the person to stop acid-reducing medications for a period of time before the test. A gastrin level that is 10 times higher than normal suggests Zollinger-Ellison syndrome.

A healthcare provider may also check for an elevated gastrin level after an infusion of secretin. Secretin is a hormone that causes gastrinomas to release more gastrin. A technician or nurse places an intravenous (IV) needle in a vein in the arm to give an infusion of secretin. A healthcare provider may suspect Zollinger-Ellison syndrome if blood drawn after the infusion shows an elevated gastrin level.

Upper Gastrointestinal Endoscopy

The healthcare provider uses an upper gastrointestinal (GI) endoscopy to check the esophagus, stomach, and duodenum for ulcers and esophagitis—a general term used to describe irritation and swelling of the esophagus. This procedure involves using an endoscope—a small, flexible tube with a light—to see the upper GI tract, which includes the esophagus, stomach, and duodenum. A gastroenterologist—a doctor who specializes in digestive diseases—performs the test at a hospital or an outpatient center. The gastroenterologist carefully feeds the endoscope down the esophagus and into the stomach and duodenum. A small camera mounted on the endoscope transmits a video image to a monitor, allowing close examination of the intestinal lining. A person may receive a liquid anesthetic that is gargled or sprayed on the back of the throat. A technician or nurse inserts an IV needle in a vein in the arm if anesthesia is given.

Imaging Tests

To help find gastrinomas, a healthcare provider may order one or more of the following imaging tests:

- **Computerized tomography (CT) scan.** A CT scan is an X-ray that produces pictures of the body. A CT scan may include the injection of a special dye, called contrast medium. CT scans use a combination of X-rays and computer technology to create images. CT scans require the person to lie on a table that slides into a tunnel-shaped device where an X-ray technician takes X-rays. A computer puts the different views together to create a model of the pancreas, stomach, and duodenum. The X-ray technician performs the procedure in an outpatient center or a hospital, and a radiologist—a doctor who specializes in medical imaging—interprets the images. The person does not need anesthesia. CT scans can show tumors and ulcers.

- **Magnetic resonance imaging (MRI).** MRI is a test that takes pictures of the body's internal organs and soft tissues without using X-rays. A specially trained technician performs the procedure in an outpatient center or a hospital, and a radiologist interprets the images. The person does not need anesthesia, though people with a fear of confined spaces may receive light sedation, taken by mouth. An MRI may include the injection of contrast medium. With most MRI machines, the person will lie on a table that slides into a tunnel-shaped device that may be open ended or closed at one end. Some machines allow the person to lie in a more open space. During an MRI, the person, although usually awake, remains perfectly still while the technician takes the images, which usually takes only a few minutes. The technician will take a sequence of images from different angles to create a detailed picture of the upper GI tract. During sequencing, the person will hear loud mechanical knocking and humming noises.

- **Endoscopic ultrasound.** This procedure involves using a special endoscope called an endoechoscope to perform ultrasound of the pancreas. The endoechoscope has a built-in miniature ultrasound probe that bounces safe, painless sound waves off organs to create an image of their structure. A gastroenterologist performs the procedure in an outpatient center or a hospital, and a radiologist interprets the images. The gastroenterologist carefully feeds the endoechoscope down the esophagus, through the stomach and duodenum, until it is near the pancreas. A person may receive a liquid anesthetic that is gargled or sprayed on the back of the throat. A sedative helps the person stay relaxed and comfortable. The images can show gastrinomas in the pancreas.

- **Angiogram.** An angiogram is a special kind of X-ray in which an interventional radiologist—a specially trained radiologist— threads a thin, flexible tube called a catheter through the large arteries, often from the groin, to the artery of interest. The radiologist injects contrast medium through the catheter so the images show up more clearly on the X-ray. The interventional radiologist performs the procedure and interprets the images in a hospital or an outpatient center. A person does not need anesthesia, though a light sedative may help reduce a person's anxiety during the procedure. This test can show gastrinomas in the pancreas.

- **Somatostatin receptor scintigraphy.** An X-ray technician performs this test, also called OctreoScan, at a hospital or an outpatient center, and a radiologist interprets the images. A person does not need anesthesia. A radioactive compound called a radiotracer, when injected into the bloodstream, selectively labels tumor cells. The labeled cells light up when scanned with a device called a gamma camera. The test can show gastrinomas in the duodenum, pancreas, and other parts of the body.

Small gastrinomas may be hard to see; therefore, healthcare providers may order several types of imaging tests to find gastrinomas.

Stomach-Acid Measurement

Using a sample of stomach juices for analysis, a healthcare provider may measure the amount of stomach acid a person produces. During the exam, a healthcare provider puts in a nasogastric tube—a tiny tube inserted through the nose and throat that reaches into the stomach. A person may receive a liquid anesthetic that is gargled or sprayed on the back of the throat. Once the tube is placed, a healthcare provider takes samples of the stomach acid. High acid levels in the stomach indicate Zollinger-Ellison syndrome.

How Is Zollinger-Ellison Syndrome Treated?

A healthcare provider treats Zollinger-Ellison syndrome with medications to reduce gastric acid secretion and with surgery to remove gastrinomas. A healthcare provider sometimes uses chemotherapy—medications to shrink tumors—when tumors are too widespread to remove with surgery.

Medications

A class of medications called proton pump inhibitors (PPIs) includes

- esomeprazole (Nexium)
- lansoprazole (Prevacid)
- pantoprazole (Protonix)
- omeprazole (Prilosec or Zegerid)
- dexlansoprazole (Dexilant)

PPIs stop the mechanism that pumps acid into the stomach, helping to relieve peptic ulcer pain and promote healing. A healthcare provider may prescribe people who have Zollinger-Ellison syndrome higher-than-normal doses of PPIs to control the acid production. Studies show that PPIs may increase the risk of hip, wrist, and spine fractures when a person takes them long term or in high doses, so it's important for people to discuss risks versus benefits with their healthcare provider.

Surgery

Surgical removal of gastrinomas is the only cure for Zollinger-Ellison syndrome. Some gastrinomas spread to other parts of the body, especially the liver and bones. Finding and removing all gastrinomas before they spread is often challenging because many of the tumors are small.

Chemotherapy

Healthcare providers sometimes use chemotherapy drugs to treat gastrinomas that cannot be surgically removed, including

- streptozotocin (Zanosar)

- 5-fluorouracil (Adrucil)

- doxorubicin (Doxil)

Part Six

Disorders of the Ovaries and Testes

Chapter 47

Hypogonadism

Female Hypogonadism

Hypogonadism is a condition in which the sex glands either under-perform or, in some cases, are absent altogether. In women, this means the ovaries produce little or no estrogen, a hormone that, among other functions, is responsible for sexual development, helps regulate the menstrual cycle, assists in the maintenance of uterine function during pregnancy, plays a role in blood clotting and brain function, helps build healthy bones, and affects mood. Hypogonadism may result in infertility and an increased risk of osteoporosis, as well other effects on overall health and quality of life.

Causes

There are two types of hypogonadism, primary and secondary. Primary hypogonadism, which under normal circumstances occurs naturally as a result of menopause, may be caused by a chromosomal disorder, such as Turner syndrome, in which the X chromosome is partially or completely missing, by surgical removal of the ovaries, or by autoimmune disorders. The causes of secondary hypogonadism include problems with the hypothalamus or pituitary gland, infection, head injury, inflammatory diseases, rapid weight loss, or drug use.

Symptoms

The signs and symptoms of hypogonadism may include:

- Lack of development of secondary sex characteristics during puberty
- Lack of (or reduced) menstruation
- Absent or decreased libido
- Reduction in vaginal lubrication
- Reduced fertility
- Hot flashes
- Loss of body hair
- Changes in energy and mood
- Sleep disturbance
- Loss of bone mass
- Frequent urination or urinary tract infections
- Inability or reduced ability to smell

Diagnosis

Diagnosing hypogonadism begins with a physical exam in which the doctor will ask about family history and the extent of symptoms, examine the genitalia, assess the development of secondary sex characteristics, and evaluate overall health. Depending on the results of the examination, tests may include:

- Measurement of estrogen levels
- Follicle-stimulating hormone (FSH) and luteinizing hormone (LH) tests to evaluate pituitary function
- Tests for anemia and iron deficiency
- Evaluation of levels of prolactin (a hormone that, among a wide range of other functions, promotes milk production)
- Thyroid tests
- Genetic tests

- Ultrasound of the ovaries

- Magnetic resonance imaging (MRI) of the head to examine the pituitary gland

Treatment

The treatment of hypogonadism depends on its cause. For example, if the problem were a tumor in the pituitary gland, surgical removal might be recommended. However, in most cases it is a chronic condition that requires lifelong management. The most common treatment involves hormone-replacement therapy to restore development and function. Estrogen and progesterone (a hormone that plays a role in maintaining pregnancy) may be administered via injection, pills, a topical gel, or slow-release skin patches.

Possible Complications

If untreated, the risks and complications of hypogonadism can include:

- Delayed puberty

- Infertility

- Sexual dysfunction

- Weakness

- Osteoporosis

- Heart disease

In addition, hormone replacement therapy, although the most effective means of treating hypogonadism, does carry some risks. These may include blood clots, stroke, heart disease, breast and endometrial cancer, and gallbladder disease.

References

1. "Hypogonadism in Females," The Woman's Clinic, n.d.

2. "Hypogonadotropic Hypogonadism," Women Health and Lifestyle, n.d.

3. Martel, Janelle. "Hypogonadism," Healthline.com, November 19, 2015.

4. Vogiatzi, Maria G., MD. "Hypogonadism," Medscape.com, October 14, 2016.

5. Wisse, Brent, MD. "Hypogonadism," Medlineplus.gov, October 25, 2014.

Male Hypogonadism

Hypogonadism is a medical term for decreased functional activity of the gonads. The gonads (ovaries or testes) produce hormones (testosterone, estradiol, antimullerian hormone, progesterone, inhibin B, activin) and gametes (eggs or sperm). Male hypogonadism is characterized by a deficiency in testosterone—a critical hormone for sexual, cognitive, and body function and development. Clinically low testosterone levels can lead to the absence of secondary sex characteristics, infertility, muscle wasting, and other abnormalities. Low testosterone levels may be due to testicular, hypothalamic, or pituitary abnormalities. In individuals who also present with clinical signs and symptoms, clinical guidelines recommend treatment with testosterone replacement therapy.

Classification of Male Hypogonadism

There are two basic types of hypogonadism that exist:

1. Primary: This type of hypogonadism—also known as primary testicular failure—originates from a problem in the testicles.

2. Secondary: This type of hypogonadism indicates a problem in the hypothalamus or the pituitary gland—parts of the brain that signal the testicles to produce testosterone. The hypothalamus produces the gonadotropin releasing hormone, which signals the pituitary gland to make the follicle-stimulating hormone (FSH) and luteinizing hormone. The luteinizing hormone then signals the testes to produce testosterone. Either type of hypogonadism may be caused by an inherited (congenital) trait or something that happens later in life (acquired), such as an injury or an infection.

Primary Hypogonadism

Common causes of primary hypogonadism include:

Klinefelter Syndrome: This condition results from a congenital abnormality of the sex chromosomes, X and Y. A male normally has one X and one Y chromosome. In Klinefelter syndrome, two or more X chromosomes are present in addition to one Y chromosome. The Y chromosome contains the genetic material that determines the sex of a child and the related development. The extra X chromosome that occurs in Klinefelter syndrome causes abnormal development of the testicles, which in turn results in the underproduction of testosterone.

Undescended Testicles: Before birth, the testicles develop inside the abdomen and normally move down into their permanent place in the scrotum. Sometimes, one or both of the testicles may not descend at birth. This condition often corrects itself within the first few years of life without treatment. If not corrected in early childhood, it may lead to malfunction of the testicles and reduced production of testosterone.

Mumps Orchitis: If a mumps infection involving the testicles in addition to the salivary glands (mumps orchitis) occurs during adolescence or adulthood, long-term testicular damage may occur. This may affect normal testicular function and testosterone production.

Hemochromatosis: Too much iron in the blood can cause testicular failure or pituitary gland dysfunction, affecting testosterone production.

Injury to the Testicles: Because of their location outside the abdomen, the testicles are prone to injury. Damage to normally developed testicles can cause hypogonadism. Damage to one testicle may not impair testosterone production.

Cancer Treatment: Chemotherapy or radiation therapy for the treatment of cancer can interfere with testosterone and sperm production. The effects of both treatments are often temporary, but permanent infertility may occur. Although many men regain their fertility within a few months after the treatment ends, preserving sperm before starting cancer therapy is an option that many men consider. Researchers reported that hypogonadism was seen in 30 percent of the men with cancer and 90 percent of these gentlemen had germinal epithelial failure.

Normal Aging: Older men generally have lower testosterone levels than younger men do. As men age, there's a slow and continuous decrease in testosterone production. The rate that testosterone declines varies greatly among men. As many as 30 percent of men older than 75 have a testosterone level that is below normal, according to the American Association of Clinical Endocrinologists (AACE). Whether or not treatment is necessary remains a matter of debate.

Secondary Hypogonadism

In secondary hypogonadism, the testicles are normal, but function improperly due to a problem with the pituitary or hypothalamus. A number of conditions can cause secondary hypogonadism, including:

Kallmann Syndrome: Abnormal development of the hypothalamus—the area of the brain that controls the secretion of pituitary hormones—can cause hypogonadism. This abnormality is also associated with the impaired development of the ability to smell (anosmia).

Pituitary Disorders: An abnormality in the pituitary gland can impair the release of hormones from the pituitary gland to the testicles, affecting normal testosterone production. A pituitary tumor or other type of brain tumor located near the pituitary gland may cause testosterone or other hormone deficiencies. Also, the treatment for a brain tumor such as surgery or radiation therapy may impair pituitary function and cause hypogonadism.

Inflammatory Disease: Certain inflammatory diseases such as sarcoidosis, Histiocytosis, and tuberculosis involve the hypothalmus and pituitary gland and can affect testosterone production, causing hypogonadism.

HIV/AIDS: This virus can cause low levels of testosterone by affecting the hypothalamus, the pituitary, and the testes.

Medications: The use of certain drugs, such as, opiate pain medications and some hormones, can affect testosterone production.

Obesity: Being significantly overweight at any age may be linked to hypogonadism.

Stress-Induced Hypogonadism: Stress, excessive physical activity, and weight loss have all been associated with hypogonadism. Some have attributed this to stress-induced hypercortisolism, which would suppress hypothalamic function.

Role of Testosterone

Throughout the male lifespan, testosterone plays a critical role in sexual, cognitive, and body development. During fetal development, testosterone aids in the determination of sex. The most visible effects of rising testosterone levels begin in the prepubertal stage. During this time, body odor develops, oiliness of the skin and hair increase, acne develops, accelerated growth spurts occur, and pubic, early facial, and axillary hair grows. In men, the pubertal effects include enlargement of the sebaceous glands, penis enlargement, increased libido, increased frequency of erections, increased muscle mass, deepening of voice, increased height, bone maturations, loss of scalp hair, and growth of facial, chest, leg, and axillary hair. Even as adults, the effects of testosterone are visible as libido, penile erections, aggression, and mental and physical energy.

Pathophysiology of Testosterone and Hypogonadism

The cerebral cortex—the layer of the brain often referred to as the gray matter—is the most highly developed portion of the human brain. This portion of the brain, encompassing about two-thirds of the brain mass, is responsible for the information processing in the brain. It is within this portion of the brain that testosterone production begins. The cerebral cortex signals the hypothalamus to stimulate production of testosterone. To do this, the hypothalamus releases the gonadotropin- releasing hormone in a pulsatile fashion, which stimulates the pituitary gland—the portion of the brain responsible for hormones involved in the regulation of growth, thyroid function, blood pressure, and other essential body functions. Once stimulated by the gonadotropin- releasing hormone, the pituitary gland produces the follicle-stimulating hormone and the luteinizing hormone. Once released into the bloodstream, the luteinizing hormone triggers activity in the Leydig cells in the testes. In the Leydig cells, cholesterol is converted to testosterone. When the testosterone levels are sufficient, the pituitary gland slows the release of the luteinizing hormone via a negative feedback mechanism, thereby, slowing testosterone production. With such a complex process, many potential problems can lead to low testosterone levels. Any changes in the testicles, hypothalamus or pituitary gland can result in hypogonadism. Such changes can be congenital or acquired, temporary, or permanent.

Certain medications are shown to reduce testosterone production. Among the medications known to alter the hypothalamic-pituitary-gonadal axis are spironolactone, corticosteroids, ketoconazole, ethanol, anticonvulsants, immunosuppressants, opiates, psychotropic medications, and hormones.

Symptoms of Hypogonadism

Hypogonadism is characterized by serum testosterone levels < 300 ng/dL in combination with at least one clinical sign or symptom. Signs of hypogonadism include absence or regression of secondary sex characteristics, anemia, muscle wasting, reduced bone mass or bone mineral density, oligospermia, and abdominal adiposity. Symptoms of post pubescent hypogonadism include sexual dysfunction

341

(erectile dysfunction, reduced libido, diminished penile sensation, difficulty attaining orgasm, and reduced ejaculate), reduced energy and stamina, depressed mood, increased irritability, difficulty concentrating, changes in cholesterol levels, anemia, osteoporosis, and hot flushes. In the prepubertal male, if treatment is not initiated, signs and symptoms include sparse body hair and delayed epiphyseal closure.

Testing of Hypogonadism

Early diagnosis and treatment can reduce risks associated with hypogonadism. Early detection in young boys can help to prevent problems due to delayed puberty. Early diagnosis in men helps protect against the development of osteoporosis and other conditions. The diagnosis of hypogonadism is based on symptoms and blood work, particularly on testosterone levels. Often the first step toward diagnosis is the Androgen Deficiency in Aging Male (ADAM) test—a 10 item questionnaire intended to identify men who exhibit signs of low testosterone. Testosterone levels vary throughout the day and are generally highest in the morning, so blood levels are typically drawn early in the morning. If low testosterone levels are confirmed, further testing is done, to identify if the cause is testicular, hypothalamic, or pituitary. These tests may include hormone testing, semen analysis, pituitary imaging, testicular biopsy, and genetic studies. Once the treatment starts, the patient may continue to have testosterone levels drawn to determine if the medication is helping to produce adequate testosterone levels.

Treatment Options

Testosterone replacement therapy is the primary treatment option for hypogonadism. Ideally, the therapy should provide physiological testosterone levels, typically in the range of 300 to 800 ng/dL. According to the guidelines from the American Association of Clinical Endocrinologists, updated in 2002, the goals of therapy are to:

- Restore sexual function, libido, well-being, and behavior

- Produce and maintain virilization

- Optimize bone density and prevent osteoporosis

- In elderly men, possibly normalize growth hormone levels

- Potentially affect the risk of cardiovascular disease

- In cases of hypogonadotropic hypogonadism, restore fertility

To achieve these goals, several testosterone delivery systems are currently available in the market. Clinical guidelines published in 2006, by the Endocrine Society, recommend reserving treatment for those patients with clinical symptoms, rather than for those with just low testosterone levels.

Transdermal Patch

Transdermal testosterone patches are available under the brand name Androderm. Transdermal patches deliver continuous levels of testosterone over a 24-hour period. Application site reactions account for the majority of adverse effects associated with transdermal patches, with elderly men proving particularly prone to skin irritation. Local reactions include pruritus, blistering under the patch, erythema, vesicle formation, indurations, and allergic contact dermatitis. Approximately 10 percent of the patients discontinue patch therapy due to skin reactions. In one study, 60 percent of the subjects discontinued the patch between weeks four and eight due to skin irritation. A small percentage of patients may also experience headache, depression, and gastrointestinal (GI) bleeding. Some patients report that the patch easily falls off and is difficult to remove from the package without good dexterity. Transdermal patches are more expensive than injections, but the convenience of use and maintenance of normal diurnal testosterone levels are advantageous. Some patients report that the patch is noisy and therefore they feel stigmatized by its presence.

Topical Gel

Currently, two topical testosterone gels—Androgel and Testim, are available. Application in the morning allows for testosterone concentrations that follow the normal circadian pattern. Topical testosterone gels also provide longer-lasting elevations in serum testosterone, compared to transdermal patches. Similar to patches, testosterone delivered via gels does not undergo first-pass metabolism. Adverse effects associated with therapy include headache, hot flushes, insomnia, increased blood pressure, acne, emotional labiality, and nervousness. Although application site reactions occur, skin irritation is approximately 10 times less frequent with gels than with transdermal patches. Advantages associated with topical gel include maintenance of normal diurnal testosterone levels and documented increases in bone density. Potential problems associated with the gel are the potential for transfer of the gel from person to person and the cost.

Buccal Tablets

Buccal testosterone tablets, marketed as Striant, release testosterone in a pulsatile manner, are similar to endogenous secretion. With this route, the peak testosterone levels are rapidly achieved and a steady state is reached by the second dose following twice-daily dosing. Similar to gel and transdermal products, buccal administration avoids first-pass metabolism. Food and beverage do not alter drug absorption. Although well-tolerated, transient gum irritation and a bitter taste are the chief adverse effects associated with this route. Gum irritation tends to resolve within the first week. Other adverse effects include dry mouth, toothache, and stomatitis. Some patients find the buccal tablet uncomfortable and report concern about the tablet shifting in the mouth while talking.

Implantable Pellet

Testosterone has also been formulated into an implantable pellet, marketed as Testopel. This surgically implanted pellet slowly releases testosterone via zero-order kinetics over many months (up to six months), although peak testosterone levels are achieved within 30 minutes. The chief complaints associated with this formulation are pellet extrusion, minor bleeding, and fibrosis at the site.

Intramuscular Injections

Intramuscular formulations are also available, sold as Depo-Testosterone (testosterone cypionate) and Delatestryl (testosterone enanthate). The testosterone is suspended in oil to prolong absorption. Peak levels occur within 72 hours of administration, but intramuscular administration is associated with the most variable pharmacokinetics of all the formulations. In the first few days after administration, supraphysiological testosterone levels are achieved, followed by subphysiological levels near the end of the dosing interval. Such fluctuations, are often associated with wide variations in mood, energy, and sexual function, and prove distressing to many patients. To reduce fluctuations, lower doses and shorter dosing intervals (two weeks) are often used. Injection site reactions are also common, but are rarely the reason for discontinuation of therapy. Despite the fluctuations in testosterone levels, intramuscular injections provide a cost-effective option and the convenience of two- to four-week dosing intervals. Disadvantages associated with injections include visits to the doctor's office, visits for dose administration, and lack of physiological testosterone patterns.

Oral Tablets

Oral testosterone tablets, under the brand name Andriol, are available in many countries. Although relatively inexpensive, oral products undergo extensive first-pass metabolism and therefore require multiple daily doses. Oral products are associated with elevated liver enzymes, GI intolerance, acne, and gynecomastia. Regardless of the treatment option, patients should be aware of the risks associated with testosterone therapy, including:

- Worsening of the prostatic hypertrophy
- Increased risk of prostate cancer
- Lower sperm count with large doses
- Swelling of ankles, feet, or body, with or without heart failure
- Gynecomastia
- Sleep apnea
- Blood clots

Patients should be educated on the signs and symptoms of these adverse effects and instructed to notify their doctor if any of these occur.

Chapter 48

Gynecomastia

What Is Gynecomastia?

Gynecomastia is a condition in which breast tissue forms in guys, usually due to normal hormonal changes during puberty. Hormones are chemicals produced by your body's glands. In a guy, hormones produced in the testicles are responsible for the physical changes that begin to take place during puberty—facial hair, muscle development, a deepening of the voice, and the lengthening of the penis, for example. Guys and girls produce both **androgens** (hormones that help develop and maintain male characteristics) and **estrogen** (a hormone that is responsible for most female characteristics).

Guys have mostly androgens in their systems, but they also have small amounts of estrogen. In girls, breast growth is caused by high levels of estrogen. Normally, when going through puberty, a guy's production of androgens increases significantly, whereas estrogen production remains low.

However, sometimes guys produce enough estrogen during puberty that some breast tissue develops. Breast tissue growth in guys can appear on one or both sides of the chest, and the breast area can feel tender. This doesn't mean you're turning into a girl or anything. It's just a minor change in your hormones as you begin to grow into adulthood.

Text in this chapter is excerpted from "Gynecomastia," © 1995–2016. The Nemours Foundation/KidsHealth®. Reprinted with permission.

How Common Is It?

It's estimated that about half of all males going through puberty experience some degree of gynecomastia in one or both breasts. Gynecomastia is almost always a temporary condition, and it's very unusual for the breasts to stay developed—they will eventually flatten out completely within a few months to a couple of years. It usually goes away on its own and no medical treatment or surgery is needed.

Even though it's just a temporary change for most teens, some guys with gynecomastia feel embarrassed or self-conscious about their appearance. Many guys find that wearing loose-fitting shirts helps make the condition less noticeable until the breast tissue shrinks over time. Surgical removal of the breast tissue is an option in some cases. If a guy finds his gynecomastia is bothering him, he can talk to a doctor about it.

Although the most common cause of gynecomastia is puberty, it can sometimes be caused by certain diseases or side effects of some medications. Using illegal drugs such as anabolic steroids, marijuana, or heroin can also disrupt hormonal balance and lead to gynecomastia.

There's also something called **pseudogynecomastia** (or false gynecomastia). This has nothing to do with puberty or hormones. It's just simply due to the fact that some guys have extra fat in the chest area, making it look like they have breasts. A doctor's exam can tell whether a guy has gynecomastia or pseudogynecomastia.

If you're concerned or have any questions about gynecomastia, talk to your doctor. Keep in mind that temporary breast tissue growth in guys is a common part of puberty that will usually go away on its own.

Chapter 49

Menstrual Problems

Chapter Contents

349

Section 49.1

Menstruation and Menstrual Irregularities

This section includes text excerpted from "Menstruation and Menstrual Problems," *Eunice Kennedy Shriver* National Institute of Child Health and Human Development (NICHD), April 16, 2013.

What Is Menstruation?

Menstruation is normal vaginal bleeding that occurs as part of a woman's monthly menstrual cycle. Menstruation occurs between menarche, a girl's first period, and menopause. Menstrual blood flows from the uterus and passes out of the body through the vagina. The average menstruation time in normally menstruating women is about 5 days. In the United States, most girls start menstruating shortly after age 12.

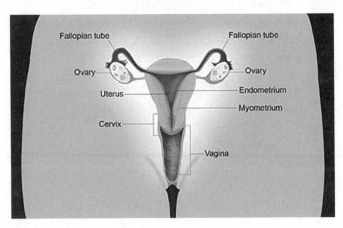

Figure 49.1. *Female Pelvis*

What Are the Symptoms of Menstruation?

The primary sign of menstruation is bleeding from the vagina. Additional symptoms include:

• abdominal or pelvic cramping

- lower back pain
- bloating and sore breasts
- food cravings
- mood swings and irritability
- headache and fatigue

What Are Menstrual Irregularities?

After a teen has been menstruating for a few years, her menstrual cycle typically becomes more regular. For most women, a normal menstrual cycle ranges from 21 to 35 days. However, up to 14 percent of women have irregular menstrual cycles or excessively heavy menstrual bleeding. Most abnormal uterine bleeding can be divided into anovulatory and ovulatory patterns.

- **Anovulatory**: Irregular/infrequent periods with absent, minimal, or excessive bleeding.

- **Ovulatory**: Periods that occur at regular intervals but are characterized by excessive bleeding or a duration of greater than 7 days.

The most common menstrual irregularities include:

Anovulatory bleeding

- Absent menstrual periods (amenorrhea): When a woman does not get her period by age 16, or when she stops getting her period for at least 3 months and is not pregnant.

- Infrequent menstrual periods (oligomenorrhea): Periods that occur more than 35 days apart.

Ovulatory bleeding

- Heavy menstrual periods (menorrhagia): Also called excessive bleeding. Although anovulatory bleeding and menorrhagia are sometimes grouped together, they do not have the same cause and require different diagnostic testing.

- Prolonged menstrual bleeding: Bleeding that exceeds 8 days in duration on a regular basis.

Dysmenorrhea: Painful periods that may include severe menstrual cramps.

Additional menstrual irregularities include:

- Polymenorrhea: Frequent menstrual periods occurring less than 21 days apart.

- Irregular menstrual periods with a cycle-to-cycle variation of more than 20 days.

- Shortened menstrual bleeding of less than 2 days in duration.

- Intermenstrual bleeding: Episodes of bleeding that occur between periods, also known as spotting.

How Many Women Are Affected by Menstrual Irregularities?

Menstrual irregularities occur in 9 percent to 14 percent of women of childbearing age.

What Causes Menstrual Irregularities?

Menstrual irregularities can be caused by a variety of conditions, including pregnancy, hormonal imbalances, infections, malignancies, diseases, trauma, and certain medications.

Common causes of anovulatory bleeding (absent, infrequent periods, and irregular periods) include:

- adolescence

- uncontrolled diabetes

- eating disorders

- hyperthyroidism or hypothyroidism

- hyperprolactinemia (an abnormally high concentration in the blood of prolactin, a protein hormone)

- medications, such as antiepileptics or antipsychotics

- perimenopause

- polycystic ovary syndrome (PCOS)

- pregnancy

Common causes of ovulatory bleeding (heavy or prolonged menstrual bleeding) include:

- structural problems, such as uterine fibroids or polyps

- bleeding disorders, such as leukemia, platelet disorders, the various factor deficiencies, or von Willebrand disease
- hypothyroidism
- advanced liver disease

Common causes of dysmenorrhea (menstrual pain) include:

- heavy menstrual flow
- smoking
- depression
- never having given birth
- endometriosis
- chronic uterine infection

Additional causes of menstrual irregularity include:

- endometriosis
- endocrine gland-related causes
  - poorly controlled diabetes
  - polycystic ovary syndrome (PCOS)
  - Cushing syndrome
  - thyroid dysfunction
  - primary ovarian insufficiency (POI)
  - late-onset congenital adrenal hyperplasia
- acquired conditions
  - stress-related hypothalamic dysfunction
  - medications
  - exercise-induced amenorrhea
  - eating disorders (both anorexia and bulimia)
- tumors
  - ovarian
  - adrenal
  - prolactinomas (a noncancerous pituitary tumor that produces prolactin)

How Do Healthcare Providers Diagnose Menstrual Irregularities?

A healthcare provider diagnoses menstrual irregularities using a combination of the following:

- medical history

- physical examination

- blood tests

- ultrasound examination

- endometrial biopsy—a small sample of the uterus's endometrial lining is taken to be examined under a microscope.

- hysteroscopy—a diagnostic scope that allows a healthcare provider to examine the inside of the uterus, typically done as an outpatient procedure.

- saline infusion sonohysterography—ultrasound imaging of the uterine cavity while it is filled with sterile saline solution.

- transvaginal ultrasonography—ultrasound imaging of the pelvic organs including the ovaries and uterus, using an ultrasound transducer that is inserted into the vagina.

What Are the Common Treatments for Menstrual Irregularities?

Treatment for menstrual irregularities that are due to anovulatory bleeding (absent periods, infrequent periods, and irregular periods) include:

- oral contraceptives

- cyclic progestin

- treatments for an underlying disorder that is causing the menstrual problem, such as counseling for an eating disorder or extreme exercise.

Treatment for menstrual irregularities that are due to ovulatory bleeding (heavy or prolonged menstrual bleeding) include:

- insertion of a hormone-releasing intrauterine device.

- use of various medications (such as those containing progestin or tranexamic acid) or nonsteroidal anti-inflammatory medications.

If the cause is structural or if medical management is ineffective, then the following may be considered:

• surgical removal of polyps or uterine fibroids

• uterine artery embolization, a procedure to block blood flow to the uterus.

• endometrial ablation, a procedure to cauterize blood vessels in the endometrial lining of the uterus.

• hysterectomy

Treatment for dysmenorrhea (painful periods) include:

• applying a heating pad to the abdomen.

• taking nonsteroidal anti-inflammatory medications.

• taking contraceptives, including injectable hormone therapy or birth control pills, using varied or less common treatment regimens.

Section 49.2

Premenstrual Syndrome (PMS) and Premenstrual Dysphoric Disorder (PMDD)

This section includes text excerpted from "Premenstrual Syndrome (PMS) Fact Sheet," Office on Women's Health (OWH), December 23, 2014.

What Is Premenstrual Syndrome (PMS)?

Premenstrual syndrome (PMS) is a group of symptoms linked to the menstrual cycle. PMS symptoms occur 1 to 2 weeks before your period (menstruation or monthly bleeding) starts. The symptoms usually go away after you start bleeding. PMS can affect menstruating women of any age and the effect is different for each woman. For some people, PMS is just a monthly bother. For others, it may be so severe that it makes it hard to even get through the day. PMS goes away when your monthly periods stop, such as when you get pregnant or go through menopause.

What Causes PMS?

The causes of PMS are not clear, but several factors may be involved. Changes in hormones during the menstrual cycle seem to be an important cause. These changing hormone levels may affect some women more than others. Chemical changes in the brain may also be involved. Stress and emotional problems, such as depression, do not seem to cause PMS, but they may make it worse. Some other possible causes include:

- low levels of vitamins and minerals

- eating a lot of salty foods, which may cause you to retain (keep) fluid

- drinking alcohol and caffeine, which may alter your mood and energy level

What Are the Symptoms of PMS?

PMS often includes both physical and emotional symptoms, such as:

- Acne

- Anxiety or depression

- Appetite changes or food cravings

- Feeling tired

- Headache or backache

- Joint or muscle pain

- Swollen or tender breasts

- Tension, irritability, mood swings, or crying spells

- Trouble sleeping

- Trouble with concentration or memory

- Upset stomach, bloating, constipation, or diarrhea

Symptoms vary from woman to woman.

How Do I Know If I Have PMS?

Your doctor may diagnose PMS based on which symptoms you have, when they occur, and how much they affect your life. If you think you have PMS, keep track of which symptoms you have and how severe they are for a few months. Record your symptoms each day on a calendar. Take this form with you when you see your doctor about your PMS.

Your doctor will also want to make sure you don't have one of the following conditions that shares symptoms with PMS:

- Anxiety
- Chronic fatigue syndrome (CFS)
- Depression
- Irritable bowel syndrome (IBS)
- Menopause
- Problems with the endocrine system, which makes hormones

What Is the Treatment for PMS?

Many things have been tried to ease the symptoms of PMS. No treatment works for every woman. You may need to try different ones to see what works for you.

Lifestyle Changes

If your PMS isn't so bad that you need to see a doctor, some lifestyle changes may help you feel better. Below are some steps you can take that may help ease your symptoms.

- Exercise regularly. Each week, you should get:
  - Two hours and 30 minutes of moderate-intensity physical activity;
  - One hour and 15 minutes of vigorous-intensity aerobic physical activity; or
  - A combination of moderate and vigorous-intensity activity; and
  - Muscle-strengthening activities on 2 or more days.
- Eat healthy foods, such as fruits, vegetables, and whole grains.

- Avoid salt, sugary foods, caffeine, and alcohol, especially when you're having PMS symptoms.

- Get enough sleep. Try to get about 8 hours of sleep each night.

- Find healthy ways to cope with stress. Talk to your friends, exercise, or write in a journal. Some women also find yoga, massage, or relaxation therapy helpful.

- Don't smoke

Medications

Over-the-counter pain relievers may help ease physical symptoms, such as cramps, headaches, backaches, and breast tenderness. These include:

- Ibuprofen (for instance, Advil, Motrin, Midol Cramp)

- Ketoprofen (for instance, Orudis KT)

- Naproxen (for instance, Aleve)

- Aspirin

In more severe cases of PMS, prescription medicines may be used to ease symptoms. One approach has been to use drugs that stop ovulation, such as birth control pills. Women on the pill report fewer PMS symptoms, such as cramps and headaches, as well as lighter periods.

Alternative Therapies

Certain vitamins and minerals have been found to help relieve some PMS symptoms. These include:

- Calcium with vitamin D

- Folic acid (400 micrograms)

- Magnesium (400 milligrams)

- Vitamin B6 (50 to 100 mg)

- Vitamin E (400 international units)

Pregnant or nursing women need the same amount of calcium as other women of the same age.

Table 49.1. Amounts of Calcium You Need Each Day

Ages	Milligrams per Day
9–18	1300
19–50	1000
51 and older	1200

Some women find their PMS symptoms relieved by taking supplements such as:

- Black cohosh
- Chasteberry
- Evening primrose oil

Talk with your doctor before taking any of these products. Many have not been proven to work and they may interact with other medicines you are taking.

What Is Premenstrual Dysphoric Disorder (PMDD)?

A brain chemical called serotonin may play a role in premenstrual dysphoric disorder (PMDD), a severe form of PMS. The main symptoms, which can be disabling, include:

- feelings of sadness or despair, or even thoughts of suicide
- feelings of tension or anxiety
- panic attacks
- mood swings or frequent crying
- lasting irritability or anger that affects other people
- lack of interest in daily activities and relationships
- trouble thinking or focusing
- tiredness or low energy
- food cravings or binge eating
- trouble sleeping
- feeling out of control
- physical symptoms, such as bloating, breast tenderness, headaches, and joint or muscle pain

You must have five or more of these symptoms to be diagnosed with PMDD. Symptoms occur during the week before your period and go away after bleeding starts.

Making some lifestyle changes may help ease PMDD symptoms.

Antidepressants called selective serotonin reuptake inhibitors (SSRIs) have also been shown to help some women with PMDD. These drugs change serotonin levels in the brain. The U.S. Food and Drug Administration (FDA) has approved three SSRIs for the treatment of PMDD:

- Sertraline (Zoloft)

- Fluoxetine (Sarafem)

- Paroxetine HCI (Paxil CR)

Yaz (drospirenone and ethinyl estradiol) is the only birth control pill approved by the FDA to treat PMDD. Individual counseling, group counseling, and stress management may also help relieve symptoms.

Section 49.3

Amenorrhea

This section includes text excerpted from "Amenorrhea," *Eunice Kennedy Shriver* National Institute of Child Health and Human Development (NICHD), March 3, 2013.

What Is Amenorrhea?

Amenorrhea is the absence of a menstrual period.

Amenorrhea is sometimes categorized as:

- **Primary amenorrhea.** This describes a young woman who has not had a period by age 16.

- **Secondary amenorrhea.** This occurs when a woman who once had regular periods experiences an absence of more than three cycles. Causes of secondary amenorrhea include pregnancy.

Having regular periods is an important sign of overall health. Missing a period, when not caused by pregnancy, breastfeeding, or menopause, is generally a sign of another health problem. If you miss your period, talk to your healthcare provider about possible causes, including pregnancy.

What Are the Symptoms of Amenorrhea?

Missing a period is the main sign of amenorrhea.

Depending on the cause, a woman might have other signs or symptoms as well, such as:

- excess facial hair
- hair loss
- headache
- lack of breast development
- milky discharge from the breasts
- vision changes

Who Is at Risk of Amenorrhea?

According to the American Society for Reproductive Medicine (ASRM), amenorrhea that is not caused by pregnancy, breastfeeding, or menopause occurs in 3 percent to 4 percent of women during their lifetime. Secondary amenorrhea is more common than primary amenorrhea.

The risk factors for amenorrhea include:

- excessive exercise
- obesity
- eating disorders such as anorexia nervosa
- a family history of amenorrhea or early menopause
- having a certain version of the *FMR1* gene, that also causes fragile X syndrome

What Causes Amenorrhea?

Amenorrhea can happen for many reasons. It most often occurs as a natural part of life, such as during pregnancy or breastfeeding, but it can also signal a more serious condition.

What Causes Primary Amenorrhea?

There are three main causes of primary amenorrhea:

- **Chromosomal or genetic abnormalities** can cause the ovaries to stop functioning normally. Turner syndrome, a condition caused by a partially or completely missing X chromosome, and androgen insensitivity syndrome, often characterized by high levels of testosterone, are two examples of genetic abnormalities that can delay or disrupt menstruation.

- **Hypothalamic or pituitary problems** in the brain and physical problems such as problems with reproductive organs can prevent periods from starting.

- **Excessive exercise, eating disorders, extreme physical or psychological stress, or a combination of these factors** can delay the onset of menstruation.

What Causes Secondary Amenorrhea?

Secondary amenorrhea can result from various causes, such as:

- **Natural causes**

  - Pregnancy is the most common cause.

  - Other natural causes include breastfeeding and menopause.

- **Medications and therapies**

  - Certain birth control pills, injectable contraceptives, and intrauterine devices (IUDs) can cause amenorrhea. It can take a few months after stopping birth control for the menstrual cycle to restart and become regular.

  - Some medications, including certain antidepressants and blood pressure medications, can increase the levels of a hormone that prevents ovulation and the menstrual cycle.

  - Chemotherapy and radiation treatments for hematologic cancer (including blood, bone marrow, and lymph nodes) and breast or gynecologic cancer can destroy estrogen-producing cells and eggs in the ovaries, leading to amenorrhea. The resulting amenorrhea may be short-term, especially in younger women.

  - Sometimes scar tissue can build up in the lining of the uterus, preventing the normal shedding of the uterine lining in the menstrual cycle. This scarring sometimes occurs after a dilation and curettage (D and C), a procedure in which tissue is removed from the uterus to diagnose or treat heavy bleeding or to clear the uterine lining after a miscarriage, a cesarean section, or treatment for uterine fibroids.

- **Hypothalamic amenorrhea.** This condition occurs when the hypothalamus, a gland in the brain that regulates body processes, slows or stops releasing gonadotropin-releasing hormone (GnRH), the hormone that starts the menstrual cycle. Common characteristics of women with hypothalamic amenorrhea include:

  - low body weight

  - low percentage of body fat

  - very low intake of calories or fat

  - emotional stress

  - strenuous exercise that burns more calories than are taken in through food

  - deficiency of leptin, a protein hormone that regulates appetite and metabolism

  - some medical conditions or illnesses

- **Gynecological conditions**. Unbalanced hormone levels are common features of certain conditions that have secondary amenorrhea as a main symptom. These can include:

  - **Polycystic ovary syndrome (PCOS).** PCOS occurs when a woman's body produces more androgens (a type of hormone) than normal. High levels of androgens can cause fluid-filled sacs or cysts to grow in the ovaries, interfering with the release of eggs (ovulation). Most women with PCOS either have amenorrhea or experience irregular periods, called oligomenorrhea.

  - **Fragile X-associated primary ovarian insufficiency (FXPOI).** The term FXPOI describes a condition in which a woman's ovaries stop functioning before normal menopause, sometimes around age 40. FXPOI results from certain changes to a gene on the X chromosome. As many as 10 percent of women who seek treatment for amenorrhea have FXPOI.

- **Thyroid problems**. The thyroid is a small butterfly-shaped gland at the base of the neck, just below the Adam's apple. The thyroid produces hormones that control metabolism and play a role in puberty and menstruation. A thyroid gland that is overactive (called hyperthyroidism) or underactive (hypothyroidism) can cause menstrual irregularities, including amenorrhea.

- **Pituitary tumor**. Noncancerous tumors in the pituitary gland in the brain, which regulates the production of hormones that affect many body functions, including metabolism and the reproductive cycle, can interfere with the body's hormonal regulation of menstruation.

How Is Amenorrhea Diagnosed?

A healthcare provider will usually ask a series of questions to begin diagnosing amenorrhea, including:

- How old were you when you started your period?

- What are your menstrual cycles like? (What is the typical length of your cycle? How heavy or light are your periods?)

- Are you sexually active?

- Could you be pregnant?

- Have you gained or lost weight recently?

- How often and how much do you exercise?

Primary Amenorrhea

If you are older than 16 and have never had a period, your healthcare provider will do a thorough medical history and physical exam, including a pelvic exam, to see if you are experiencing other signs of puberty. Depending on the findings and on your answers to the questions above, other tests may be ordered to determine the cause of your amenorrhea.

Secondary Amenorrhea

If you are sexually active, your healthcare provider will likely order a pregnancy test. He or she will also perform a complete physical exam, including a pelvic exam.

You should contact your healthcare provider as soon as possible after you miss a period.

Other Tests You May Need:

- **Thyroid function test.** This test measures the amount of thyroid-stimulating hormone (TSH) in your blood, which can help determine if your thyroid is working properly. A thyroid gland that is overactive (hyperthyroidism) or underactive (hypothyroidism) can cause menstrual irregularities, including amenorrhea.

- **Ovary function test.** This test measures the amount of follicle-stimulating hormone (FSH) or luteinizing hormone (LH)—hormones made by the pituitary gland—in your blood to determine if your ovaries are working properly. Your healthcare provider may also evaluate the level of anti-Mullerian hormone (AMH), which is produced by the ovarian follicles. Higher levels of AMH may be associated with polycystic ovary syndrome (PCOS). Low or undetectable amounts of AMH may be associated with menopause or primary ovarian insufficiency.

- **Androgen test.** Androgens are sometimes called "male hormones" because men need higher levels of these hormones than woman do for overall health. However, both men and women need androgens to stay healthy. Your healthcare provider may want to check the level of androgens in your blood. High levels of androgens may indicate a woman has PCOS.

- **Hormone challenge test.** With this test, you will take a hormonal medication for seven to 10 days in an effort to trigger a menstrual cycle. Results from the test can tell your healthcare provider whether your periods have stopped because of a lack of estrogen.

- **Screening for a premutation of the *FMR1* gene.** Changes in this gene can cause the ovaries to stop functioning properly, leading to amenorrhea.

- **Chromosome evaluation.** This test, also known as a karyotype, involves counting and evaluating the chromosomes from cells in the body to identify any missing, extra, or rearranged cells. Results from this evaluation can help determine the cause of the chromosomal abnormality causing primary or secondary amenorrhea.

- **Ultrasound.** This painless test uses sound waves to produce images of internal organs. This test can help determine if your reproductive organs are all present and shaped normally.

- **Computed tomography (CT).** CT scans combine many X-ray images taken from different directions to create cross-sectional views of internal structures. A CT scan can indicate whether your uterus, ovaries, and kidneys look normal.

- **Magnetic resonance imaging (MRI).** MRI uses radio waves with a strong magnetic field to produce detailed images of soft tissues within the body. Your healthcare provider may order an MRI to check for a pituitary tumor or to examine your reproductive organs.

- **Hysteroscopy.** In this procedure a thin, lighted camera is passed through your vagina and cervix to allow your healthcare provider to look at the inside of your uterus.

Your healthcare provider might use several of these tests to attempt to diagnose the cause of amenorrhea. In some cases, no specific cause for the amenorrhea can be found. This situation is called idiopathic amenorrhea.

What Are the Treatments for Amenorrhea?

The treatment for amenorrhea depends on the underlying cause, as well as the health status and goals of the individual.

If primary or secondary amenorrhea is caused by lifestyle factors, your healthcare provider may suggest changes in the areas below:

- **Weight.** Being overweight or severely underweight can affect your menstrual cycle. Attaining and maintaining a healthy weight often helps balance hormone levels and restore your menstrual cycle.

- **Stress.** Assess the areas of stress in your life and reduce the things that are causing stress. If you can't decrease stress on your own, ask for help from family, friends, your healthcare provider, or a professional listener such as a counselor.

- **Level of physical activity.** You may need to change or adjust your physical activity level to help restart your menstrual cycle. Talk to your healthcare provider and your coach or trainer about how to train in a way that maintains your health and menstrual cycles.

Be aware of changes in your menstrual cycle and check with your healthcare provider if you have concerns. Keep a record of when your periods occur. Note the date your period starts, how long it lasts, and any problems you experience. The first day of bleeding is considered the first day of your menstrual cycle.

For **primary amenorrhea**, depending on your age and the results of the ovary function test, healthcare providers may recommend watchful waiting. If an ovary function test shows low follicle-stimulating hormone (FSH) or luteinizing hormone (LH) levels, menstruation may just be delayed. In females with a family history of delayed menstruation, this kind of delay is common.

Primary amenorrhea caused by chromosomal or genetic problems may require surgery. Women with a genetic condition called 46, XY gonadal dysgenesis have one X and one Y chromosome, but their ovaries do not develop normally. This condition increases the risk for cancer developing in the ovaries. The gonads (ovaries) are often removed through laparoscopic surgery to prevent or reduce the risk of cancer.

Treatment for **secondary amenorrhea**, depending on the cause, may include medical or surgical treatments or a combination of the two.

Medical Treatments for Secondary Amenorrhea

Common medical treatments for secondary amenorrhea include:

- **Birth control pills or other types of hormonal medication.** Certain oral contraceptives may help restart the menstrual cycle.

- **Medications to help relieve the symptoms of PCOS.** Clomiphene citrate (CC) therapy is often prescribed to help trigger ovulation.

- **Estrogen replacement therapy (ERT).** ERT may help balance hormonal levels and restart the menstrual cycle in women with primary ovarian insufficiency (POI) or fragile X-associated primary ovarian insufficiency (FXPOI). Women with FXPOI often experience symptoms of menopause, such as hot flashes and night sweats. ERT replaces the estrogen a woman's body should be making naturally for a normal menstrual cycle. In addition, ERT may help women with FXPOI lower their risk for the bone disease osteoporosis. ERT can increase the risk for uterine cancer, so your healthcare provider may also prescribe progestin or progesterone to reduce this risk.

In general, medications are safe, but they can have side effects, some of which may be serious. You should discuss side effects and risks with your healthcare provider before deciding on any specific medical treatment.

Surgical Treatments for Secondary Amenorrhea

Surgical treatment for amenorrhea is not common, but may be recommended in certain conditions. These include:

- **Uterine scarring**. This scarring sometimes occurs after removal of uterine fibroids, a Cesarean section, or a dilation and curettage (D and C), a procedure in which tissue is removed from the uterus to diagnose or treat heavy bleeding or to clear the uterine lining after a miscarriage. Removal of the scar tissue during a procedure called a hysteroscopic resection can help restore the menstrual cycle.

- **Pituitary tumor**. Medications may be recommended to shrink the tumor. If this does not work, surgery may be necessary to remove the tumor. Pituitary tumors are not cancerous, but they can cause problems as they grow. Pituitary tumors can put pressure on surrounding blood vessels and nerves such as the optic nerve and may result in loss of vision.

- Most of the time, pituitary tumors are removed through the nose and sinuses. Radiation therapy may be used to shrink the tumor, either in combination with surgery or, for those who cannot have surgery, by itself.

Other FAQs

How Does Amenorrhea Affect Bone Health?

An important part of the menstrual cycle is the production of the hormone estrogen. Estrogen also plays a role in bone health. If amenorrhea is caused by low estrogen or problems with estrogen production, a woman may be at risk for loss of bone mass.

Some common causes of estrogen deficiency are excessive exercise and eating disorders. These can have a negative effect on bone density. Adolescent girls in particular need a combination of calcium, vitamin D, and physical activity to build strong bones during this critical time. Years ago, researchers found that girls with amenorrhea who diet are at risk for low bone density and that this condition increases their risk for osteoporosis later in life.

Amenorrhea that results from Fragile X-associated primary ovarian insufficiency (FXPOI) also increases the risk for osteoporosis. It is important to see your healthcare provider as early as possible to begin investigating the cause of amenorrhea. According to one study, two-thirds of adolescent girls who reported FXPOI also had osteopenia, an early stage of osteoporosis, at their first visit.

When Should I Talk to My Healthcare Provider about a Missed Period or Several Missed Periods?

If you have had regular periods or if there is any chance you may be pregnant, check with your healthcare provider about a missed period right away.

If you are just beginning to menstruate, keep in mind that it may take several months for your menstrual cycle to become regular. As you age, the time from the beginning of one cycle to the beginning of the next will likely range from 21 to 35 days, but your periods should become more regular over time.

See your healthcare provider right away if:

- You have not started menstruating by the age of 16.

- You have not started menstruating within 3 years after you developed breasts, or if you have not started developing breasts by age 13.

- You have not had a period for more than 3 months.

- Your periods become very irregular after you previously had regular, monthly cycles.

Can I Still Get Pregnant If I Have Amenorrhea?

Yes, you can still get pregnant even if you do not have regular periods. Although some of the conditions that cause amenorrhea can also contribute to infertility, there is still a chance for pregnancy.

In addition, certain medical treatments for amenorrhea can increase the chances of pregnancy. If you do not want to become pregnant and you have amenorrhea, you should use contraception to prevent pregnancy.

Some women believe that they cannot get pregnant if they are breastfeeding and they aren't having menstrual periods. Unless a woman has gone through menopause, there is always the chance that she could get pregnant. If you are breastfeeding and want to prevent pregnancy, you should use a form of birth control to do so.

369

Chapter 50

Polycystic Ovarian Syndrome

Polycystic ovary syndrome (PCOS) is a health problem that affects one in 10 women of childbearing age. Women with PCOS have a hormonal imbalance and metabolism problems that may affect their overall health and appearance. PCOS is also a common and treatable cause of infertility.

What Is Polycystic Ovary Syndrome (PCOS)?

Polycystic ovary syndrome (PCOS), also known as polycystic ovarian syndrome, is a common health problem caused by an imbalance of reproductive hormones. The hormonal imbalance creates problems in the ovaries. The ovaries make the egg that is released each month as part of a healthy menstrual cycle. With PCOS, the egg may not develop as it should or it may not be released during ovulation as it should be.

PCOS can cause missed or irregular menstrual periods. Irregular periods can lead to:

- Infertility (inability to get pregnant). In fact, PCOS is one of the most common causes of female infertility.

- Development of cysts (small fluid-filled sacs) in the ovaries.

This chapter includes text excerpted from "Polycystic Ovary Syndrome," Office on Women's Health (OWH), June 8, 2016.

Who Gets PCOS?

Between 5 percent and 10 percent of women of childbearing age (between 15 and 44) have PCOS. Most often, women find out they have PCOS in their 20s and 30s, when they have problems getting pregnant and see their doctor. But PCOS can happen at any age after puberty.

Women of all races and ethnicities are at risk for PCOS, but your risk for PCOS may be higher if you are obese or if you have a mother, sister, or aunt with PCOS.

What Are the Symptoms of PCOS?

Some of the symptoms of PCOS include:

- **Irregular menstrual cycle.** Women with PCOS may miss periods or have fewer periods (fewer than eight in a year). Or, their periods may come every 21 days or more often. Some women with PCOS stop having menstrual periods.

- **Too much hair** on the face, chin, or parts of the body where men usually have hair. This is called "hirsutism." Hirsutism affects up to 70 percent of women with PCOS.

- **Acne** on the face, chest, and upper back.

- **Thinning hair** or hair loss on the scalp; male-pattern baldness.

- **Weight gain** or difficulty losing weight.

- **Darkening of skin**, particularly along neck creases, in the groin, and underneath breasts.

- **Skin tags**, which are small excess flaps of skin in the armpits or neck area.

What Causes PCOS?

The exact cause of PCOS is not known. Most experts think that several factors, including genetics, play a role:

- **High levels of androgens.** Androgens are sometimes called "male hormones," although all women make small amounts of androgens. Androgens control the development of male traits, such as male-pattern baldness. Women with PCOS have more androgens than estrogens. Estrogens are also called "female hormones." Higher than normal androgen levels in women can prevent the ovaries from releasing an egg (ovulation) during each menstrual cycle, and can cause extra hair growth and acne, two signs of PCOS.

- **High levels of insulin.** Insulin is a hormone that controls how the food you eat is changed into energy. Insulin resistance is when the body's cells do not respond normally to insulin. As a result, your insulin blood levels become higher than normal. Many women with PCOS have insulin resistance, especially those who are overweight or obese, have unhealthy eating habits, do not get enough physical activity, and have a family history of diabetes (usually type 2 diabetes). Over time, insulin resistance can lead to type 2 diabetes.

Can I Still Get Pregnant If I Have PCOS?

Yes. Having PCOS does not mean you can't get pregnant. PCOS is one of the most common, but treatable, causes of infertility in women. In women with PCOS, the hormonal imbalance interferes with the growth and release of eggs from the ovaries (ovulation). If you don't ovulate, you can't get pregnant.

Your doctor can talk with you about ways to help you ovulate and to raise your chance of getting pregnant.

Does PCOS Raise My Risk for Other Health Problems?

Yes, studies have found links between PCOS and other health problems, including:

- **Diabetes.** More than half of women with PCOS will have diabetes or pre-diabetes (glucose intolerance) before the age of 40.

- **High blood pressure.** Women with PCOS are at greater risk of having high blood pressure compared with women of the same age without PCOS. High blood pressure is a leading cause of heart disease and stroke.

- **Unhealthy cholesterol.** Women with PCOS often have higher levels of LDL (bad) cholesterol and low levels of HDL (good) cholesterol. High cholesterol raises your risk for heart disease and stroke.

- **Sleep apnea.** This is when momentary and repeated stops in breathing interrupt sleep. Many women with PCOS are overweight or obese, which can cause sleep apnea. Sleep apnea raises your risk for heart disease and diabetes.

373

- **Depression and anxiety.** Depression and anxiety are common among women with PCOS.

- **Endometrial cancer.** Problems with ovulation, obesity, insulin resistance, and diabetes (all common in women with PCOS) increase the risk of developing cancer of the endometrium (lining of the uterus or womb).

Will My PCOS Symptoms Go Away at Menopause?

Yes and no. PCOS affects many systems in the body. Many women with PCOS find that their menstrual cycles become more regular as they get closer to menopause. However, their PCOS hormonal imbalance does not change with age, so they may continue to have symptoms of PCOS.

Also, the risks of PCOS-related health problems, such as diabetes, stroke, and heart attack, increase with age. These risks may be higher in women with PCOS than those without.

How Is PCOS Diagnosed?

There is no single test to diagnose PCOS. To help diagnose PCOS and rule out other causes of your symptoms, your doctor may talk to you about your medical history and do a physical exam and different tests:

- **Physical exam.** Your doctor will measure your blood pressure, body mass index (BMI), and waist size. He or she will also look at your skin for extra hair on your face, chest or back, acne, or skin discoloration. Your doctor may look for any hair loss or signs of other health conditions (such as an enlarged thyroid gland).

- **Pelvic exam.** Your doctor may do a pelvic exam for signs of extra male hormones (for example, an enlarged clitoris) and check to see if your ovaries are enlarged or swollen.

- **Pelvic ultrasound (sonogram).** This test uses soundwaves to examine your ovaries for cysts and check the endometrium (lining of the uterus or womb).

- **Blood tests.** Blood tests check your androgen hormone levels, sometimes called "male hormones." Your doctor will also check for other hormones related to other common health problems that can be mistaken for PCOS, such as thyroid disease. Your doctor may also test your cholesterol levels and test you for diabetes.

Once other conditions are ruled out, you may be diagnosed with PCOS if you have at least two of the following symptoms:

- Irregular periods, including periods that come too often, not often enough, or not at all.

- Signs that you have high levels of androgens:

  - extra hair growth on your face, chin, and body (hirsutism)

  - acne

  - thinning of scalp hair

- Higher than normal blood levels of androgens.

- Multiple cysts on one or both ovaries.

How Is PCOS Treated?

There is no cure for PCOS, but you can manage the symptoms of PCOS. You and your doctor will work on a treatment plan based on your symptoms, your plans for children, and your risk for long-term health problems such as diabetes and heart disease. Many women will need a combination of treatments, including:

- steps you can take at home to help relieve your symptoms

- medicines

What Steps Can I Take at Home to Improve My PCOS Symptoms?

You can take steps at home to help your PCOS symptoms, including:

- **Losing weight.** Healthy eating habits and regular physical activity can help relieve PCOS-related symptoms. Losing weight may help to lower your blood glucose levels, improve the way your body uses insulin, and help your hormones reach normal levels. Even a 10 percent loss in body weight (for example, a 150-pound woman losing 15 pounds) can help make your menstrual cycle more regular and improve your chances of getting pregnant.

- **Removing hair.** You can try facial hair removal creams, laser hair removal, or electrolysis to remove excess hair. You can find hair removal creams and products at drugstores. Procedures like laser hair removal or electrolysis must be done by a doctor and may not be covered by health insurance.

- **Slowing hair growth.** A prescription skin treatment (eflornithine HCl cream) can help slow down the growth rate of new hair in unwanted places.

What Types of Medicines Treat PCOS?

The types of medicines that treat PCOS and its symptoms include:

- **Hormonal birth control, including the pill, patch, shot, vaginal ring, and hormone intrauterine device (IUD).** For women who don't want to get pregnant, hormonal birth control can:

  - make your menstrual cycle more regular

  - lower your risk of endometrial cancer

  - help improve acne and reduce extra hair on the face and body (Ask your doctor about birth control with both estrogen and progesterone.)

- **Anti-androgen medicines.** These medicines block the effect of androgens and can help reduce scalp hair loss, facial and body hair growth, and acne. They are not approved by the U.S. Food and Drug Administration (FDA) to treat PCOS symptoms. These medicines can also cause problems during pregnancy.

- **Metformin.** Metformin is often used to treat type 2 diabetes and may help some women with PCOS symptoms. It is not approved by the FDA to treat PCOS symptoms. Metformin improves insulin's ability to lower your blood sugar and can lower both insulin and androgen levels. After a few months of use, metformin may help restart ovulation, but it usually has little effect on acne and extra hair on the face or body. Recent research shows that metformin may have other positive effects, including lowering body mass and improving cholesterol levels.

What Are My Treatment Options for PCOS If I Want to Get Pregnant?

You have several options to help your chances of getting pregnant if you have PCOS:

- **Losing weight.** If you are overweight or obese, losing weight through healthy eating, including eating the right amount of calories for you, and regular physical activity can help make your menstrual cycle more regular and improve your fertility.

- **Medicine.** After ruling out other causes of infertility in you and your partner, your doctor might prescribe medicine to help you ovulate, such as clomiphene (Clomid).

- **In vitro fertilization (IVF).** IVF may be an option if medicine does not work. In IVF, your egg is fertilized with your partner's sperm in a laboratory and then placed in your uterus to implant and develop. Compared to medicine alone, IVF has higher pregnancy rates and better control over your risk for twins and triplets (by allowing your doctor to transfer a single fertilized egg into your uterus).

- **Surgery.** Surgery is also an option, usually only if the other options do not work. The outer shell (called the *cortex*) of ovaries is thickened in women with PCOS and thought to play a role in preventing spontaneous ovulation. Ovarian drilling is a surgery in which the doctor makes a few holes in the surface of your ovary using lasers or a fine needle heated with electricity. Surgery usually restores ovulation, but only for six to eight months.

How Does PCOS Affect Pregnancy?

PCOS can cause problems during pregnancy for you and for your baby. Women with PCOS have higher rates of:

- miscarriage

- gestational diabetes

- preeclampsia

- Cesarean section (C-section)

Your baby also has a higher risk of being heavy (macrosomia) and of spending more time in a neonatal intensive care unit (NICU).

How Can I Prevent Problems from PCOS during Pregnancy?

You can lower your risk of problems during pregnancy by:

- Reaching a healthy weight before you get pregnant. Use this interactive tool to see your healthy weight before pregnancy and what to gain during pregnancy.

- Reaching healthy blood sugar levels before you get pregnant. You can do this through a combination of healthy eating habits, regular physical activity, weight loss, and medicines such as metformin.

- Taking folic acid. Talk to your doctor about how much folic acid you need.

Chapter 51

Primary Ovarian Insufficiency

What Is Primary Ovarian Insufficiency (POI)?

Healthcare providers use the term primary ovarian insufficiency (POI) when a woman's ovaries stop working normally before she is 40 years of age.

Many women naturally experience reduced fertility when they are around 40 years old. This age may mark the start of irregular menstrual periods that signal the onset of menopause. For women with POI, irregular periods and reduced fertility occur before the age of 40, sometimes as early as the teenage years.

In the past, POI used to be called "premature menopause" or "premature ovarian failure," but those terms do not accurately describe what happens in a woman with POI. A woman who has gone through menopause will never have another normal period and cannot get pregnant. A woman with POI may still have periods, even though they might not come regularly, and she may still get pregnant.

What Are the Symptoms of POI?

The first sign of POI is usually menstrual irregularities or missed periods, which is sometimes called amenorrhea.

This chapter includes text excerpted from "Primary Ovarian Insufficiency (POI)," *Eunice Kennedy Shriver* National Institute of Child Health and Human Development (NICHD), April 12, 2013.

In addition, some women with POI have symptoms similar to those experienced by women who are going through natural menopause, including:

- Decreased sex drive

- Hot flashes

- Irritability

- Night sweats

- Pain during sex

- Poor concentration

- Vaginal dryness

For many women with POI, trouble getting pregnant or infertility is the first symptom they experience and is what leads them to visit their healthcare provider. This is sometimes called "occult" (hidden) or early POI.

What Causes POI?

In about 90 percent of cases, the exact cause of POI is a mystery.

Research shows that POI is related to problems with the follicles—the small sacs in the ovaries in which eggs grow and mature.

Follicles start out as microscopic seeds called primordial follicles. These seeds are not yet follicles, but they can grow into them. Normally, a woman is born with approximately 2 million primordial follicles, typically enough to last until she goes through natural menopause, usually around age 50.

For a woman with POI, there are problems with the follicles:

- **Follicle depletion.** A woman with follicle depletion runs out of working follicles earlier than normal or expected. In the case of POI, the woman runs out of working follicles before natural menopause occurs around age 50. Presently there is no safe way for scientists today to make primordial follicles.

- **Follicle dysfunction.** A woman with follicle dysfunction has follicles remaining in her ovaries, but the follicles are not working properly. Scientists do not have a safe and effective way to make follicles start working normally again.

Although the exact cause is unknown in a majority of cases, some causes of follicle depletion and dysfunction have been identified:

- **Genetic and chromosomal disorders.** Disorders such as Fragile X syndrome and Turner syndrome can cause follicle depletion.

- **Low number of follicles.** Some women are born with fewer primordial follicles, so they have a smaller pool of follicles to use throughout their lives. Even though only one mature follicle releases an egg each month, less mature follicles usually develop along with that mature follicle and egg. Scientists don't understand exactly why this happens, but these "supporting" follicles seem to help the mature follicle function normally. If these extra follicles are missing, the main follicle will not mature and release an egg properly.

- **Autoimmune diseases.** Typically, the body's immune cells protect the body from invading bacteria and viruses. However, in autoimmune diseases, immune cells turn on healthy tissue. In the case of POI, the immune system may damage developing follicles in the ovaries. It could also damage the glands that make the hormones needed for the ovaries and follicles to work properly. Recent studies suggest that about 20 percent of women with POI have an autoimmune disease.

  - Thyroiditis is the autoimmune disorder most commonly associated with POI. It is an inflammation of the thyroid gland, which makes hormones that control metabolism, or the pace of body processes.

  - Addison disease is also associated with POI. Addison disease affects the adrenal glands, which produce hormones that help the body respond to physical stress, such as illness and injury; the hormones also affect ovary function. About 3 percent of women with POI have Addison disease.

- **Chemotherapy or radiation therapy.** These strong treatments for cancer may damage the genetic material in cells, including follicle cells.

- **Metabolic disorders.** These disorders affect the body's ability to create, store, and use the energy it needs. For example, galactosemia affects how your body processes galactose, a type of sugar. More than 80 percent of women and girls with galactosemia also have POI.

- **Toxins.** Cigarette smoke, chemicals, and pesticides can speed up follicle depletion. In addition, viruses have been shown to affect follicle function.

How Do Healthcare Providers Diagnose POI?

The key signs of POI are:

- missed or irregular periods for 4 months, typically after having had regular periods for a while
- high levels of follicle-stimulating hormone (FSH)
- low levels of estrogen

If a woman is younger than age 40 and begins having irregular periods or stops having periods for 4 months or longer, her healthcare provider may take these steps to diagnose the problem:

- **Do a pregnancy test.** This test will rule out an unexpected pregnancy as the reason for missed periods.

- **Do a physical exam.** During the physical exam, the healthcare provider looks for signs of other disorders. In some cases, the presence of these other disorders will rule out POI. Or, if the other disorders are associated with POI, such as Addison disease, a healthcare provider will know that POI may be present.

- **Collect blood.** The healthcare provider will collect your blood and send it to a lab, where a technician will run several tests, including:

  - **Follicle-stimulating hormone (FSH) test.** FSH signals the ovaries to make estrogen, sometimes called the "female hormone" because women need high levels of it for fertility and overall health. If the ovaries are not working properly, as is the case in POI, the level of FSH in the blood increases. The healthcare provider may do two FSH tests, at least a month apart. If the FSH level in both tests is as high as it is in women who have gone through menopause, then POI is likely.

  - **Luteinizing hormone (LH) test.** LH signals a mature follicle to release an egg. Women with POI have high LH levels, more evidence that the follicles are not functioning normally.

  - **Estrogen test.** In women with POI, estrogen levels are usually low, because the ovaries are not functioning properly in their role as estrogen producers.

  - **Karyotype test.** This test looks at all 46 of your chromosomes to check for abnormalities. The karyotype test could reveal genetic changes in the structure of chromosomes that might be associated with POI and other health problems.

- **Do a pelvic ultrasound.** In this test, the healthcare provider uses a sound wave (sonogram) machine to create and view pictures of the inside of a woman's pelvic area. A sonogram can show whether or not the ovaries are enlarged or have multiple follicles.

If they do not do tests to rule out POI, some healthcare providers might assume missed periods are related to stress. However, this approach is problematic because it will lead to a delay in diagnosis; further evaluation is needed.

Are There Disorders or Conditions Associated with POI?

Because POI results in lower levels of certain hormones, women with POI are at greater risk for a number of health conditions, including:

- **Osteoporosis.** The hormone estrogen helps keep bones strong. Without enough estrogen, women with POI often develop osteoporosis. Osteoporosis is a bone disease that causes weak, brittle bones that are more likely to break and fracture.

- **Low thyroid function.** This problem also is called hypothyroidism. The thyroid is a gland that makes hormones that control your body's metabolism and energy level. Low levels of the hormones made by the thyroid can affect your metabolism and can cause very low energy and mental sluggishness. Cold feet and constipation are also features of low thyroid function. Researchers estimate that between 14 percent and 27 percent of women with POI also have low thyroid function.

- **Anxiety and depression.** Hormonal changes caused by POI can contribute to anxiety or lead to depression. Women diagnosed with POI can be shy, anxious in social settings, and may have low self-esteem more often than women without POI. It is possible that depression may contribute to POI.

- **Cardiovascular (heart) disease.** Lower levels of estrogen, as seen in POI, can affect the muscles lining the arteries and can increase the buildup of cholesterol in the arteries. Both factors increase the risk of atherosclerosis—or hardening of the arteries—which can slow or block the flow of blood to the heart.

Women with POI have higher rates of illness and death from heart disease than do women without POI.

- **Dry eye syndrome and ocular (eye) surface disease.** Some women with POI have one of these conditions, which cause discomfort and may lead to blurred vision. If not treated, these conditions can cause permanent eye damage.

Addison disease is also associated with POI. Addison disease is a life-threatening condition that affects the adrenal glands, which produce hormones that help the body respond to physical stress, such as illness and injury. These hormones also affect ovary function. About 3 percent of women with POI have Addison disease.

What Are the Treatments for POI?

Currently, there is no proven treatment to restore normal function to a woman's ovaries. But there are treatments for some of the symptoms of POI, as well as treatments and behaviors to reduce health risks and conditions associated with POI.

It is also important to note that between 5 percent and 10 percent of women with POI get pregnant without medical intervention after they are diagnosed with POI. Some research suggests that these women go into what is known as "spontaneous remission" of POI, meaning that the ovaries begin to function normally on their own. When the ovaries are working properly, fertility is restored and the women can get pregnant.

Hormone Replacement Therapy (HRT)

HRT is the most common treatment for women with POI. It gives the body the estrogen and other hormones that the ovaries are not making. HRT improves sexual health and decreases the risks for cardiovascular disease (including heart attacks, stroke, and high blood pressure) and osteoporosis.

If a woman with POI begins HRT, she is expected to start having regular periods again. In addition, HRT is expected to reduce other symptoms, such as hot flashes and night sweats, and help maintain bone health. HRT will not prevent pregnancy, and evidence suggests it might improve pregnancy rates for women with POI by lowering high levels of luteinizing hormone—which stimulates ovulation—to normal in some women.

HRT is usually a combination of an estrogen and a progestin. A progestin is a form of progesterone. Sometimes, the combination might also include testosterone, although this approach is controversial. HRT comes in several forms: pills, creams, gels, patches that stick onto the skin, an intrauterine device, or a vaginal ring. Estradiol is the natural form of human estrogen. The optimal method of providing estradiol to women with POI is by a skin patch or vaginal ring. These methods are linked with a lower risk of potentially fatal blood clots developing. Most women require a dose of 100 micrograms of estradiol per day. It is important to take a progestin along with estradiol to balance out the effect of estrogen on the lining of the womb. Women who do not take a progestin along with estradiol are at increased risk of developing endometrial cancer. The progestin with the best evidence available to support use in women with POI is 10 mg of medroxyprogesterone acetate by mouth per day for the first 12 calendar days of each month.

A healthcare provider may suggest that a woman with POI take HRT until she is about 50 years old, the age at which menopause usually begins.

After that time, she should talk with her healthcare provider about stopping the treatment because of risks associated with using this type of therapy in the years after the normal age of menopause.

Calcium and Vitamin D Supplements

Because women with POI are at higher risk for osteoporosis, they should get at least 1,200 to 1,500 mg of elemental calcium and 1000 IU (international units) of vitamin D, which helps the body absorb calcium, every day. These nutrients are important for bone health. A healthcare provider may do a bone mineral density test to check for bone loss.

Regular Physical Activity and Healthy Body Weight

Weight-bearing physical activity, such as walking, jogging, and stair climbing, helps build bone strength and prevents osteoporosis. Maintaining a healthy body weight and getting regular physical activity are also important for reducing the risk of heart disease. These factors can affect cholesterol levels, which in turn can change the risk for heart disease.

Treatments for Associated Conditions

POI is associated with other health conditions, including (but not limited to) Addison disease, Fragile X permutation, thyroid dysfunction, depression, anxierty, and certain other genetic, metabolic, and auto-immune disorders.

Women who have POI as well as one of these associated conditions will require additional treatment for the associated condition. In some cases, treatment involves medication or hormone therapy. Other types of treatments might also be needed.

Emotional Support

For many women who experience infertility, including those with POI, feelings of loss are common. In one study, almost 9 out of 10 women reported feeling moderate to severe emotional distress when they learned of their POI diagnosis. Several organizations offer help finding these types of professionals.

POI in Teens

Receiving a diagnosis of POI can be emotionally difficult for teenagers and their parents. A teen may have a similar emotional experience as an adult who receives the diagnosis, but there are many aspects of the experience that are unique to being a teenager. It is important for parents, the teenager, and healthcare providers to work closely together to ensure that the teenager gets the right treatment and maintains her emotional and physical health in the long term. There are resources to provide advice and support for parents, teenagers, and healthcare providers.

Chapter 52

Precocious Puberty

What Are Normal Puberty, Precocious Puberty, and Delayed Puberty?

Normal Puberty

The time in one's life when sexual maturity takes place is known as puberty. The physical changes that mark puberty typically begin in girls between ages 8 and 13 and in boys between ages 9 and 14.

Precocious Puberty

Precocious puberty is a condition that occurs when sexual maturity begins earlier than normal. Precocious (meaning prematurely developed) puberty begins before age 8 for girls and before age 9 for boys.

Children affected by precocious puberty may experience problems such as:

- Failure to reach their full height because their growth halts too soon.

- Psychological and social problems, such as anxiety over being "different" from their peers. However, many children do not

---

This chapter includes text excerpted from "Puberty and Precocious Puberty," *Eunice Kennedy Shriver* National Institute of Child Health and Human Development (NICHD), December 16, 2013.

experience major psychological or social problems, particularly when the onset of puberty is only slightly early.

Delayed Puberty

Delayed puberty is the term for a condition in which the body's timing for sexual maturity is later than the normal range of ages.

Many children with delayed puberty will eventually go through an otherwise normal puberty, just at a late age. Other children have a long-lasting condition known as hypogonadism in which the sex glands (the testes in men and the ovaries in women) produce few or no hormones. For example, hypogonadism can occur in girls with Turner syndrome or in individuals with hypogonadotropic hypogonadism, which occurs when the hypothalamus produces little to no gonadotropin-releasing hormone (GnRH).

What Are the Symptoms of Puberty, Precocious Puberty, and Delayed Puberty?

Normal Puberty

In Girls

The signs of puberty include:

- growth of pubic and other body hair
- growth spurt
- breast development
- onset of menstruation (after puberty is well advanced)
- acne

In Boys

The signs of puberty include:

- growth of pubic hair, other body hair, and facial hair
- enlargement of testicles and penis
- muscle growth
- growth spurt
- acne
- deepening of the voice

Precocious Puberty

The symptoms of precocious puberty are similar to the signs of normal puberty but they manifest earlier—before the age of 8 in girls and before age 9 in boys.

Delayed Puberty

Delayed puberty is characterized by the lack of onset of puberty within the normal range of ages.

How Many Children Are Affected by/at Risk of Precocious Puberty?

Precocious puberty affects about 1 percent of the U.S. population (roughly 3 million children). Many more girls are affected than boys. One study suggests that African American girls have some early breast development or some early pubic hair more often than white girls or Hispanic girls.

Who Is at Risk?

There is a greater chance of being affected by precocious puberty if a child is:

- female

- African American

- obese

What Causes Normal Puberty, Precocious Puberty, and Delayed Puberty?

Normal Puberty

Puberty is the body's natural process of sexual maturation. Puberty's trigger lies in a small part of the brain called the hypothalamus, a gland that secretes gonadotropin-releasing hormone (GnRH). GnRH stimulates the pituitary gland, a pea-sized organ connected to the bottom of the hypothalamus, to emit two hormones: luteinizing hormone (LH) and follicle-stimulating hormone (FSH). These two hormones signal the female and male sex organs (ovaries and testes, respectively) to begin releasing the appropriate sex hormones, including estrogens and testosterone, which launch the other signs of puberty in the body.

389

Precocious Puberty

In approximately 90 percent of girls who experience precocious puberty, no underlying cause can be identified—although heredity and being overweight may contribute in some cases. When a cause cannot be identified, the condition is called idiopathic precocious puberty. In boys with precocious puberty, approximately 50 percent of cases are idiopathic. In the remaining 10 percent of girls and 50 percent of boys with precocious puberty, an underlying cause can be identified.

Sometimes the cause is an abnormality involving the brain. In other children, the signs of puberty occur because of a problem such as a tumor or genetic abnormality in the ovaries, testes, or adrenal glands, causing overproduction of sex hormones.

Precocious puberty can be divided into two categories, depending on where in the body the abnormality occurs—*central precocious puberty* and *peripheral precocious puberty*.

1. Central Precocious Puberty

This type of early puberty, also known as gonadotropin-dependent precocious puberty, occurs when the abnormality is located in the brain. The brain signals the pituitary gland to begin puberty at an early age. Central precocious puberty is the most common form of precocious puberty and affects many more girls than boys. The causes of central precocious puberty include:

- brain tumors
- prior radiation to the brain
- prior infection of the brain
- other brain abnormalities

Often, however, there is no identifiable abnormality in the brain; this is called *idiopathic central precocious puberty.*

2. Peripheral Precocious Puberty

This form of early puberty is also called gonadotropin-independent precocious puberty. In peripheral precocious puberty, the abnormality is not in the brain but in the testicles, ovaries, or adrenal glands, causing overproduction of sex hormones, like testosterone and estrogens. Peripheral precocious puberty may be caused by:

- tumors of the ovary, testis, or adrenal gland

- in boys, tumors that secrete a hormone called hCG, or human chorionic gonadotropin

- certain rare genetic syndromes, such as McCune-Albright syndrome or familial male precocious puberty

- severe hypothyroidism, in which the thyroid gland secretes abnormally low levels of hormones

- disorders of the adrenal gland, such as congenital adrenal hyperplasia

- exposure of the child to medicines or creams that contain estrogens or androgens

Delayed Puberty

Many children with delayed puberty will eventually go through an otherwise normal puberty, just at a late age. Sometimes, this delay occurs because the child is just maturing more slowly than average, a condition called *constitutional delay of puberty*. This condition often runs in families.

Puberty can be delayed in children who have not gotten proper nutrition due to long-term illnesses. Also, some young girls who undergo intense physical training for a sport, such as running or gymnastics, start puberty later than normal.

In other cases, the delay in puberty is not just due to slow maturation but occurs because the child has a long-term medical condition known as hypogonadism, in which the sex glands (the testes in men and the ovaries in women) produce few or no hormones. Hypogonadism can be divided into two categories: *secondary hypogonadism* and *primary hypogonadism*.

- *Secondary hypogonadism* (also known as central hypogonadism or hypogonadotropic hypogonadism), is caused by a problem with the pituitary gland or hypothalamus (part of the brain). In secondary hypogonadism, the hypothalamus and the pituitary gland fail to signal the gonads to properly release sex hormones. Causes of secondary hypogonadism include:

  - Kallmann syndrome, a genetic problem that also diminishes the sense of smell

  - isolated hypogonadotropic hypogonadism, a genetic condition that only affects sexual development but not the sense of smell

391

- prior radiation, trauma, surgery, or other injury to the brain or pituitary

- tumors of the brain or pituitary

- In *primary hypogonadism*, the problem lies in the ovaries or testes, which fail to make sex hormones normally. Some causes include:

  - genetic disorders, especially Turner syndrome (in women) and Klinefelter syndrome (in men)

  - certain autoimmune disorders

  - developmental disorders

  - radiation or chemotherapy

  - infection

  - surgery

How Do Healthcare Providers Diagnose Precocious Puberty and Delayed Puberty?

To identify whether a child is entering puberty, a pediatrician (a physician specializing in the treatment of children) will carefully examine the following:

- in girls, the growth of pubic hair and breasts

- in boys, the increase in size of the testicles and penis and the growth of pubic hair

The pediatrician will compare what he or she finds against the Tanner scale, a 5-point scale that gauges the extent of puberty development in children.

Precocious Puberty

After giving a child a complete physical examination and analyzing his or her medical history, a healthcare provider may perform tests to diagnose precocious puberty, including:

- A blood test to check the level of hormones, such as the gonadotropins (LH and FSH), estradiol, testosterone, dehydroepiandrosterone sulfate (DHEAS), and thyroid hormones.

- A gonadotropin-releasing hormone agonist (GnRHa) stimulation test, which can tell whether a child's precocious puberty is gonadotropin-dependent or gonadotropin-independent.

- Measuring blood 17-hydroxyprogesterone to test for congenital adrenal hyperplasia.

- A "bone age" X-ray to determine if bones are growing at a normal rate.

The healthcare provider may also use imaging techniques to rule out a tumor or other organ abnormality as a cause. These imaging methods may include:

- Ultrasound (sonography) to examine the gonads. An ultrasound painlessly creates an image on a computer screen of blood vessels and tissues, allowing a healthcare provider to monitor organs and blood flow in real time.

- An MRI (magnetic resonance imaging) scan of the brain and pituitary gland using an instrument that produces detailed images of organs and bodily structures.

Delayed Puberty

To diagnose hypogonadotropic hypogonadism, a healthcare provider may prescribe these tests:

- blood tests to measure hormone levels

- blood tests to measure if the pituitary gland can correctly respond to GnRH

- an MRI of the brain and pituitary gland.

What Are Common Treatments for Problems of Puberty?

Precocious Puberty

There are a number of reasons to treat precocious puberty.

Treatment for precocious puberty can help stop puberty until the child is closer to the normal time for sexual development. One reason to consider treating precocious puberty is that rapid growth and bone maturation, caused by precocious puberty, can prevent a child from reaching his or her full height potential. Children grow rapidly in height during puberty and reach their final adult height after puberty. Children who go through puberty too early may not reach their full adult height potential because their growth stops too soon.

Another reason to consider treating precocious puberty is that a young child may not be psychologically ready for the physical and hormonal changes that occur in puberty.

However, not all children with precocious puberty require treatment, particularly if the onset of puberty is only slightly early. The goal of treatment is to prevent the production of sex hormones to prevent the early halt of growth, short stature in adulthood, emotional effects, social problems, and problems with libido (especially in boys).

If precocious puberty is caused by a specific medical problem, treating the underlying problem can often stop the progression of precocious puberty. In addition, precocious puberty can often be stopped by medical treatment to block the hormones that cause puberty. For example, medications called gonadotropin-releasing hormone agonists (GnRHa) are used to treat central precocious puberty. These medications, some of which are injected, suppress production of LH and FSH.

Delayed Puberty

With delayed puberty or hypogonadism, treatment varies with the origin of the problem but may involve:

- in males, testosterone injections, skin patches, or gel

- in females, estrogen and/or progesterone given as pills or skin patches

Part Seven

Other Disorders of Endocrine and Metabolic Functioning

Chapter 53

Inborn Errors of Metabolism

Chapter Contents

Section 53.1

Inborn Errors of Metabolism: Overview

This section includes text excerpted from "The NIH
MINI Study: Metabolism, Infection and Immunity in Inborn
Errors of Metabolism," National Human Genome Research
Institute (NHGRI), February 22, 2013.

What Are Inborn Errors of Metabolism?

Metabolism is a sequence of chemical reactions that take place
in cells in the body. These reactions are responsible for the breakdown of nutrients and the generation of energy in our bodies. Inborn
errors of metabolism (IEM) are a group of disorders that causes
a block in a metabolic pathway leading to clinically significant
consequences.

Specific chemical compounds, called enzymes, are responsible for
the reactions that make up metabolism. There are also 'co-factors', or
compounds that help enzymes carry out their reactions.

What Are the Different Forms of IEM?

The different IEM are usually named for the enzyme that is not
working properly. For example, if the enzyme carbamoyl phosphate
synthetase 1 (CPS1) is not working, the IEM is called "CPS1 deficiency." A list of broad categories of IEM and some examples are listed
below.

Table 53.1. Broad Categories of IEM

IEM	Examples
Urea cycle disorders	Ornithine transcarbamylase deficiency, citrullinemia, argininosuccinic aciduria, argininemia
Organic acidemias	Propionic acidemia, methylmalonic aciduria, isovaleric acidemia, glutaric acidemia, maple syrup urine disease

Table 53.1. Continued

IEM	Examples
Fatty acid oxidation defects	Medium chain acyl-CoA dehydrogenase deficiency, carnitine palmitoyl transferase 1 deficiency, long chain hydroxyacyl-CoA dehydrogenase deficiency
Amino acidopathies	Tyrosinemia, phenylketonuria, homocysteinuria
Carbohydrate disorders	Galactosemia, fructosemia
Mitochondrial disorders	MELAS, MERFF, pyruvate dehydrogenase deficiency

What Causes the IEM and How Are the Different Forms Inherited?

The IEM are caused by mutations (or alterations) in the genes that tell our cells how to make the enzymes and the co-factors for metabolism. A mutation causes a gene to not function at all or not to function as well as it should. Most often these altered genes are inherited from parent(s), but they may also occur spontaneously.

When discussing how genetic conditions are passed on in a family, it is important to understand that we have two copies of most genes, with one copy inherited from our mother and one copy inherited from our father. This is not the case for the genes that are on our sex chromosomes (the "X" and "Y" chromosomes). These are different in men and women: men have only one X chromosome and therefore only one copy of the genes on that chromosome, while women have two X chromosomes and therefore have two copies of the genes on that chromosome. A father passes on his X chromosome to all of his daughters and his Y chromosome on to all of his sons. A mother passes on an X chromosome to each child.

What Is the Chance of Having an IEM If Someone Else in the Family Has It?

The chance that someone else in the family has the same IEM as their relative depends on the inheritance pattern of the IEM, whether the at-risk family member is male or female, and the rest of the family history (how many relatives have been diagnosed with the disorder already and whether genetic testing has been performed in other relatives). In some cases, the age of the at-risk family member and whether or not they have shown any signs or symptoms of the disorder is helpful in estimating the chances that they also have the disorder.

It is recommended talking to your metabolic specialist and/or genetic counselor to determine those relatives who may be at risk for having an IEM and for coordination of genetic testing, when appropriate.

What Are the Symptoms of IEM and How Are They Diagnosed?

In general, the earlier someone develops symptoms of an IEM, the more severe their disorder. The severity of symptoms is generally based on

1. the position of the defective enzyme within the metabolic pathway and

2. whether or not there is any functional enzyme or co-factor being produced.

However, other environmental and genetic factors may play a role in determining the severity of symptoms for a given patient.

IEM are multisystemic diseases and thus patients may present with a variety of symptoms, many of which depend on the specific metabolic pathway(s) involved. Some findings in patients with IEM may include elevated acid levels in the blood, low blood sugar, high blood ammonia, abnormal liver function tests, and blood cell abnormalities. Certain patients may also have neurologic abnormalities such as seizures and developmental delays. Growth may also be affected.

How Are IEM Treated?

Treatment of IEM is tailored to the specific disorder once a diagnosis is made. In general, the goals of treatment are to minimize or eliminate the buildup of toxic metabolites that result from the block in metabolism while maintaining growth and development. This may be accomplished by special modified diets, supplements and medications.

A doctor who specializes in metabolic disorders should see IEM patients on a regular basis. Severely affected patients will likely be seen on a more frequent basis than mild or moderately affected patients.

Section 53.2

Galactosemia

This section includes text excerpted from "Galactosemia," Genetic
and Rare Diseases Information Center (GARD), National Center for
Advancing Translational Sciences (NCATS), June 25, 2015.

What Is Galactosemia?

Galactosemia, which means "galactose in the blood," is a rare inherited condition. People with galactosemia have problems digesting a
type of sugar called galactose from the food they eat. Because they
cannot break galactose down properly, it builds up in their blood.
Galactose is found in milk and all foods that contain milk. Galactosemia occurs when an enzyme, called 'galactose-1-phosphate uridyl
transferase' (GALT), is either missing or not working properly. Without
enough GALT enzyme activity, galactose cannot be changed to glucose
so it builds up in the blood in large amounts.

There are different types of galactosemia: classic galactosemia (also
known as type I, is the most common and most severe form of the condition), galactosemia type II (also called galactokinase deficiency), and type
III (also called galactose epimerase deficiency). The different types of
galactosemia are caused by mutations in the *GALT*, *GALE*, and *GALK1*
genes. The condition is inherited in an autosomal recessive fashion.

Symptoms

If infants with classic galactosemia are not treated promptly with a
low-galactose diet, life-threatening complications appear within a few
days after birth. Affected infants typically develop feeding difficulties,
a lack of energy, failure to grow and gain weight as expected (failure
to thrive), yellowing of the skin and whites of the eyes (jaundice),
liver damage, and abnormal bleeding. Other serious complications can
include overwhelming bacterial infections (sepsis) and shock. Affected
children are also at increased risk of developmental delay, clouding
of the lens of the eye (cataract), speech difficulties, and intellectual
disability. Females with classic galactosemia may experience reproductive problems caused by premature ovarian failure.

Signs and Symptoms

- Chronic hepatic failure
- Cognitive impairment
- Feeding difficulties in infancy
- Hepatic failure
- Nausea and vomiting
- Reduced bone mineral density
- Reduced consciousness/ confusion
- Weight loss
- Abnormality of coagulation
- Abnormality of the voice
- Ascites
- Cataract
- Decreased fertility
- Edema of the lower limbs
- Hepatomegaly
- Muscular hypotonia
- Neurological speech impairment
- Sepsis
- Tremor
- Abnormality of the genital system

- Hemolytic anemia
- Hypoglycemia
- Incoordination
- Microcephaly
- Renal insufficiency
- Seizures
- Visual impairment
- Aminoaciduria
- Autosomal recessive inheritance
- Cirrhosis
- Decreased liver function
- Diarrhea
- Failure to thrive
- Galactosuria
- Hyperchloremic metabolic acidosis
- Hypergalactosemia
- Hypergonadotropic hypogonadism
- Intellectual disability
- Metabolic acidosis
- Premature ovarian failure
- Vomiting

Diagnosis

Newborn screening programs in many states will test for galactosemia. The diagnosis of this condition is usually established by measurement of erythrocyte galactose-1-phosphate uridyltransferase (GALT) enzyme activity, erythrocyte galactose-1-phosphate (gal-1-P) concentration, and genetic testing looking for mutations in the GALT gene. In classic galactosemia, GALT enzyme activity is less than 5 percent of control values and erythrocyte gal-1-P is higher than 10 mg/dL.

Treatment

When treatment starts before a baby is 10 days old, there is a much better chance for normal growth, development and intelligence. Affected individuals must avoid all milk, milk-containing products (including dry milk), and other foods that contain galactose for life. It is essential to read product labels and be an informed consumer. Infants can be fed with soy formula, meat-based formula or Nutramigen (a protein hydrolysate formula), or another lactose-free formula. Calcium supplements are also recommended.

Because the body also makes some galactose, symptoms cannot be completely avoided by removing all lactose and galactose from the diet. Researchers are working on finding a treatment to lower the amount of galactose made by the body, but there is no effective method to do so at this time.

The Screening, Technology, and Research in Genetics (STAR-G) Project is a U.S.-based organization that provides information on newborn screening. They provide comprehensive information for treatment on galactosemia.

Sugars that are simple are known as monosaccharides and include glucose, galactose and fructose. When the sugar contain two monosaccharides is called disaccharide. The disaccharides include sucrose (formed by glucose and fructose), maltose (formed by two glucoses) and lactose (formed by galactose and glucose).

Basically, any food or beverage or medication containing galactose or lactose should be avoided by the patients with galactosemia.The main source of galactose is from the lactose contained in the diet.

Sucralose is an artificial sweetener. During processing, sucrose (sugar) is broken down to a compound that has the word galactose in it, but it is not broken down to simple galactose, therefore it is acceptable for patients with galactosemia.

A guide offered by the Biochemical Genetics Program, Waisman Center University of Wisconsin-Madison entitled: *Understanding Galactosemia—A Diet Guide* has detailed information about diet management, galactose content of foods, medicines and supplements, and tools for day-to-day food choices and meal planning.

Section 53.3

Maple Syrup Urine Disease

This section contains text excerpted from the following sources: Text
under headings marked 1 are excerpted from "Maple Syrup Urine
Disease," Genetic and Rare Diseases Information Center (GARD),
National Center for Advancing Translational Sciences (NCATS),
October 1, 2016; Text under headings marked 1 are excerpted from
"Maple Syrup Urine Disease," Genetic Home Reference (GHR),
National Institutes of Health (NIH), September 28, 2016.

What Is Maple Syrup Urine Disease?[1]

Maple syrup urine disease is an inherited disorder in which the
body is unable to process certain protein building blocks (amino acids)
properly. Beginning in early infancy, this condition is characterized
by poor feeding, vomiting, lack of energy (lethargy), seizures, and
developmental delay. The urine of affected infants has a distinctive
sweet odor, much like burned caramel, that gives the condition its
name. Maple syrup urine disease can be life-threatening if untreated.

Symptoms[1]

Signs and Symptoms

- Abnormality of the pharynx
- Abnormality of the voice
- Aminoaciduria
- Cognitive impairment
- Flexion contracture
- Muscular hypotonia
- Nausea and vomiting
- Reduced consciousness/ confusion
- Respiratory insufficiency

- Seizures
- Attention deficit hyperactivity disorder
- Chorea
- Hallucinations
- Hemiplegia/hemiparesis
- Incoordination
- Recurrent respiratory infections
- Recurrent urinary tract infections

- Pancreatitis
- Reduced bone mineral density
- Ataxia
- Autosomal recessive inheritance
- Cerebral edema
- Coma
- Elevated plasma branched chain amino acids

- Feeding difficulties in infancy
- Growth abnormality
- Hypertonia
- Hypoglycemia
- Intellectual disability
- Ketosis
- Lactic acidosis
- Lethargy
- Vomiting

Frequency[2]

Maple syrup urine disease affects an estimated 1 in 185,000 infants worldwide. The disorder occurs much more frequently in the Old Order Mennonite population, with an estimated incidence of about 1 in 380 newborns.

Genetic Changes[2]

Mutations in the *BCKDHA, BCKDHB,* and *DBT* genes can cause maple syrup urine disease. These three genes provide instructions for making proteins that work together as a complex. The protein complex is essential for breaking down the amino acids leucine, isoleucine, and valine, which are present in many kinds of food, particularly protein-rich foods such as milk, meat, and eggs.

Mutations in any of these three genes reduce or eliminate the function of the protein complex, preventing the normal breakdown of leucine, isoleucine, and valine. As a result, these amino acids and their byproducts build up in the body. Because high levels of these substances are toxic to the brain and other organs, their accumulation leads to the serious health problems associated with maple syrup urine disease.

Inheritance[1]

Maple syrup urine disease is inherited in an autosomal recessive pattern. This means that both copies of a gene in each cell have mutations. The parents of an individual who has the condition each carry one copy of the mutated gene.

Diagnosis[1]

Carrier testing is available on a clinical basis in families with a history of maple syrup urine disease once the mutations have been identified in the affected individual.

GeneTests lists laboratories offering clinical genetic testing for this condition. Clinical genetic tests are ordered to help diagnose a person or family and to aid in decisions regarding medical care or reproductive issues. Individuals interested in pursuing genetic testing, including carrier testing, are encouraged to work with a genetics professional who can discuss testing options, arrange for testing, and discuss test results and their implications.

Section 53.4

Phenylketonuria (PKU)

This section includes text excerpted from "Phenylketonuria (PKU),"
Eunice Kennedy Shriver National Institute of Child Health and
Human Development (NICHD), August 23, 2013.

Phenylketonuria, often called PKU, is an inherited disorder that that can cause intellectual and developmental disabilities (IDDs) if not treated. In PKU, the body can't process a portion of a protein called phenylalanine, which is in all foods containing protein. If the phenylalanine level gets too high, the brain can become damaged.

All children born in U.S. hospitals are tested routinely for PKU soon after birth, making it easier to diagnose and treat affected children early.

Children and adults who are treated early and consistently develop normally.

Depending on the level of phenylalanine and tolerance for phenylalanine in the diet, PKU is classified into two different types: classic, which is the severe form, and moderate. Therefore, each patient needs an individualized treatment plan. Some people may benefit from a medication called sapropterin dihydrochloride (brand name Kuvan®) that treats the disorder.

What Are Common Symptoms of Phenylketonuria (PKU)?

Children with untreated PKU appear normal at birth. But by age 3 to 6 months, they begin to lose interest in their surroundings. By age 1 year, children are developmentally delayed and their skin has less pigmentation than someone without the condition. If people with PKU do not restrict the phenylalanine in their diet, they develop severe intellectual and developmental disabilities.

Other symptoms include:

- behavioral or social problems

- seizures, shaking, or jerking movements in the arms and legs

- stunted or slow growth

- skin rashes, like eczema

- small head size, called microcephaly

- a musty odor in urine, breath, or skin that is a result of the extra phenylalanine in the body

- fair skin and blue eyes, due to the body's failure to transform phenylalanine into melanin, the pigment responsible for a person's coloring

What Causes Phenylketonuria (PKU)?

PKU is caused by mutations in the gene that helps make an enzyme called phenylalanine hydroxylase, or PAH. This enzyme is needed to convert the amino acid phenylalanine into other substances the body needs. When this gene, known as the *PAH* gene, is defective, the body cannot break down phenylalanine.

Amino acids help build protein, but phenylalanine can cause harm when it builds up in a person's body. In particular, nerve cells in the brain are sensitive to phenylalanine.

Many different PAH mutations result in problems with breaking down phenylalanine. Some mutations cause PKU, others cause non-PKU hyperphenylalaninemia and others are silent mutations that do not have an effect.

Is PKU Inherited?

PKU is inherited from a person's parents. The disorder is passed down in a recessive pattern, which means that for a child to develop

PKU, both parents have to contribute a mutated version of the *PAH* gene. If both parents have PKU, their child will have PKU as well.

Sometimes, a parent does not have PKU but is a carrier, which means the parent carries a mutated PAH gene. If only one parent carries the mutated gene, the child will not develop PKU.

Even if both parents carry the mutated *PAH* gene, their child still may not develop PKU. This is because a child's parents each carry two versions of the *PAH* gene, only one of which they will pass on during conception.

If both of a child's parents are carriers, there is a 25 percent chance that each parent will pass on the normal *PAH* gene. In this case, the child will not have the disorder. Conversely, there also is a 25 percent chance that the carrier parents will both pass along the mutated gene, causing the child to have PKU. However, there is a 50 percent chance that a child will inherit one normal gene from one parent and one abnormal one from the other, making the child a carrier.

How Do Healthcare Providers Diagnose Phenylketonuria (PKU)?

Nearly all cases of PKU are diagnosed through a blood test done on newborns.

Newborn Screening for PKU

All 50 U.S. states and territories require that newborns get screened for PKU. In addition to the United States, many other countries routinely screen infants for PKU.

Before screening for PKU was possible, most infants with the disorder developed severe intellectual disabilities. In the 1960s, researchers supported by the federal Children's Bureau determined that a test for PKU given to newborns was safe and effective. Later, the *Eunice Kennedy Shriver* National Institute of Child Health and Human Development (NICHD) led research on the safety and effectiveness of a restricted diet to treat PKU. Since then, PKU has been almost completely eliminated as a cause of intellectual disabilities.

How Are Newborns Tested for PKU?

Healthcare providers conduct a PKU screening test using a few drops of blood from a newborn's heel. The blood sample, which can be used to screen for other conditions as well, is tested in a laboratory to determine if it has too much phenylalanine in it. The newborn screening test should be performed by the child's pediatrician if the mother did not give birth in a hospital or is discharged from the hospital before the test is performed.

What If My Newborn Tests Positive for PKU?

If your newborn's screening test comes back positive for PKU, your child will need additional tests to confirm that he or she definitely has the disorder. It is very important to follow your healthcare providers' instructions for further tests. These tests may be blood or urine tests that may show whether or not the child has PKU. If your child does have PKU, getting treatment quickly will help protect your child's health.

Your healthcare providers may also suggest genetic testing to look at the mutations in genes that cause PKU. This testing is not required to figure out whether your child has PKU, but it will help identify the specific type of genetic mutation causing the disorder. This information may be useful for determining the best treatment plan going forward.

Screening for PKU Later in Life

In the United States, newborn screening identifies nearly all people born with PKU. However, there are concerns that cases of PKU could be missed due to errors at any step of the screening process — specimen collection, laboratory procedures, treatment initiation, or clinical follow-up. Missed cases are considered to be extremely rare. Because of these rare cases, health professionals recommend PKU testing if a person of any age has developmental delays or an intellectual disability.

Testing during Pregnancy

A pregnant woman can request a prenatal DNA test to learn whether or not her child will be born with PKU. To perform this test, a healthcare provider takes some cells, either through a needle inserted into the abdomen or a small tube inserted into the vagina. A genetic counselor who understands the risks and benefits of genetic testing can help explain the choices available for testing. This discussion may be particularly useful for parents who already have one child with PKU, because they have a higher-than-average chance of conceiving another child with the disorder.

What Are Common Treatments for Phenylketonuria (PKU)?

There is no cure for PKU, but treatment can prevent intellectual disabilities and other health problems. A person with PKU should receive treatment at a medical center that specializes in the disorder.

The PKU Diet

People with PKU need to follow a diet that limits foods with phenylalanine. The diet should be followed carefully and be started as soon after birth as possible. In the past, experts believed that it was safe for people to stop following the diet as they got older. However, they now recommend that people with PKU stay on the diet throughout their lives for better physical and mental health.

It is especially important for a pregnant woman with PKU to strictly follow the low-phenylalanine diet throughout her pregnancy to ensure the healthy development of her infant.

People with PKU need to avoid various high-protein foods, including:

- milk and cheese
- eggs
- nuts
- soybeans
- beans

- chicken, beef, or pork
- fish
- peas
- beer

People with PKU also need to avoid the sweetener aspartame, which is in some foods, drinks, medications, and vitamins. Aspartame releases phenylalanine when it is digested, so it raises the level of phenylalanine in a person's blood.

Often, people with PKU also have to limit their intake of lower-protein foods, such as certain fruits and vegetables. However, a PKU diet can include low-protein noodles and other special products.

The amount of phenylalanine that is safe to consume differs for each person. Therefore, a person with PKU needs to work with a healthcare professional to develop an individualized diet. The goal is to eat only the amount of phenylalanine necessary for healthy growth and body processes but not any extra. Frequent blood tests and doctor visits are necessary to help determine how well the diet is working. Some relaxation of the diet may be possible as a child gets older, but the recommendation today is lifelong adherence to the diet. Following the diet is especially important during pregnancy.

However, the PKU diet can be very challenging. Getting support from friends and family or a support group can help. Sticking with the diet ensures better functioning and improved overall health.

A PKU Formula

People who follow the PKU diet will not get enough essential nutrients from food. Therefore, they must drink a special formula.

A newborn who is diagnosed with PKU should receive special infant formula. The formula may be mixed with a small amount of breast milk or regular infant formula to make sure the child gets enough phenylalanine for normal development but not enough to cause harm.

Older children and adults receive a different formula to meet their nutritional needs. This formula should be consumed every day throughout a person's life.

In addition to the formula, healthcare professionals may recommend other supplements. For example, fish oil may be recommended to help with fine motor coordination and other aspects of development.

Medication for PKU

The U.S. Food and Drug Administration (FDA) has approved the drug sapropterin dihydrochloride (Kuvan®) for the treatment of PKU. Kuvan® is a form of BH (hydrobiopterin), which is a substance in the body that helps break down phenylalanine. However, having too little BH is only one reason a person may not break down phenylalanine. Therefore, Kuvan® only helps some people reduce the phenylalanine in their blood. Even if the medication helps, it will not decrease the phenylalanine to the desired amount and must be used together with the PKU diet.

When the FDA approved Kuvan®, the agency suggested that research on the medication continue to determine its long-term safety and effectiveness.

Other Treatments for PKU

NICHD-supported researchers and other scientists are exploring additional treatments for PKU. These treatments include large neutral amino acid supplementation, which may help prevent phenylalanine from entering the brain, and enzyme replacement therapy, which uses a substance similar to the enzyme that usually breaks down phenylalanine. Researchers are also investigating the possibility of using gene therapy, which involves injecting new genes to break down phenylalanine. That would result in the breakdown of phenylalanine and decreased blood phenylalanine levels.

If Phenylketonuria (PKU) Is Not Treated, What Problems Occur?

Children and adults who do not receive treatment for PKU may develop a variety of symptoms.

- **Children with PKU** who are not treated may develop symptoms including behavioral problems, seizures, and severe intellectual and developmental disabilities.

- **Adults with PKU** who do not follow a special diet may develop unstable moods and take longer to process information. Adults with high phenylalanine levels who go back on a PKU diet may be able to improve their mental functioning and slow down any damage to their central nervous systems.

- **Pregnant Women with PKU** who do not strictly follow a low-phenylalanine diet may give birth to a child with serious problems, including intellectual and developmental disabilities, a head that is too small (microcephaly), heart defects, and low birth weight. Women with PKU and uncontrolled phenylalanine levels also have an increased risk of pregnancy loss.

Phenylketonuria (PKU): Other FAQs

Is Genetic Testing for PKU Available?

A blood sample can be used to test for the mutations that cause PKU.

Testing an Infant

A blood test that measures the phenylalanine in an infant's blood is enough to help make a PKU diagnosis. Therefore, DNA testing is not necessary. However, if a child tests positive for PKU, healthcare providers may recommend genetic testing because identifying the type of mutation involved can help guide selection of the most appropriate treatment plan.

A DNA test also should be performed on a child if both parents are PKU carriers and the standard newborn blood test does not show the condition. The test will definitively indicate or rule out PKU, if the disease-causing mutations in the family have been identified.

Testing during Pregnancy

A pregnant woman can request a prenatal DNA test to learn whether or not her child will be born with PKU. To perform this test, a healthcare provider takes some cells, either through a needle inserted into the abdomen or a small tube inserted into the vagina. A genetic counselor who understands the risks and benefits of genetic testing can help explain the choices available for testing. This discussion may be particularly useful for parents who already have one child with PKU, because they have a higher-than-average chance of conceiving another child with the disorder. The disease causing mutations must have been identified before prenatal testing can be performed.

Testing Possible PKU Carriers

If a child is diagnosed with PKU, other family members may be more likely to conceive children who also will have PKU. The parents' siblings and other close blood relatives should be told that the child has PKU so that they can decide whether or not they should have DNA testing as well.

What Is Maternal PKU?

Maternal PKU is the term used when a woman who has PKU becomes pregnant. Most children born to PKU mothers do not have the disorder. But if a pregnant woman who has PKU does not strictly follow a low-phenylalanine diet, her child can develop serious problems. These include:

- intellectual disabilities

- having a head that is too small (microcephaly)

- heart defects

- low birth weight

- behavioral problems

The newborn's problems from untreated maternal PKU are caused by the high phenylalanine levels present in the mother's blood during pregnancy—not by PKU itself. The infant does not have PKU and does not need a PKU diet. The PKU diet will not help these health problems.

Women with PKU and uncontrolled phenylalanine levels also have an increased risk of pregnancy loss.

If I Have PKU, What Steps Should I Take during Pregnancy to Protect My Infant?

If you have PKU, it is very important to follow a strict low-phenylalanine diet before becoming pregnant and throughout your pregnancy. In addition to staying on a PKU diet, also make sure to:

• Visit a PKU clinic on a regular basis.

• Have your blood checked often for phenylalanine.

• Ask your healthcare provider how much PKU formula to drink.

Keep in mind that untreated maternal PKU can cause serious problems for a developing fetus.

A newborn's problems from untreated maternal PKU are caused by the high phenylalanine levels present in the mother's blood during pregnancy—not PKU itself. The infant does not have PKU and does not need a PKU diet. The PKU diet will not help these health problems.

Women with PKU and uncontrolled phenylalanine levels also have an increased risk of pregnancy loss.

What Determines the Severity of PKU?

A number of factors influence whether a person with PKU has mild symptoms or more severe problems.

Genetic Factors

Many different mutations of the *PAH* gene can cause PKU. The type of mutation greatly affects the severity of the person's symptoms.

Some mutations cause classic PKU, the most severe form of the disorder. In these cases, the enzyme that breaks down phenylalanine barely works or does not work at all. If it is not treated, classic PKU can cause severe brain damage and other serious medical problems. Some mutations allow the enzyme to work a little better than it does in classic PKU. This is sometimes called non-PKU hyperphenylalaninemia, and is also known as non-PKU HPA. Such cases come with a smaller risk of brain damage. People with very mild cases may not require treatment with a low-phenylalanine diet.

Non-Genetic Factors

Genes are not the only factor that influences the severity of PKU symptoms. For example, strictly following a PKU diet greatly reduces the chances that a person will have intellectual disabilities and other problems caused by PKU. Other factors include the person's age at diagnosis and how quickly the person's blood levels of phenylalanine are brought under control.

Does a Child with PKU Need Repeated Testing?

Infants and children with PKU need frequent blood tests to measure the phenylalanine in their blood. The healthcare provider may suggest changes to the diet or formula the child receives if there is evidence of too much or too little phenylalanine.

Infants with PKU will be tested about once a week for the first year of their lives. After the first year, children may be tested once or twice a month. Adults also need to be checked regularly throughout their lives. Often, blood samples can be taken at home and mailed to a laboratory.

Section 53.5

Urea Cycle Disorders

This section includes text excerpted from "Urea Cycle Disorders," Genetic and Rare Diseases Information Center (GARD), National Center for Advancing Translational Sciences (NCATS), September 10, 2013.

What Is Urea Cycle Disorders?

A urea cycle disorder (UCD) is a genetic disorder that results in a deficiency of one of the six enzymes in the urea cycle. These enzymes are responsible for removing ammonia from the blood stream. The urea cycle involves a series of biochemical steps in which nitrogen, a waste product of protein metabolism, is changed to a compound called urea and removed from the blood. Normally, the urea is removed from the body through the urine. In UCDs, nitrogen builds up in the blood in the form of ammonia, a highly toxic substance, resulting in hyperammonemia (elevated blood ammonia). Ammonia then reaches the brain through the blood, where it can cause irreversible brain damage, coma and/or death. The onset and severity of UCDs is highly variable. The severity correlates with the amount of urea cycle enzyme function.

415

Treatment

The medication(s) listed below have been approved by the U.S. Food and Drug Administration (FDA) as orphan products for treatment of this condition.

- **Benzoate and phenylacetate (Brand name: Ammonul®)**

  FDA-approved indication: Adjunctive therapy in the treatment of acute hyperammonemia and associated encephalopathy in patients with deficiencies in enzymes of the urea cycle.

- **Sodium phenylbutyrate (Brand name: Buphenyl®)**

  FDA-approved indication: Adjunctive therapy in the chronic managment of patients with UCDs involving deficiencies of carbamylphosphate synthetase, ornithine transcarbamylase, or argininosuccinic acid synthetase.

- **Glycerol phenylbutyrate (Brand name: Ravicti)**

  FDA-approved indication: Use as a nitrogen-binding adjunctive therapy for chronic management of adult and pediatric patients > or = to 2 years of age with UCDs that cannot be managed by dietary protein restriction and/or amino acid supplementation alone. Ravicti must be used with dietary protein restriction and, in some cases, dietary supplements (e.g., essential amino acids, arginine, citrulline, protein-free calorie supplements).

- **Benzoate and phenylacetate (Brand name: Ucephan)**

  FDA-approved indication: For adjunctive therapy in the prevention and treatment of hyperammonemia in patients with urea cycle enzymopathy due to carbamylphosphate synthetase, ornithine, transcarbamylase, or argininosuccinate synthetase deficiency.

Related Diseases

The following diseases are related to UCDs.

- Adult-onset citrullinemia type II
- Arginase deficiency
- Argininosuccinic aciduria
- Carbamoyl phosphate synthetase 1 deficiency

- Citrullinemia type I
- N-acetylglutamate synthetase deficiency
- Ornithine transcarbamylase deficiency
- Ornithine translocase deficiency syndrome

Chapter 54

Glycogen-Storage Diseases (GSDs)

Chapter Contents

Section 54.1

Type 0

This section includes text excerpted from "Glycogen
Storage Disease Type 0, Liver," Genetic and Rare Diseases
Information Center (GARD), National Center for Advancing
Translational Sciences (NCATS), June 11, 2015.

What Is Glycogen Storage Disease Type 0, Liver?

Glycogen storage disease type 0, liver (liver GSD 0), a form of glycogen storage disease (GSD), is a rare abnormality of glycogen metabolism (how the body uses and stores glycogen, the storage form of glucose). Unlike other types of GSD, liver GSD 0 does not involve excessive or abnormal glycogen storage, and causes moderately decreased glycogen stores in the liver. Symptoms typically begin in infancy or in early childhood and may include drowsiness, sweating, lack of attention, fasting hypoglycemia associated with hyperketonemia, seizures, and other findings. It is caused by a deficiency of the enzyme glycogen synthetase in the liver, due to mutations in the *GYS2* gene. It is inherited in an autosomal recessive manner. Treatment involves a specific diet that includes frequent meals with high protein intake during the day, and uncooked starch in the evening. The prognosis is usually favorable when the disease is correctly managed. This condition differs from another form of GSD 0 which chiefly affects the muscles and heart (Glycogen storage disease type 0, muscle) and is thought to be caused by mutations in the *GYS1* gene.

Signs and Symptoms

- Fasting hypoglycemia
- Increased serum lactate
- Ketosis
- Neonatal hypoglycemia
- Postprandial hyperglycemia
- Seizures

Other Names

- Liver GSD 0

- Liver glycogen storage disease 0

- Hepatic glycogen synthase deficiency

- Liver glycogen synthase deficiency

Section 54.2

Type 1 with 1A and 1B

This section contains text excerpted from the following sources: Text beginning with the heading "What Is Glycogen Storage Disease Type 1A?" is excerpted from "Glycogen Storage Disease Type 1A," Genetic and Rare Diseases Information Center (GARD), National Center for Advancing Translational Sciences (NCATS), October 1, 2016; Text beginning with the heading "What Is Glycogen Storage Disease Type 1B?" is excerpted from "Glycogen Storage Disease Type 1B," Genetic and Rare Diseases Information Center (GARD), National Center for Advancing Translational Sciences (NCATS), October 1, 2016.

What Is Glycogen Storage Disease Type 1A?

Glycogen storage disease type 1 is an inherited disorder caused by the buildup of a complex sugar called glycogen in the body's cells. The accumulation of glycogen in certain organs and tissues, especially the liver, kidneys, and small intestines, impairs their ability to function normally. Researchers have described two types of glycogen storage disease type 1, which differ in their signs and symptoms and genetic cause. These types are known as glycogen storage disease type IA and glycogen storage disease type IB.

Glycogen storage disease type 1A is characterized by growth retardation leading to short stature and accumulation of glycogen and fat in the liver and kidneys. Although some newborns present with severe hypoglycemia, it is more common for infants to present at age three to four months with hepatomegaly, lactic acidosis, hyperuricemia,

421

hyperlipidemia, and/or hypoglycemic seizures. Untreated children typically have doll-like faces with fat cheeks and relatively thin extremities. Xanthoma and diarrhea may be present. Impaired platelet function can lead to a bleeding tendency, making epistaxis a frequent problem. Glycogen storage disease type 1A is caused by the deficiency of glucose-6-phosphatase (G6Pase) catalytic activity which results from mutations in the *G6PC* gene. This condition is inherited in an autosomal recessive pattern.

Signs and Symptoms

- Abnormality of lipid metabolism
- Cognitive impairment
- Full cheeks
- Hyperuricemia
- Hypoglycemia
- Muscular hypotonia
- Recurrent respiratory infections
- Seizures
- Short stature
- Multiple lipomas
- Abnormal bleeding
- Decreased glomerular filtration rate
- Decreased muscle mass
- Delayed puberty
- Doll-like facies
- Elevated hepatic transaminases
- Enlarged kidneys
- Focal segmental glomerulosclerosis
- Gout
- Hepatocellular carcinoma
- Hepatomegaly
- Hyperlipidemia
- Hypertension
- Intermittent diarrhea
- Lactic acidosis
- Lipemia retinalis
- Nephrolithiasis
- Osteoporosis
- Pancreatitis
- Proteinuria
- Protuberant abdomen
- Xanthomatosis

Other Names

- GSD1
- Glycogen storage disease 1A

- Von Gierke disease

- Glycogenosis type 1

- Hepatorenal form of glycogen storage disease

- Glucose-6-phosphatase deficiency

- Hepatorenal glycogenosis

- Glucose-6-phosphatase deficiency glycogen storage disease

What Is Glycogen Storage Disease Type 1B?

Glycogen storage disease type 1B (GSD1B) is an inherited condition in which the body is unable to break down a complex sugar called glycogen. As a result, glycogen accumulates in cells throughout the body. In GSD1B, specifically, glycogen and fats build up within the liver and kidneys which can cause these organs to be enlarged and not function properly. Signs and symptoms of the condition generally develop at age 3 to 4 months and may include hypoglycemia, seizures, lactic acidosis, hyperuricemia (high levels of a waste product called uric acid in the body), and hyperlipidemia. Affected people may also have short stature; thin arms and legs; a protruding abdomen; neutropenia (which may lead to frequent infections); inflammatory bowel disease and oral health problems. GSD1B is caused by changes (mutations) in the *SLC37A4* gene and is inherited in an autosomal recessive manner. Although there is currently no cure for the condition, symptoms can often be managed with a special diet in combination with certain medications.

Signs and Symptoms

- Decreased glomerular filtration rate

- Delayed puberty

- Doll-like facies

- Elevated hepatic transaminases

- Enlarged kidneys

- Focal segmental glomerulosclerosis

- Gout

- Hepatocellular carcinoma

- Hepatomegaly

- Hyperlipidemia

- Hypertension

- Hypoglycemia

- Lactic acidosis

- Lipemia retinalis

- Nephrolithiasis
- Neutropenia
- Oral ulcer
- Osteoporosis
- Pancreatitis

- Proteinuria
- Protuberant abdomen
- Recurrent bacterial infections
- Short stature
- Xanthomatosis

Other Name

- Glucose-6-phosphate transport defect

Section 54.3

Pompe Disease (Glycogen Storage Disease Type 2)

This section includes text excerpted from "Glycogen Storage Disease Type 2," Genetic and Rare Diseases Information Center (GARD), National Center for Advancing Translational Sciences (NCATS), May 14, 2015.

What Is Glycogen Storage Disease Type 2?

Glycogen storage disease type 2, also known as Pompe disease or acid maltase deficiency disease, is an inherited metabolic disorder caused by an inborn lack of the enzyme acid alpha-glucosidase (also known as acid maltase), which is necessary to break down glycogen, a substance that is a source of energy for the body. This enzyme deficiency causes excess amounts of glycogen to accumulate in the lysosomes, which are structures within cells that break down waste products within the cell. This accumulation of glycogen in certain tissues, especially muscles, impairs their ability to function normally. Glycogen storage disease type 2 is a single disease continuum with variable rates of disease progression. In 2006, the U.S. Food and Drug Administration (FDA) approved the enzyme replacement therapy Myozyme as a treatment for all patients with glycogen storage disease type 2.

Another similar drug called Lumizyme has recently been approved for the treatment this disease.

Symptoms

The classic infantile form of glycogen storage disease type 2 is characterized by severe muscle weakness (myopathy) and abnormally diminished muscle tone (hypotonia) without muscle wasting, and usually manifests within the first few months of life. Additional abnormalities may include enlargement of the heart (cardiomegaly), the liver (hepatomegaly), and/or the tongue (macroglossia). Affected infants may also have poor feeding, failure to gain weight and grow at the expected rate (failure to thrive), breathing problems, and hearing loss. Most infants with glycogen storage disease type 2 cannot hold up their heads or move normally. Without treatment, progressive cardiac failure usually causes life-threatening complications by the age of 12 to 18 months.

The non-classic infantile form of glycogen storage disease type 2 usually presents within the first year of life. Initial symptoms may include delayed motor skills (crawling, sitting) and myopathy. Cardiomegaly may be present, but unlike the classic infantile form, cardiac failure does not typically occur. Muscle weakness may lead to serious, life-compromising breathing problems by early childhood.

In the late onset form of glycogen storage disease type 2, symptoms may not be evident until childhood, adolescence, or adulthood. This form is usually milder than the infantile-onset form of the disorder. Most individuals experience progressive muscle weakness, especially in the legs and the trunk, including the muscles that control breathing.

Signs and Symptoms

- Aplasia/Hypoplasia of the abdominal wall musculature
- Cardiomegaly
- Cognitive impairment
- EEG abnormality
- EMG abnormality
- Emphysema
- Feeding difficulties in infancy
- Gait disturbance
- Hypertrophic cardiomyopathy

- Neurological speech impairment
- Seizures
- Type II diabetes mellitus
- Arrhythmia
- Muscular hypotonia
- Abnormality of the tongue
- Hepatomegaly
- Myopathy
- Recurrent respiratory infections
- Abnormal CNS myelination
- Areflexia
- Cerebral aneurysm
- Diaphragmatic paralysis
- Dyspnea
- Elevated serum creatine phosphokinase
- Fever
- Firm muscles
- Hearing impairment
- Macroglossia
- Proximal muscle weakness
- Respiratory insufficiency due to muscle weakness
- Shortened PR interval
- Splenomegaly
- Wolff-Parkinson-White syndrome

Cause

Mutations in the *GAA* gene cause glycogen storage disease type 2. The *GAA* gene provides instructions for producing an enzyme called acid alpha-glucosidase (commonly called acid maltase). This enzyme is active in lysosomes, which are structures that serve as the cell's recycling center. The enzyme normally breaks down glycogen into a simpler sugar called glucose, which is the main energy source for most cells. Mutations in the *GAA* gene prevent acid alpha-glucosidase from breaking down glycogen, allowing it to build up in the body's cells. Over time, this buildup damages cells throughout the body, particularly muscle cells.

Inheritance

Glycogen storage disease type 2 is inherited in an autosomal recessive pattern, which means both copies of the gene in each cell have mutations. The parents of an individual with an autosomal recessive condition each carry one copy of the mutated gene, but they typically do not show signs and symptoms of the condition.

Treatment

Individuals with glycogen storage disease type 2 are best treated by a team of specialists (such as cardiologist, neurologist, and respiratory therapist) knowledgeable about the disease, who can offer supportive and symptomatic care. The discovery of the *GAA* gene has led to rapid progress in understanding the biological mechanisms and properties of the GAA enzyme. As a result, an enzyme replacement therapy has been developed that has shown, in clinical trials with infantile-onset patients, to decrease heart size, maintain normal heart function, improve muscle function, tone, and strength, and reduce glycogen accumulation. A drug called alglucosidase alfa (Myozyme©) has received FDA approval for the treatment of glycogen storage disease type 2. Myozyme is a form of *GAA*—the enzyme that is absent or reduced in this condition. The drug is usually administered via intravenous infusion every other week. Myozyme has been remarkably successful in reversing cardiac muscle damage and in improving life expectancy in those with the infantile form of the disease.

The medication(s) listed below have been approved by the FDA as orphan products for treatment of this condition.

- **Recombinant human acid alpha-glucosidase; alglucosidase alfa (Brand name: Lumizyme)**

  FDA-approved indication: Lumizyme for patients 8 years and older with late (non-infantile) onset Pompe disease (*GAA* deficiency) who do not have evidence of cardiac hypertrophy. The safety and efficacy of Lumizyme (alglucosidase alfa) have not been evaluated in controlled clinical trials in infantile-onset patients, or in late (non-infantile) onset patients less than 8 years of age.

- **Recombinant human acid alpha-glucosidase (Brand name: Myozyme®)**

  FDA-approved indication: For use in patients with Pompe disease (*GAA* deficiency). Alglucosidase alfa has been shown to improve ventilator-free survival in patients with infantile onset Pompe disease as compared to an untreated historical control, whereas use of Alphaglucosidase in patients with other forms of Pompe disease has not been adequately studied to assure safety and efficacy.

Other Names

- Aglucosidase alfa
- Alpha-1,4-glucosidase deficiency
- Cardiomegalia glycogenica diffusa
- Deficiency of alpha-glucosidase
- GSD II
- Deficiency of lysosomal alpha-glucosidase

Section 54.4

Forbes Disease (Glycogen Storage Disease Type 3)

This section includes text excerpted from "Glycogen Storage Disease Type 3," Genetic and Rare Diseases Information Center (GARD), National Center for Advancing Translational Sciences (NCATS), February 13, 2012. Reviewed November 2016.

What Is Glycogen Storage Disease Type 3 (Forbes Disease)?

Glycogen storage disease type 3 (GSDIII) is an inherited disorder caused by the buildup of glycogen in the body's cells. This buildup impairs the function of certain organs and tissues, especially the liver and muscles. Symptoms typically begin in infancy and may include hypoglycemia, hyperlipidemia (excess of fats in the blood), and elevated blood levels of liver enzymes; later symptoms may include hepatomegaly, chronic liver disease (cirrhosis) and liver failure later in life. Some individuals have short stature and noncancerous (benign) tumors called adenomas in the liver. GSDIII is cause by mutations in the *AGL* gene and is inherited in an autosomal recessive manner. Treatment typically includes a high-protein diet with cornstarch supplementation to maintain a normal level of glucose in the blood. GSDIII is divided into types IIIa, IIIb, IIIc, and IIId.

Symptoms

In infancy, individuals with GSDIII may have low blood sugar (hypoglycemia), increased amounts of fats in the blood (hyperlipidemia), and elevated levels of liver enzymes in the blood. Hypoglycemia may cause occasional seizures in some individuals. As they age, children usually develop an enlarged liver (hepatomegaly), which can cause the abdomen to protrude. Liver size may return to normal during adolescence, but some affected individuals develop chronic liver disease and subsequent liver failure years later. Individuals often have delayed growth due to their liver problems, which can lead to short stature.

They may also have difficulty fighting infections, and may experience unusually frequent nosebleeds. A small percentage of individuals develop benign (non-cancerous) tumors in the liver called adenomas.

GSD types IIIa and IIIc typically affect both the liver and muscles, while types IIIb and IIId typically affect only the liver. Individuals with type IIIa may develop myopathy in both the heart and skeletal muscles later in life. The first signs and symptoms of this are typically poor muscle tone (hypotonia) and mild myopathy in early childhood. The myopathy may become severe by early to mid-adulthood.

Signs and Symptoms

- Abnormality of immune system physiology
- Abnormality of lipid metabolism
- Cognitive impairment
- Full cheeks
- Hypoglycemia
- Short stature
- Myopathy
- Broad nasal tip
- Cardiomyopathy
- Deeply set eye
- Depressed nasal bridge
- Distal amyotrophy
- Elevated hepatic transaminases
- Elevated serum creatine phosphokinase
- Hepatic fibrosis
- Hepatomegaly
- Hyperlipidemia
- Malar flattening
- Midface retrusion
- Muscle weakness
- Ventricular hypertrophy

Cause

GSDIII is caused by changes (mutations) in the *AGL* gene. This gene provides instructions for making the glycogen debranching enzyme, which is involved in the breakdown of glycogen—an important source of stored energy in the body. Most mutations in the *AGL* gene lead to production of a non-working form of the glycogen debranching enzyme; these mutations are usually responsible for causing GSD types IIIa and IIIb. The mutations in the *AGL* gene that cause types IIIc and IIId presumably lead to the production of glycogen debranching enzyme with reduced function. All *AGL* mutations, however, lead to the increased buildup of abnormal, partially broken down glycogen within cells. This buildup damages tissues and organs in the body, thereby causing the signs and symptoms of GSDIII.

Inheritance

GSDIII is inherited in an autosomal recessive manner. This means that mutations in both copies of the disease-causing gene (usually one inherited from each parent) are necessary to cause the condition. Individuals with one abnormal copy of the gene are referred to as carriers; carriers are unaffected and typically do not show any signs or symptoms of the condition. When two carriers for an autosomal recessive condition have children together, each child has a 25 percent (1 in 4) risk to have the condition, a 50 percent (1 in 2) risk to be a carrier like each of his/her parents, and a 25 percent chance to not be a carrier *and* not have the condition.

Diagnosis

GSDIII should be suspected when three main features are present: hepatomegaly (enlarged liver), ketotic hypoglycemia (low blood sugar accompanied by ketosis), and elevated serum concentration of transaminases (a type of enzyme) and CK. Debranching enzyme activity (which is deficient in individuals with the condition) can be measured in a liver biopsy, but this is now not typically necessary for diagnosis. Genetic testing of the *AGL* gene, the only gene known to be associated with GSDIII, confirms the diagnosis.

Treatment

There is not currently a cure for for GSDIII. In some cases, diet therapy is helpful. Strict adherence to a dietary regimen may reduce liver size, prevent hypoglycemia (low blood sugar), help to reduce symptoms, and allow for growth and development. Management typically includes a high-protein diet with cornstarch supplementation to maintain a normal level of glucose in the blood. In infancy, feeding every three to four hours is typically recommended. Toward the end of the first year of life, cornstarch is usually tolerated and can be used to avoid hypoglycemia. A high-protein diet prevents breakdown of muscle protein in times of glucose need and preserves skeletal and cardiac muscles. Skeletal and cardiac myopathies may be improved with high-protein diet and avoiding excessive carbohydrate intake. Liver transplantation may be indicated for patients with hepatic cancers.

Individuals seeking personal treatment advice should speak with their healthcare provider.

Other Names

- Forbes disease

- Cori disease

- Limit dextrinosis

- Amylo-1,6-glucosidase deficiency

- Glycogen debrancher deficiency

Section 54.5

McArdle Disease (Glycogen Storage Disease Type 5)

This section includes text excerpted from "Glycogen Storage Disease Type 5," Genetic and Rare Diseases Information Center (GARD), National Center for Advancing Translational Sciences (NCATS), October 1, 2016.

What Is Glycogen Storage Disease Type 5?

Glycogen storage disease type 5 (GSDV) is a genetic disorder that prevents the body from breaking down glycogen. Glycogen is an important source of energy that is stored in muscle tissue. People with GSDV typically experience fatigue, muscle pain, and cramps during the first few minutes of exercise (exercise intolerance). Usually, when people with this disease rest after brief exercise they can resume exercising with little or no discomfort (a characteristic phenomenon known as "second wind"). The signs and symptoms can vary significantly and may include burgundy-colored urine, fatigue, exercise intolerance, muscle cramps, muscle pain, muscle stiffness, and muscle weakness. It is caused by mutations in the *PYGM* gene and is inherited in an autosomal recessive fashion. There is no cure or specific treatment but

432

the disease can be managed with moderate-intensity aerobic training (e.g., walking or brisk walking, bicycling) and diet.

Signs and Symptoms

- Myopathy
- Abnormality of the cardiovascular system
- Renal insufficiency
- Adult onset
- Elevated serum creatine phosphokinase
- Exercise-induced muscle cramps
- Exercise-induced myalgia
- Muscle weakness
- Myoglobinuria
- Rhabdomyolysis

Other Names

- GSD 5
- McArdle disease
- McArdle type glycogen storage disease
- PYGM deficiency
- Muscle glycogen phosphorylase deficiency
- Myophosphorylase deficiency

Section 54.6

Hers Disease (Glycogen Storage Disease Type 6)

This section includes text excerpted from "Glycogen Storage Disease Type 6," Genetic and Rare Diseases Information Center (GARD), National Center for Advancing Translational Sciences (NCATS), October 1, 2016.

What Is Glycogen Storage Disease Type 6?

Glycogen storage disease type 6 is a genetic disease in which the liver cannot process sugar properly. Symptoms usually begin in infancy or childhood and include low blood sugar (hypoglycemia), an enlarged liver (hepatomegaly), or an increase in the amount of lactic acid in the blood (lactic acidosis) particularly when an individual does not eat for a long time. Symptoms improve significantly as individuals with this condition get older. Glycogen storage disease type 6 is caused by mutations in the *PYGL* gene and is inherited in an autosomal recessive manner.

Signs and Symptoms

- Hypoglycemia
- Short stature
- Hepatomegaly
- Increased hepatic glycogen content
- Postnatal growth retardation

Other Names

- GSD6
- Glycogen storage disease 6
- Hers disease
- Phosphorylase deficiency glycogen-storage disease of liver

Section 54.7

Tarul Disease (Glycogen-Storage Disease Type 7)

This section includes text excerpted from "Glycogen Storage Disease Type 7," Genetic and Rare Diseases Information Center (GARD), National Center for Advancing Translational Sciences (NCATS), October 1, 2016.

What Is Glycogen Storage Disease Type 7?

Glycogen storage disease type 7 (GSD7) is an inherited condition in which the body is unable to break down glycogen (a complex sugar) in the muscle cells. Because glycogen is an important source of energy, this can interfere with the normal functioning of muscle cells. The severity of the condition and the associated signs and symptoms vary, but may include muscle weakness and stiffness; painful muscle cramps; nausea and vomiting; and/or myoglobinuria (the presence of myoglobin in the urine) following moderate to strenuous exercise. Symptoms typically resolve with rest. GSD7 is most commonly diagnosed during childhood; however, some affected people may rarely develop symptoms during infancy or later in adulthood. Those who develop the condition during infancy may experience additional symptoms such as hypotonia (poor muscle tone), cardiomyopathy and breathing difficulties that often lead to a shortened lifespan (less than 1 year). This condition is caused by changes (mutations) in the *PFKM* gene and is inherited in an autosomal recessive manner. There is no specific treatment for GSD7; however, affected people are generally advised to avoid vigorous exercise and high-carbohydrate meals.

Signs and Symptoms

- Myotonia
- Skeletal muscle atrophy
- Cholelithiasis
- Exercise intolerance

435

- Exercise-induced muscle cramps
- Exercise-induced myoglobinuria
- Gout
- Hemolytic anemia
- Increased muscle glycogen content
- Increased total bilirubin
- Jaundice
- Muscle weakness
- Reduced erythrocyte 2,3-diphosphoglycerate concentration
- Reticulocytosis
- Variable expressivity

Other Names

- Muscle phosphofructokinase deficiency
- Tarui disease
- GSD7
- PFKM deficiency

Section 54.8

Fanconi Bickel Syndrome
(Glycogen Storage Disease XI)

This section includes text excerpted from "Fanconi Bickel
Syndrome," Genetic and Rare Diseases Information Center (GARD),
National Center for Advancing Translational Sciences (NCATS),
December 12, 2012. Reviewed November 2016.

What Is Fanconi Bickel Syndrome?

Fanconi Bickel syndrome (FBS) is a rare glycogen storage disease characterized by glycogen accumulation in the liver and kidneys;

severe renal tubular dysfunction; and impaired glucose and galactose metabolism. Signs and symptoms begin in the first few months of life and include failure to thrive, excessive urination (polyuria) and rickets, followed by short stature and hepatosplenomegaly in early childhood. Puberty is delayed. FBS is inherited in an autosomal recessive manner and is caused by mutations in the *SLC2A2* gene. Treatment is generally symptomatic.

Signs and Symptoms

- Abdominal distention
- Chronic acidosis
- Elevated alkaline phosphatase
- Failure to thrive
- Generalized aminoaciduria
- Glycosuria
- Hyperphosphaturia
- Hypokalemia
- Hypophosphatemia
- Hypouricemia
- Impairment of galactose metabolism
- Malabsorption
- Obsolete decreased subcutaneous fat
- Osteomalacia
- Poor appetite
- Renal tubular dysfunction

Treatment

Management of FBS generally focuses on the signs and symptoms of the condition. Treatment includes replacement of water and electrolytes, and vitamin D and phosphate supplements for prevention of hypophosphatemic rickets. Although there is limited data on the effectiveness of dietary treatment for this condition, it is recommended that affected individuals follow a galactose-restricted diabetic diet, with fructose as the main source of carbohydrate. Diet and supplements may alleviate some of the signs and symptoms of the condition but generally do not improve growth, resulting in short stature in adulthood.

Other Names

- Hepatorenal glycogenosis with renal Fanconi syndrome
- Hepatic glycogenosis with amino aciduria and glucosuria
- Fanconi syndrome with intestinal malabsorption and galactose intolerance

- Pseudo-Phlorizin diabetes
- Glycogenosis Fanconi type
- Glycogen storage disease XI
- GLUT2 deficiency
- Glycogen storage disease due to GLUT2 deficiency

Section 54.9

Glycogen Storage Disease 13

This section includes text excerpted from "Glycogen Storage Disease Type 13," Genetic and Rare Diseases Information Center (GARD), National Center for Advancing Translational Sciences (NCATS), June 24, 2012. Reviewed November 2016.

What Is Glycogen Storage Disease Type 13?

Glycogen storage disease type 13 (GSD13), also known as β-enolase deficiency, is an inherited disease of the muscles. The muscles of an affected individual are not able to produce enough energy to function properly, causing muscle weakness and pain. GSD13 is caused by changes (mutations) in the *ENO3* gene and is inherited in an autosomal recessive pattern.

Symptoms

GSD13 causes muscle pain (myalgia). Individuals with GSD13 also experience exercise intolerance, which means they have difficulty exercising because they may have muscle weakness and tire easily.

Signs and Symptoms

- Adult onset
- Elevated serum creatine phosphokinase
- Exercise intolerance
- Increased muscle glycogen content
- Myalgia

Cause

GSD13 is caused by changes (mutations) in the *ENO3* gene. Glycogen is a substance that is stored in muscle tissue and is used as an important source of energy for the muscles during movement and exercise. The *ENO3* gene makes a chemical called enolase, which is an enzyme that helps the muscles use glycogen for energy. In GSD13, the *ENO3* genes do not work properly such that the body cannot make enolase, and as a result, the muscles do not have enough energy to work properly.

Diagnosis

GSD13 is diagnosed by taking a sample of muscle tissue (muscle biopsy) to determine if there is enough of the chemical enolase working in the muscle cells. Genetic testing can also be done to look for changes (mutations) in the *ENO3* gene.

Other Names

- Glycogen storage disease 13
- Enolase-beta deficiency
- Enolase 3 deficiency

Chapter 55

Inherited Metabolic Storage Disorders

Chapter Contents

Section 55.1

Lipid Storage Diseases

This section includes text excerpted from "Lipid Storage Diseases," National Institute of Neurological Disorders and Stroke (NINDS), February 23, 2016.

What Are Lipid Storage Diseases?

Lipid storage diseases, or the lipidoses, are a group of inherited metabolic disorders in which harmful amounts of fatty materials (lipids) accumulate in various cells and tissues in the body. People with these disorders either do not produce enough of one of the enzymes needed to break down (metabolize) lipids or they produce enzymes that do not work properly. Over time, this excessive storage of fats can cause permanent cellular and tissue damage, particularly in the brain, peripheral nervous system, liver, spleen, and bone marrow.

What Are Lipids?

Lipids are fat-like substances that are important parts of the membranes found within and between each cell and in the myelin sheath that coats and protects the nerves. Lipids include oils, fatty acids, waxes, steroids (such as cholesterol and estrogen), and other related compounds.

These fatty materials are stored naturally in the body's cells, organs, and tissues. Minute bodies within cells called lysosomes regularly convert, or metabolize, the lipids and proteins into smaller components to provide energy for the body. Disorders in which intracellular material is stored are called lysosomal storage diseases. In addition to lipid storage diseases, other lysosomal storage diseases include the mucolipidoses, in which excessive amounts of lipids and sugar molecules are stored in the cells and tissues, and the mucopolysaccharidoses, in which excessive amounts of sugar molecules are stored.

How Are Lipid Storage Diseases Inherited?

Lipid storage diseases are inherited from one or both parents who carry a defective gene that regulates a particular protein in a class of the body's cells. They can be inherited two ways:

- *Autosomal recessive* inheritance occurs when both parents carry and pass on a copy of the faulty gene, but neither parent is affected by the disorder. Each child born to these parents has a 25 percent chance of inheriting both copies of the defective gene, a 50 percent chance of being a carrier like the prents, and a 25 percent chance of not inheriting either copy of the defective gene. Children of either gender can be affected by an autosomal recessive this pattern of inheritance.

- *X-linked* inheritance occurs when the mother carries the affected gene on the X chromosome that determines the child's gender and passes it to her son. Sons of carriers have a 50 percent chance of inheriting the disorder. Daughters have a 50 percent chance of inheriting the X-linked chromosome but usually are not severely affected by the disorder. Affected men do not pass the disorder to their sons but their daughters will be carriers for the disorder.

How Are These Disorders Diagnosed?

Diagnosis is made through clinical examination, enzyme assays (which measure enzyme activity), biopsy, genetic testing, and molecular analysis of cells or tissues. In some forms of the disorder, a urine analysis can identify the presence of stored material. Some tests can also determine if a person carries the defective gene that can be passed on to her or his children. This process is known as genotyping.

Biopsy for lipid storage disease involves removing a small sample of the liver or other tissue and studying it under a microscope. In this procedure, a physician will administer a local anesthetic and then remove a small piece of tissue either surgically or by needle biopsy (a small piece of tissue is removed by inserting a thin, hollow needle through the skin). The latter biopsy is usually performed at an outpatient testing facility.

Genetic testing can help individuals who have a family history of lipid storage disease determine if they are carrying a mutated gene that causes the disorder. Other genetic tests can determine if a fetus has the disorder or is a carrier of the defective gene. Prenatal testing is usually done by *chorionic villus sampling*, in which a very small sample of the placenta is removed and tested during early pregnancy. The sample, which contains the same DNA as the fetus, is removed by catheter or fine needle inserted through the cervix or by a fine needle inserted through the abdomen. Results are usually available within 2 weeks.

What Are the Types of Lipid Storage Disease?

- Gaucher disease

- Niemann-Pick disease

- Fabry disease (also known as alpha-galactosidase-A deficiency)

- Farber disease (also known as Farber lipogranulomatosis)

- GM1 gangliosidoses

- GM2 gangliosidoses

  - Tay-Sachs disease (also known as GM2 gangliosidosis-variant B)

  - Sandhoff disease (variant AB)

- Krabbe disease (also known as globoid cell leukodystrophy and galactosylceramide lipidosis)

- Metachromatic leukodystrophy, or MLD

- Wolman disease (also known as acid lipase deficiency)

How Are These Disorders Treated?

Currently, there is no specific treatment available for most of the lipid storage disorders but highly effective enzyme replacement therapy is available for patients with type 1 Gaucher disease and some patients with type 3 Gaucher disease. Patients with anemia may require blood transfusions. In some patients, the enlarged spleen must be removed to improve cardiopulmonary function. Medications such as gabapentin and carbamazepine may be prescribed to help treat pain (including bone pain) for patients with Fabry disease. Restricting one's diet does not prevent lipid buildup in cells and tissues.

Section 55.2

Gaucher Disease

This section includes text excerpted from "Gaucher
Disease," National Institute of Neurological Disorders and
Stroke (NINDS), August 22, 2016.

What Is Gaucher Disease?

Gaucher disease is one of the inherited metabolic disorders known as
lipid storage diseases. Lipids are fatty materials that include oils, fatty
acids, waxes, and steroids (such as cholesterol and estrogen). Gaucher
disease is caused by a deficiency of the enzyme *glucocerebrosidase*. Fatty
materials can accumulate in the brain, spleen, liver, lungs, bone marrow,
and kidneys. Symptoms may begin in early life or adulthood and include
skeletal disorders and bone lesions that may cause pain and fractures,
enlarged spleen and liver, liver malfunction, anemia, and yellow spots in
the eyes. There are three common clinical subtypes of Gaucher disease.
The first category, called **type 1** (or nonneuropathic), typically does not
affect the brain. Symptoms may begin early in life or in adulthood. People
in this group usually bruise easily due to low blood platelets and experience fatigue due to anemia They also may have an enlarged liver and
spleen. Many individuals with a mild form of the disorder may not show
any symptoms. In **type 2** Gaucher disease (acute infantile neuropathic
Gaucher disease), symptoms usually begin by 3 months of age and include
extensive brain damage, seizures, spasticity, poor ability to suck and swallow, and enlarged liver and spleen. Affected children usually die before 2
years of age. In the third category, called **type 3** (or chronic neuropathic
Gaucher disease), signs of brain involvement such as seizures gradually
become apparent. Major symptoms also include skeletal irregularities,
eye movement disorders, cognitive deficit, poor coordination, enlarged
liver and spleen, respiratory problems, and blood disorders.

Is There Any Treatment?

Enzyme replacement therapy is available for most people with
types 1 and **3** Gaucher disease. Given intravenously every two weeks,

this therapy decreases liver and spleen size, reduces skeletal abnormalities, and reverses other symptoms of the disorder. The U.S. Food and Drug Administration (FDA) has approved eligustat tartrate for Gaucher treatment, which works by administering small molecules that reduce the action of the enzyme that catalyzes glucose to ceramide. Surgery to remove the whole or part of the spleen may be required on rare occasions, and blood transfusions may benefit some anemic individuals. Other individuals may require joint replacement surgery to improve mobility and quality of life. There is no effective treatment for severe brain damage that may occur in persons with **types 2** and **3** Gaucher disease.

What Is the Prognosis?

Enzyme replacement therapy is very beneficial for **type 1** and most type 3 individuals with this condition. Successful bone marrow transplantation can reverse the non-neurological effects of the disease, but the procedure carries a high risk and is rarely performed in individuals with Gaucher disease.

Section 55.3

Mucopolysaccharidoses

This section includes text excerpted from
"Mucopolysaccharidoses," National Institute of Neurological
Disorders and Stroke (NINDS), February 23, 2016.

What Are the Mucopolysaccharidoses?

The mucopolysaccharidoses are a group of inherited metabolic diseases caused by the absence or malfunctioning of certain enzymes needed to break down molecules called glycosaminoglycans—long chains of sugar carbohydrates in each of our cells that help build bone, cartilage, tendons, corneas, skin, and connective tissue. Glycosaminoglycans (formerly called mucopolysaccharides) are also found in the fluid that lubricates our joints.

People with a mucopolysaccharidosis either do not produce enough of one of the 11 enzymes required to break down these sugar chains into proteins and simpler molecules or they produce enzymes that do not work properly. Over time, these glycosaminoglycans collect in the cells, blood, and connective tissues. The result is permanent, progressive cellular damage that affects the individual's appearance, physical abilities, organ and system functioning, and, in most cases, cognitive development.

Who Is at Risk?

It is estimated that one in every 25,000 babies born in the United States will have some form of the mucopolysaccharidoses. They are autosomal recessive disorders, meaning that only individuals inheriting the defective gene from both parents are affected. (The exception is MPS II, or Hunter syndrome, in which the mother alone passes along the defective gene to a son.) When both people in a couple have the defective gene, each pregnancy carries with it a one in four chance that the child will be affected. The parents and siblings of an affected child may have no sign of the disorder. Unaffected siblings and select relatives of a child with one of the mucopolysaccharidoses may carry the recessive gene and could pass it to their own children.

In general, the following factors may increase the chance of getting or passing on a genetic disease:

- A family history of a genetic disease.

- Parents who are closely related or part of a distinct ethnic or geographic circle.

- Parents who do not show disease symptoms but carry a disease gene.

The mucopolysaccharidoses are classified as lysosomal storage diseases. These are conditions in which large numbers of molecules that are normally broken down or degraded into smaller pieces by intracellular units called lysosomes accumulate in harmful amounts in the body's cells and tissues, particularly in the lysosomes.

What Are the Signs and Symptoms?

The mucopolysaccharidoses share many clinical features but have varying degrees of severity. These features may not be apparent at

447

birth but progress as storage of glycosaminoglycans affects bone, skeletal structure, connective tissues, and organs. Neurological complications may include damage to neurons (which send and receive signals throughout the body) as well as pain and impaired motor function. This results from compression of nerves or nerve roots in the spinal cord or in the peripheral nervous system, the part of the nervous system that connects the brain and spinal cord to sensory organs such as the eyes and to other organs, muscles, and tissues throughout the body.

Depending on the mucopolysaccharidoses subtype, affected individuals may have normal intellect or may be profoundly impaired, may experience developmental delay, or may have severe behavioral problems. Many individuals have hearing loss, either conductive (in which pressure behind the ear drum causes fluid from the lining of the middle ear to build up and eventually congeal), neurosensitive (in which tiny hair cells in the inner ear are damaged), or both. Communicating hydrocephalus, in which the normal circulation of cerebrospinal fluid becomes blocked over time and causes increased pressure inside the head, is common in some of the mucopolysaccharidoses. Surgically inserting a shunt into the brain can drain fluid. The eye's cornea often becomes cloudy from intracellular storage, and degeneration of the retina and glaucoma also may affect the patient's vision.

Physical symptoms generally include coarse or rough facial features (including a flat nasal bridge, thick lips, and enlarged mouth and tongue), short stature with disproportionately short trunk (dwarfism), dysplasia (abnormal bone size and/or shape) and other skeletal irregularities, thickened skin, enlarged organs such as liver or spleen, hernias, and excessive body hair growth. Short and often claw-like hands, progressive joint stiffness, and carpal tunnel syndrome can restrict hand mobility and function. Recurring respiratory infections are common, as are obstructive airway disease and obstructive sleep apnea. Many affected individuals also have heart disease, often involving enlarged or diseased heart valves.

Another lysosomal storage disease often confused with the mucopolysaccharidoses is *mucolipidosis*. In this disorder, excessive amounts of fatty materials known as lipids (another principal component of living cells) are stored, in addition to sugars. Persons with mucolipidosis may share some of the clinical features associated with the mucopolysaccharidoses (certain facial features, bony structure abnormalities, and damage to the brain), and increased amounts of the enzymes needed to break down the lipids are found in the blood.

What Are the Different Types of the Mucopolysaccharidoses?

Seven distinct clinical types and numerous subtypes of the mucopolysaccharidoses have been identified. Although each mucopolysaccharidosis (MPS) differs clinically, most patients generally experience a period of normal development followed by a decline in physical and/ or mental function.

- MPS I
- MPS II, Hunter syndrome
- MPS III, Sanfilippo syndrome
  - MPS IIIA
  - MPS IIIB
  - MPS IIIC
  - MPS IIID
- MPS IV, Morquio syndrome
- MPS VI, Maroteaux-Lamy syndrome
- MPS VII, Sly syndrome

How Are the Mucopolysaccharidoses Diagnosed?

Clinical examination and urine tests (excess mucopolysaccharides are excreted in the urine) are the first steps in the diagnosis of an MPS disease. Enzyme assays (testing a variety of cells or blood in culture for enzyme deficiency) are also used to provide definitive diagnosis of one of the mucopolysaccharidoses. Prenatal diagnosis using amniocentesis and chorionic villus sampling can verify if a fetus is affected with the disorder. Genetic counseling can help parents who have a family history of the mucopolysaccharidoses determine if they are carrying the mutated gene that causes the disorders.

How Are the Mucopolysaccharidoses Treated?

Currently there is no cure for these disorders. Medical care is directed at treating systemic conditions and improving the person's quality of life. Physical therapy and daily exercise may delay joint problems and improve the ability to move.

Changes to the diet will not prevent disease progression, but limiting milk, sugar, and dairy products has helped some individuals experiencing excessive mucus.

Surgery to remove tonsils and adenoids may improve breathing among affected individuals with obstructive airway disorders and sleep apnea. Sleep studies can assess airway status and the possible need for nighttime oxygen. Some patients may require surgical insertion of an endotrachial tube to aid breathing. Surgery can also correct hernias, help drain excessive cerebrospinal fluid from the brain, and free nerves and nerve roots compressed by skeletal and other abnormalities. Corneal transplants may improve vision among patients with significant corneal clouding.

Enzyme replacement therapies are currently in use for MPS I, MPS II, and MPS VI, and are being tested in the other MPS disorders. Enzyme replacement therapy has proven useful in reducing non-neurological symptoms and pain.

Bone marrow transplantation (BMT) and umbilical cord blood transplantation (UCBT) have had limited success in treating the mucopolysaccharidoses. Abnormal physical characteristics, except for those affecting the skeleton and eyes, may be improved, but neurologic outcomes have varied. BMT and UCBT are high-risk procedures and are usually performed only after family members receive extensive evaluation and counseling.

Section 55.4

Globoid-Cell Leukodystrophy (Krabbe Disease)

This section includes text excerpted from "Krabbe Disease," Genetic and Rare Diseases Information Center (GARD), National Center for Advancing Translational Sciences (NCATS), October 9, 2015.

What Is Krabbe Disease?

Krabbe disease is an inherited condition that affects the nervous system. The signs and symptoms of the condition and the disease severity differ by type. Babies affected by early-onset (infantile) Krabbe disease, the most common and severe form of the condition, typically develop features in the first six months of life. Symptoms of infantile Krabbe disease may include irritability; failure to thrive; slowed development; unexplained fevers; and progressive muscle weakness, hearing loss and vision loss. People affected by the late-onset forms may not develop symptoms until later in childhood, early adolescence or even into adulthood. Signs and symptoms of these forms are extremely variable but may include muscle weakness and rigidity; walking difficulties; vision loss; intellectual regression; and/or seizures. Krabbe disease is caused by changes (mutations) in the *GALC* gene and is inherited in an autosomal recessive manner. Treatment is generally based on the signs and symptoms present in each person; however, preliminary studies suggest that it may be beneficial to use hematopoietic stem cell transplantation (i.e., umbilical cord blood stem cells) as a treatment for patients in the early stages of infantile Krabbe disease and older people with mild symptoms.

Symptoms

The signs and symptoms of Krabbe disease can develop at different ages. Babies affected by early-onset (infantile) Krabbe disease typically develop features in the first six months of life, while people affected by the late-onset forms may not develop symptoms until later in childhood, early adolescence or even into adulthood.

Approximately 85–90 percent of people affected by Krabbe disease have the infantile form which is characterized by the following features:

- Developmental delay and/or regression
- Failure to thrive
- Hearing loss
- Hypertonia
- Irritability
- Peripheral neuropathy
- Seizures
- Sensitivity to loud sounds
- Unexplained fevers
- Vision loss
- Vomiting and other feeding difficulties

Signs and symptoms of the later-onset forms are extremely variable but may include muscle weakness and rigidity; walking difficulties; vision loss; intellectual regression; and/or seizures.

Cause

Krabbe disease is caused by changes (mutations) in the *GALC* gene. This gene provides instructions for making an enzyme called galactosylceramidase, which breaks down a certain type of fat that is primarily found in the brain and kidneys. Mutations in the *GALC* gene lead to reduced levels of the galactosylceramidase enzyme which can cause a build up of toxic fats in the cells of the brain and other tissues. This may result in the progressive loss of myelin, the protective covering around certain nerve cells that ensures the rapid transmission of nerve impulses. Without myelin, nerves in the brain and other parts of the body cannot function properly, leading to the signs and symptoms of Krabbe disease.

Inheritance

Krabbe disease is inherited in an autosomal recessive manner. This means that to be affected, a person must have a mutation in both copies of the responsible gene in each cell. The parents of an affected person usually each carry one mutated copy of the gene and are referred to as carriers. Carriers typically do not show signs or symptoms of the condition. When two carriers of an autosomal recessive condition have children, each child has a 25 percent (1 in 4) risk to have the condition, a 50 percent (1 in 2) risk to be a carrier like each of the parents, and a 25 percent chance to not have the condition *and* not be a carrier.

Diagnosis

A diagnosis of Krabbe disease may be suspected based on the presence of characteristic signs and symptoms or in certain states of the United States, due to an abnormal newborn screen. Additional testing can then be ordered to confirm the diagnosis. This testing generally includes a blood test and/or skin biopsy to evaluate the levels of galactosylceramidase, the enzyme that is low in people with Krabbe disease. Genetic testing for changes (mutations) in the *GALC* gene can also confirm the diagnosis.

Treatment

Unfortunately, there is no cure for Krabbe disease. However, preliminary studies suggest hematopoietic stem cell transplantation (i.e., umbilical cord blood stem cells) may be an effective treatment in affected babies who have not yet developed symptoms and in older people with mild symptoms. For example, there is evidence that this treatment may delay disease progression and improve survival and quality of life. Although both short-term and long-term benefits have been reported, the data comes primarily from small clinical trials; thus, additional research is needed to more clearly define the outcomes of this treatment.

When a diagnosis is made after a person has already developed symptoms, treatment is focused on the symptoms present and may include various medications, adaptive equipment and therapies— including physical, respiratory, occupational, and speech.

The advocacy organization, Hunter's Hope, offers a family resource guide that includes information on the supportive treatment of Krabbe disease as well as tips for caring for an affected child. Please click on the link to access this resource.

Prognosis

The long-term outlook (prognosis) for people with Krabbe disease varies by type. Infantile Krabbe disease is generally fatal before age two. However, prognosis may be better for children who receive umbilical cord blood stem cells prior to disease onset or early bone marrow transplantation.

People with later-onset Krabbe disease generally have a milder course of the disease. However, the progression of disease and lifespan reduction can vary significantly.

Section 55.5

Metachromatic Leukodystrophy (MLD)

This section includes text excerpted from "Metachromatic Leukodystrophy," Genetics Home Reference (GHR), National Institutes of Health (NIH), September 28, 2016.

What Is Metachromatic Leukodystrophy?

Metachromatic leukodystrophy is an inherited disorder characterized by the accumulation of fats called sulfatides in cells. This accumulation especially affects cells in the nervous system that produce myelin, the substance that insulates and protects nerves. Nerve cells covered by myelin make up a tissue called white matter. Sulfatide accumulation in myelin-producing cells causes progressive destruction of white matter (leukodystrophy) throughout the nervous system, including in the brain and spinal cord (the central nervous system) and the nerves connecting the brain and spinal cord to muscles and sensory cells that detect sensations such as touch, pain, heat, and sound (the peripheral nervous system).

In people with metachromatic leukodystrophy, white matter damage causes progressive deterioration of intellectual functions and motor skills, such as the ability to walk. Affected individuals also develop loss of sensation in the extremities (peripheral neuropathy), incontinence, seizures, paralysis, an inability to speak, blindness, and hearing loss. Eventually they lose awareness of their surroundings and become unresponsive. While neurological problems are the primary feature of metachromatic leukodystrophy, effects of sulfatide accumulation on other organs and tissues have been reported, most often involving the gallbladder.

The most common form of metachromatic leukodystrophy, affecting about 50 to 60 percent of all individuals with this disorder, is called the late infantile form. This form of the disorder usually appears in the second year of life. Affected children lose any speech they have developed, become weak, and develop problems with walking (gait disturbance). As the disorder worsens, muscle tone generally first decreases, and then increases to the point of rigidity. Individuals with the late infantile form of metachromatic leukodystrophy typically do not survive past childhood.

In 20 to 30 percent of individuals with metachromatic leukodystrophy, onset occurs between the age of 4 and adolescence. In this juvenile form, the first signs of the disorder may be behavioral problems and increasing difficulty with schoolwork. Progression of the disorder is slower than in the late infantile form, and affected individuals may survive for about 20 years after diagnosis.

The adult form of metachromatic leukodystrophy affects approximately 15 to 20 percent of individuals with the disorder. In this form, the first symptoms appear during the teenage years or later. Often behavioral problems such as alcoholism, drug abuse, or difficulties at school or work are the first symptoms to appear. The affected individual may experience psychiatric symptoms such as delusions or hallucinations. People with the adult form of metachromatic leukodystrophy may survive for 20 to 30 years after diagnosis. During this time there may be some periods of relative stability and other periods of more rapid decline.

Metachromatic leukodystrophy gets its name from the way cells with an accumulation of sulfatides appear when viewed under a microscope. The sulfatides form granules that are described as metachromatic, which means they pick up color differently than surrounding cellular material when stained for examination.

Frequency

Metachromatic leukodystrophy is reported to occur in 1 in 40,000 to 160,000 individuals worldwide. The condition is more common in certain genetically isolated populations: 1 in 75 in a small group of Jews who immigrated to Israel from southern Arabia (Habbanites), 1 in 2,500 in the western portion of the Navajo Nation, and 1 in 8,000 among Arab groups in Israel.

Inheritance Pattern

This condition is inherited in an autosomal recessive pattern, which means both copies of the gene in each cell have mutations. The parents of an individual with an autosomal recessive condition each carry one copy of the mutated gene, but they typically do not show signs and symptoms of the condition.

Other Names for This Condition

- ARSA deficiency
- arylsulfatase A deficiency disease

- cerebral sclerosis, diffuse, metachromatic form
- cerebroside sulphatase deficiency disease
- Greenfield disease
- metachromatic leukoencephalopathy
- MLD
- sulfatide lipidosis
- sulfatidosis

Section 55.6

X-Linked Adrenoleukodystrophy (ALD)

This section includes text excerpted from "X-Linked
Adrenoleukodystrophy," Genetics Home Reference (GHR),
National Institutes of Health (NIH), September 28, 2016.

What Is X-Linked Adrenoleukodystrophy?

X-linked adrenoleukodystrophy is a genetic disorder that occurs primarily in males. It mainly affects the nervous system and the adrenal glands, which are small glands located on top of each kidney. In this disorder, the fatty covering (myelin) that insulates nerves in the brain and spinal cord is prone to deterioration (demyelination), which reduces the ability of the nerves to relay information to the brain. In addition, damage to the outer layer of the adrenal glands (adrenal cortex) causes a shortage of certain hormones (adrenocortical insufficiency). Adrenocortical insufficiency may cause weakness, weight loss, skin changes, vomiting, and coma.

There are three distinct types of X-linked adrenoleukodystrophy: a childhood cerebral form, an adrenomyeloneuropathy type, and a form called Addison disease only.

Children with the cerebral form of X-linked adrenoleukodystrophy experience learning and behavioral problems that usually begin between the ages of 4 and 10. Over time the symptoms worsen, and these children may have difficulty reading, writing, understanding speech, and comprehending written material. Additional signs and symptoms of the cerebral form include aggressive behavior, vision problems, difficulty swallowing, poor coordination, and impaired adrenal gland function. The rate at which this disorder progresses is variable but can be extremely rapid, often leading to total disability within a few years. The life expectancy of individuals with this type depends on the severity of the signs and symptoms and how quickly the disorder progresses. Individuals with the cerebral form of X-linked adrenoleukodystrophy usually survive only a few years after symptoms begin but may survive longer with intensive medical support.

Signs and symptoms of the adrenomyeloneuropathy type appear between early adulthood and middle age. Affected individuals develop progressive stiffness and weakness in their legs (paraparesis), experience urinary and genital tract disorders, and often show changes in behavior and thinking ability. Most people with the adrenomyeloneuropathy type also have adrenocortical insufficiency. In some severely affected individuals, damage to the brain and nervous system can lead to early death.

People with X-linked adrenoleukodystrophy whose only symptom is adrenocortical insufficiency are said to have the Addison disease only form. In these individuals, adrenocortical insufficiency can begin anytime between childhood and adulthood. However, most affected individuals develop the additional features of the adrenomyeloneuropathy type by the time they reach middle age. The life expectancy of individuals with this form depends on the severity of the signs and symptoms, but typically this is the mildest of the three types.

Rarely, individuals with X-linked adrenoleukodystrophy develop multiple features of the disorder in adolescence or early adulthood. In addition to adrenocortical insufficiency, these individuals usually have psychiatric disorders and a loss of intellectual function (dementia). It is unclear whether these individuals have a distinct form of the condition or a variation of one of the previously described types.

For reasons that are unclear, different forms of X-linked adrenoleukodystrophy can be seen in affected individuals within the same family.

Frequency

The prevalence of X-linked adrenoleukodystrophy is 1 in 20,000 to 50,000 individuals worldwide. This condition occurs with a similar frequency in all populations.

Inheritance Pattern

X-linked adrenoleukodystrophy is inherited in an X-linked pattern. A condition is considered X-linked if the mutated gene that causes the disorder is located on the X chromosome, one of the two sex chromosomes in each cell. In males (who have only one X chromosome), one altered copy of the *ABCD1* gene in each cell is sufficient to cause X-linked adrenoleukodystrophy. Because females have two copies of the X chromosome, one altered copy of the *ABCD1* gene in each cell usually does not cause any features of X-linked adrenoleukodystrophy; however, some females with one altered copy of the gene have health problems associated with this disorder. The signs and symptoms of X-linked adrenoleukodystrophy tend to appear at a later age in females than in males. Affected women usually develop features of the adrenomyeloneuropathy type.

Other Names for This Condition

- Addison disease and cerebral sclerosis
- melanodermic leukodystrophy
- Schilder-Addison Complex
- Schilder disease
- Siemerling-Creutzfeldt disease
- X-ALD

Chapter 56

McCune-Albright Syndrome

What Is McCune-Albright Syndrome?

McCune-Albright Syndrome (MAS) is a genetic disorder that affects the skin, bones, and the production of certain hormones. Because of its effects on hormones, MAS often causes early puberty in girls. There are also other distinctive symptoms, such as light-brown birthmarks and unusual formations of the bones.

What Are the Symptoms of McCune-Albright Syndrome?

MAS symptoms can vary from mild to severe. They may begin at birth or later in childhood.

Main Symptoms

Many people with MAS have the following symptoms:

- **Café-au-lait spots**

  - Café-au-lait (French for "coffee with milk") spots, which are light-brown birthmarks. The birthmarks:

This chapter includes text excerpted from "McCune-Albright Syndrome (MAS)," *Eunice Kennedy Shriver* National Institute of Child Health and Human Development (NICHD), January 14, 2014.

- are usually are present at birth

- may be hard to see on dark skin

- often appear on one side of the body

- have jagged edges sometimes referred to as the "coast of Maine"

- **Polyostotic fibrous dysplasia**

  A person with polyostotic fibrous dysplasia (PFD) has scar-like tissue, or fibrous tissue, in his or her bones. PFD usually occurs on one side of the body in weight-bearing bones, such as leg bones. PFD may cause:

  - bone pain

  - cancer of the bone (very rare)

  - abnormal bone growth

  - fractures

  - limping

  - scoliosis, a curvature of the spine

  - uneven growth, including uneven growth of the face

  In addition, bone lesions in the skull may pinch nerves that affect a person's ability to see and hear.

- **Precocious puberty**

  Precocious puberty is when sexual and physical changes occur earlier than normal.

  Girls with MAS may experience such symptoms as:

  - early menstrual bleeding, usually before 2 years of age

  - early breast growth

  - beginning to grow faster

  Boys with MAS are less likely to experience early puberty. Symptoms in boys include:

  - faster than normal growth of penis or testicles

  - premature sexual behavior

  - early growth of armpit or pubic hair

Additional Symptoms

Additional features of MAS may include (but are not limited to):

- overproduction of growth hormone from the pituitary gland
- Cushing syndrome, overactivity of the adrenal glands, leading to an increase in stress hormone levels
- formation of benign (noncancerous) tumors in the testicles, called Sertoli cell hyperplasia and Leydig cell hyperplasia
- hyperthyroidism, an overactive thyroid gland
- loss of phosphate in the urine, leading to low blood phosphorus levels
- liver disease

How Many People Are Affected/at Risk by McCune-Albright Syndrome?

Number of People Affected

MAS is rare, affecting between 1 in every 100,000 to 1 million live births worldwide.

Who Is at Risk?

Because the genetic change or mutation that causes MAS occurs at random very early in fetal development, MAS is not an inherited disease, meaning parents do not pass it on to their children.

MAS likely occurs equally in males and females.

What Causes McCune-Albright Syndrome?

MAS is a genetic disorder, which means that a change, also called a mutation, in a gene causes it. Genes are in the chromosomes of almost all human cells, and they code for each cell's specialized actions. The mutation that causes MAS leads to errors in the functioning of certain cells.

MAS is not an inherited disease, meaning parents do not pass it on to their child, because the mutation occurs randomly while an embryo is developing.

GNAS Gene Mutation

MAS is caused by a mutation in the *GNAS* gene. The *GNAS* gene codes for one part of the G protein, which is short for guanine nucleotide-binding protein. This protein plays an important role in triggering many other cell processes. One of these processes is to turn off an enzyme called the adenylate cyclase enzyme. The mutated form of the G protein cannot turn this enzyme off, so the constantly active adenylate cyclase enzyme causes excess production of other hormones, resulting in the symptoms of MAS.

Mosaicism

The *GNAS* mutation happens after an embryo begins to form, and not when the mother's egg or the father's sperm is formed. Therefore, not all of the embryo's cells have the mutation. This is called mosaicism. The severity of MAS symptoms depends on the number and location of cells containing the mutated *GNAS* gene.

MAS is caused by a mutation in the *GNAS* gene. The mutation leads to errors in the functioning of certain cells.

The *GNAS* gene codes for one part of the G protein, which is short for guanine nucleotide-binding protein. This protein plays an important role in triggering many cell processes, including the process that "turns off" an enzyme called the adenylate cyclase enzyme. The mutated form of the G protein cannot turn off the enzyme. High levels of active adenylate cyclase cause excess production of other hormones, resulting in the symptoms of MAS.

Not every cell in the body is exactly the same, so some cells may have the *GNAS* mutation while others do not. This is called mosaicism. The severity of MAS symptoms depends on the number of cells with the mutated *GNAS* gene and the location of those cells in the body.

How Do HealthCare Providers Diagnose McCune-Albright Syndrome?

A person is diagnosed with MAS if he or she has a combination of any of the following symptoms:

- café-au-lait (French for "coffee with milk") spots, which are light brown birthmarks

- PFD, which is a bone irregularity

- precocious puberty, which is premature development in a child

- hyperthyroidism, which is an overactive thyroid gland

- growth hormone excess

- Cushing syndrome, an overactivity of the adrenal glands

- Sertoli cell hyperplasia and Leydig cell hyperplasia, which are tumors in the testicles

A healthcare provider may use X-rays to examine bones for PFD. He or she may perform ultrasounds to look for an abnormal appearance of the thyroid or testicles. Blood tests may be done to check for abnormal hormone levels. He or she may take a small sample or biopsy of abnormal bone tissue and analyze it to confirm PFD, thereby confirming MAS.

A genetic test is also available to detect the *GNAS* gene mutation, but it is often not reliable for diagnosing MAS. The diagnosis of MAS is made clinically, based on the presence of characteristic features.

Symptoms and severity of MAS vary, so diagnosis may occur at birth or later in childhood.

What Are the Treatments for McCune-Albright Syndrome?

Treatment for MAS depends on the extent and the severity of a person's symptoms. For example, healthcare providers may recommend medication for endocrine problems, or surgery for bone issues.

- Medications, including agents that block the production of certain hormones, may help address several conditions associated with MAS, including:

  - Cushing syndrome

  - hyperthyroidism

  - growth hormone excess

  - low blood phosphates

  - precocious puberty

  - bone pain

- Surgery may help address:

  - bone deformities or uneven growth

  - Cushing syndrome, by removing adrenal glands

  - hyperthyroidism, by removing the thyroid gland

  - hearing and vision problems, such as by relieving pinched nerves

Healthcare providers may also recommend bisphosphonates, or drugs that help prevent bone loss. More research is needed to determine the role of these medications in MAS; at present, they are often recommended to treat pain from the PFD caused by MAS. In addition, strengthening exercises may help build muscle around bones affected by PFD, which can reduce the risk of bone fractures.

Chapter 57

Metabolic Diseases of the Muscle

Metabolism is a term used to describe the system by which the body breaks down food into sugars and acids, which it uses for energy. A metabolic disorder takes place when abnormal chemical reactions interrupt this process causing an individual to have too much or too little of certain substances needed for optimal health. When such disorders affect muscles they can be called metabolic myopathy (from the Greek *myo*—"muscle" and *pathos*—"suffering"), or simply metabolic muscle diseases.

This group of rare disorders is caused by genetic defects that are usually the result of enzyme defects in the body that make it difficult for the muscles to maintain adequate levels of adenosine triphosphate (ATP) a molecule that stores the energy we need to do work. Some of the metabolic muscle diseases that begin in infancy can be very serious, or even fatal, while those that affect older children or adults are often (although not always) less severe, tend to progress more slowly, and are generally more treatable, sometimes through adjustments in lifestyle, physical activity, or diet.

Types of Metabolic Muscle Diseases

Metabolic muscle diseases are a very large and diverse group of conditions. And although some of these disorders don't fit neatly into

"Metabolic Diseases of the Muscle," © 2017 Omnigraphics. Reviewed November 2016.

categories, the majority of them are often organized into three major types:

1. **Glycogen metabolic disorders.** The body needs glucose (sugar) to generate energy, and most glucose is stored in the liver and muscles as a substance called glycogen. When the body is unable to convert sufficient amounts of this material into a usable form of energy, glycogen metabolic disorders are the result. There are numerous glycogen metabolic disorders, some of which include McArdle disease, Pompe disease, and Tarui disease.

2. **Lipid metabolic diseases.** Lipids are water-insoluble fatty molecules that, among other biological functions, are responsible for storing energy. When abnormalities occur in the enzymes that break down lipids, the result can be a buildup of fatty acids, which can cause muscle weakness and pain. Some lipid metabolic disorders include carnitine palmitoyltransferase II deficiency (CPT II), very long-chain acyl-CoA dehydrogenase deficiency (VLCAD), and trifunctional protein deficiency (TFP).

3. **Mitochondrial myopathies.** Mitochondria are rod-shaped organelles (specialized cell structures) that convert nutrients into ATP and produce energy. Because they are found in all cells, problems with mitochondria, generally caused by genetic mutations, may result in disorders in many systems, including the muscles. Mitochondrial myopathies include Myoclonus Epilepsy with Ragged-Red Fibers (MERFF), Mitochondrial DNA depletion syndrome (MDS), and Progressive external ophthalmoplegia (PEO).

Symptoms

Since the group of metabolic muscle diseases is so large and varied, symptoms may be specific to the particular disorder. But, in general, they can be broken down into two groups.

1. Dynamic, or activity-related symptoms, such as:

   - pain after exercise

   - cramps

   - myoglobinuria (myoglobin in the urine, usually from muscle deterioration)

- weakness after exercise or in response to cold

2. Static, or fixed symptoms, which include:

- progressive muscle weakness
- swollen and tender muscles
- systemic involvement, such as with disorders of the endocrine system or the brain
- general malaise

Diagnosis

Because metabolic muscle diseases are both rare and diverse, diagnosing them can be a challenge, especially since many symptoms are common to all three major types. In general, doctors use biopsies and various blood tests to narrow down a diagnosis. And as with most medical conditions, the process begins with a thorough patient history and physical examination, then proceeds to various diagnostic tests.

- Blood tests, such as:
  - complete blood count (CBC)
  - serum electrolytes
  - glucose levels
  - ammonia levels
  - liver transaminases (an enzyme whose level may indicate muscle damage)
  - creatinine and blood urea nitrogen levels
  - creatine kinase (an enzyme found in the muscles and brain)
  - thyroid function test
- Other diagnostic tests, including:
  - urinalysis
  - forearm ischemic lactate test (which measures lactate and ammonia levels after forearm exercise)
  - electromyography (in which needle electrodes measure electrical currents in a muscle as it contracts)
  - muscle biopsy (the removal of a small piece of muscle tissue for analysis)

- electrocardiogram, or EKG (a test of heart function)

- DNA analysis (used especially in tests for mitochondrial myopathies)

- magnetic resonance imaging, or MRI (generally used to test for complications)

Treatments

Not surprisingly, treatments for metabolic muscle diseases vary widely depending upon the disorder's type and underlying cause. Common treatments include medication, physical therapy, braces and other devices, lifestyle changes, and diet restrictions. More specific treatments are recommended based on the classification of disease:

- Glycogen metabolic muscular disorders

  - Patients are often advised to engage in regular aerobic exercise while avoiding isometric, or muscle-straining, activities. Studies show that those who follow such an exercise routine have a much better long-term outcome and quality of life, so physical therapy is frequently recommended.

  - Maintaining blood glucose levels during the daytime has been shown to help alleviate exercise intolerance. This can be accomplished through diet or by consuming the equivalent of 40 grams of sugar about 30–40 minutes before exercise.

  - Depending on the specific type of disorder, a high-protein diet may prove beneficial, as will eating several small meals throughout the day, rather fewer large meals.

  - Certain medications, such as statins, should be avoided. Typically prescribed to reduce blood pressure, statins are a class of drug that have muscle aches as a known side effect. There is also evidence that patients with an underlying metabolic muscular disorder have a predisposition to even more serious statin myopathy.

  - Some glycogen disorders result in a build-up of high levels of uric acid in the body, resulting in muscle and joint pain, as with gout. To counter this, a doctor may prescribe corticosteroids or other medications. In addition, patients are also often advised to increase their water intake, modify their diet, and take citric acid or other supplements.

- In some cases, doctors advise that young children with glycogen metabolic muscular disorders be given a mixture of uncooked cornstarch and water or soy milk.

- Lipid metabolic muscular disorders

  - Treatment often involves avoiding prolonged strenuous activity, since this can trigger muscle aches or weakness, cramps, and the breakdown of muscle fibers. Exposure to extremes of heat and cold should also be avoided.

  - Meals should be eaten frequently to prevent hypoglycemia, or low blood sugar, which can cause headache, nausea, anxiety, impaired judgement, and possibly coma, as well as metabolic crisis, a serious condition that results from the build-up of toxic substances in the blood.

  - Doctors often recommend a low-fat, high-carbohydrate diet, which provides the body with sugars that can be readily converted to energy. Long-chain fatty acids should be replaced with medium-chain fatty acids (the so-called "good fat"), which provide a number of health benefits, including lower cholesterol, easier digestion, and improved cardiac health.

  - Supplementing the diet with medium-chain triglyceride oil (MCT oil) may be prescribed for some patients. This product, generally made from coconut and palm kernel oils, can help make up for certain deficiencies and provide extra energy.

  - L-Carnitine supplements may help some individuals with lipid metabolic disorders. These are intended to boost a natural substance responsible for creating energy and helping the body eliminate waste. Riboflavin (vitamin B2) and coenzyme (a natural antioxidant) supplements are sometimes prescribed, as well.

  - Other treatments for some serious cases of certain disorders may include enzyme-replacement therapy, bone-marrow transplant, or LDL apheresis, a procedure in which blood is regularly cleaned of cholesterol by circulating it through a machine.

- Mitochondrial metabolic muscular disorders

  - Some of the dietary and lifestyle changes recommended for other types of metabolic muscle diseases may also apply to certain mitochondrial disorders, including high-protein food.

regular aerobic exercise, and avoiding activities that strain muscles.

- Since these disorders are associated with muscle weakness and problems with balance and coordination, a regimen of physical therapy can help improve muscle tone and range of motion, relieve pain, and help with balance issues.

- As with other types of muscular diseases, supplements are often recommended. These can include coenzyme Q-10, L-carnitine, B-vitamins, and riboflavin, as well as antioxidants to help to reduce free radical accumulation, which in some patients may improve energy and function.

- Other supplements have also been used with some success, including Pyruvate, which helps break down fats, and N-acetylcysteine, which affects glucose levels and works as an antioxidant.

- Since this group of disorders is made up of inherited conditions and genetic mutations, a number of treatments based on gene-therapy are undergoing experimentation. Future therapies could include substituting faulty genetic material with healthy replacements.

References

1. Katirji, Bashar, MD, FACP. "Metabolic Myopathies," Medscape.com, December 10, 2014.

2. Kimpton, Kimberly, PT. "Metabolic Myopathies," The Rheumatologist, December 1, 2007.

3. Muscular Dystrophy Association. "Metabolic Diseases of Muscle," n.d.

4. Kennedy Krieger Institute. "Metabolic Myopathies," n.d.

5. Wortmann, Robert L., MD. "Metabolic Myopathies," American College of Rheumatology, August 2013.

Chapter 58

Metabolic Neuropathies

Metabolic neuropathies are a range of peripheral nerve disorders that have a metabolic origin. "Metabolic" is a term used to describe the process through which the body breaks down food into sugars and acids, which it uses for energy, and "neuropathy" refers to nerve problems. Some of these conditions are inherited and some are caused by various diseases, but one thing they have in common is nerve damage that results from problems with myelin (the protective coating around nerve fibers) and axons (nerve fibers) as a result of dysfunction of the metabolic pathways within cells.

Causes of Metabolic Neuropathies

There are a very large number of possible origins for metabolic neuropathies but they are generally caused either by the body's inability to use energy (often the result of a nutritional deficiency) or by a buildup of toxins in the body. Some of the most common causes include:

- **Diabetes.** Probably the most common cause of metabolic neuropathy, diabetes refers to a group of disorders characterized by high glucose (blood sugar) levels, either because of inadequate insulin production or the inability to respond to insulin. Glucose will be present in large quantities in the blood but they will not reach the cells, and the cells undergo starvation. Some serious long-term complications may include heart disease, kidney failure, stroke and eye damage.

- **Uremia.** Another common cause of metabolic neuropathy, uremia is a serious condition that results from kidney disease or damage. With this disorder, the kidneys are unable to function normally, causing a buildup of urea and other waste products, which become toxic in high enough concentrations.

- **Hypoglycemia.** Also called low blood sugar, hypoglycemia is a condition in which the body doesn't have enough glucose to produce the energy it needs. This can lead to heart palpitations, fatigue, blurred vision, and in extreme cases, seizures and loss of consciousness.

- **Liver disease.** Liver disease can be inherited or may be acquired through such factors as infection, immune system problems, cancer, excessive alcohol or drug use, and exposure to toxins. Untreated, liver disease can progress to liver failure, which could be life-threatening.

- **Polycythemia.** This is a condition in which red-blood-cell count is abnormally high. It can be hereditary or may be caused by long-term cigarette smoking, exposure to carbon monoxide, or hypoxia (oxygen deficiency). It can make the patient susceptible to blood clots, stroke, or heart attack.

- **COPD.** Chronic obstructive pulmonary disease is a progressive inflammatory lung disorder that makes it hard to breathe. Exposure to cigarette smoke is one of its primary causes, but long-term exposure to other irritants, such as air pollution, dust, or chemical fumes, may also be contributing factors.

There are many other possible causes for metabolic neuropathies, some of which include hypothyroidism, amyloidosis, vitamin deficiency, porphyria, mitochondrial disorders, sepsis, Refsum disease, and Krabbe disease. Note that in many cases no specific cause for the metabolic neuropathy can be found. In these instances, the condition is called idiopathic, and treatment would focus on relief of symptoms.

Symptoms

The symptoms of metabolic neuropathy, which develop because nerves are damaged and are unable to transmit signals to the brain effectively, can vary considerably depending on the type and location of the affected nerve fibers. Some typical symptoms include:

- pain, which could arise in any part of the body

- numbness or a tingling sensation
- tremors
- difficult walking
- loss of balance
- muscle weakness in any area of the body
- difficulty using arms or hands
- cramps
- tics or twitches

Pain, numbness, or tingling often begin at the ends of the longest nerves in the body, those in the feet and legs, and then progresses upward. At some point, if the condition affects nerves in the autonomous nervous system (which controls unconscious functions such as heartbeat and breathing), symptoms might also include dizziness, difficulty urinating, difficulty swallowing, or constipation.

Diagnosis

Diagnosing metabolic myopathy begins with a discussion, in which the doctor will ask the patient about details of the symptoms and past episodes of similar symptoms. In the physical examination, the doctor will attempt to determine the exact nature, location, and extent of the disorder. Depending on the findings, other diagnostic tests and procedures are likely to be required, including:

- complete blood count (CBC)
- blood glucose and glucose tolerance
- serum protein
- vitamin B-12 and vitamin E
- creatinine level
- cryoglobulins
- various antibodies
- thyroid and liver function
- ischemic forearm exercise test (measured after forearm exercise)

- urine tests

- leukocyte glycogen levels

- enzyme assays of muscle, platelets, liver, and fibroblasts

- serum mitochondrial DNA deletion and mutation tests

Treatment

The treatment plan for metabolic neuropathy depends on its underlying cause, but in general the goals include addressing the bothersome and often painful symptoms and attempting to control the originating condition. Treatments may include:

- **Pain management.** Mild pain can be treated with over-the-counter medication, such as nonsteroidal anti-inflammatories. If the pain is more serious, the doctor may prescribe a variety of drugs, including opioids, as necessary. With some patients, topical patches and sprays containing lidocaine or capsaicin might help.

- **Muscle weakness.** Physical therapy is often recommended to help exercise and strengthen muscles. The use of a cane or walker can help some patients who have balance issues, and leg or angle braces may be needed for those experiencing difficulty walking.

- **Nutrition.** Depending on the underlying condition, a nutrition counselor is likely to recommend diet modifications. For example, patients with diabetes will benefit from a low-calorie diet, and those with vitamin deficiencies may be advised to eat certain foods or take supplements.

- **Surgery.** In some cases, surgery may be an option, such as vascular or plastic surgery for patients experiencing foot issues related to diabetes, liver transplants for those with conditions like familial amyloid neuropathy, and kidney transplants to address renal failure.

Treatment for the conditions that cause metabolic neuropathy can vary widely depending on the disorder and may be extremely complicated, especially in the case of systemic diseases. But once the condition is treated, in some cases nerves can regenerate or recover to a large extent and resolve the neuropathy.

References

1. Campellone, Joseph V., MD. "Metabolic Neuropathies," Med-linePlus.com, January 5, 2016.

2. Jasmin, Luc, MD, PhD, "Metabolic Neuropathies," New York Times Health Guide, February 16, 2012.

3. National Institute of Neurological Disorders and Stroke (NINDS). "Peripheral Neuropathy Fact Sheet," March 9, 2016.

4. Ramachandran, Tarakad S., MBBS, MBA, MPH, FAAN, FACP. "Metabolic Neuropathy," Medscape.com, October 27, 2014.

Chapter 59

Metabolic Syndrome

What Is Metabolic Syndrome?

Metabolic syndrome is the name for a group of risk factors that raises your risk for heart disease and other health problems, such as diabetes and stroke.

The term "metabolic" refers to the biochemical processes involved in the body's normal functioning. Risk factors are traits, conditions, or habits that increase your chance of developing a disease.

In this chapter, "heart disease" refers to coronary heart disease (CHD). CHD is a condition in which a waxy substance called plaque builds up inside the coronary (heart) arteries.

Plaque hardens and narrows the arteries, reducing blood flow to your heart muscle. This can lead to chest pain, a heart attack, heart damage, or even death.

Metabolic Risk Factors

The five conditions described below are metabolic risk factors. You can have any one of these risk factors by itself, but they tend to occur together. You must have at least three metabolic risk factors to be diagnosed with metabolic syndrome.

- A large waistline. Excess fat in the stomach area is a greater risk factor for heart disease than excess fat in other parts of the body, such as on the hips.

This chapter includes text excerpted from "Metabolic Syndrome," National Heart, Lung, and Blood Institute (NHLBI), June 22, 2016.

- A high triglyceride level (or you're on medicine to treat high triglycerides). Triglycerides are a type of fat found in the blood.

- A low high-density lipoprotein (HDL) cholesterol level (or you're on medicine to treat low HDL cholesterol). HDL sometimes is called "good" cholesterol. This is because it helps remove cholesterol from your arteries. A low HDL cholesterol level raises your risk for heart disease.

- High blood pressure (or you're on medicine to treat high blood pressure). Blood pressure is the force of blood pushing against the walls of your arteries as your heart pumps blood. If this pressure rises and stays high over time, it can damage your heart and lead to plaque buildup.

- High fasting blood sugar (or you're on medicine to treat high blood sugar). Mildly high blood sugar may be an early sign of diabetes.

Other Names for Metabolic Syndrome

- Dysmetabolic syndrome

- Hypertriglyceridemic waist

- Insulin resistance syndrome

- Obesity syndrome

- Syndrome X

What Causes Metabolic Syndrome?

Metabolic syndrome has several causes that act together. You can control some of the causes, such as overweight and obesity, an inactive lifestyle, and insulin resistance.

You can't control other factors that may play a role in causing metabolic syndrome, such as growing older. Your risk for metabolic syndrome increases with age.

You also can't control genetics (ethnicity and family history), which may play a role in causing the condition. For example, genetics can increase your risk for insulin resistance, which can lead to metabolic syndrome.

People who have metabolic syndrome often have two other conditions: excessive blood clotting and constant, low-grade inflammation throughout the body. Researchers don't know whether these conditions cause metabolic syndrome or worsen it.

Researchers continue to study conditions that may play a role in metabolic syndrome, such as:

- a fatty liver (excess triglycerides and other fats in the liver)
- polycystic ovarian syndrome, or PCOS (a tendency to develop cysts on the ovaries)
- gallstones
- breathing problems during sleep (such as sleep apnea)

Who Is at Risk for Metabolic Syndrome?

People at greatest risk for metabolic syndrome have these underlying causes:

- abdominal obesity (a large waistline)
- an inactive lifestyle
- insulin resistance

Some people are at risk for metabolic syndrome because they take medicines that cause weight gain or changes in blood pressure, blood cholesterol, and blood sugar levels. These medicines most often are used to treat inflammation, allergies, HIV, and depression and other types of mental illness.

Populations Affected

Some racial and ethnic groups in the United States are at higher risk for metabolic syndrome than others. Mexican Americans have the highest rate of metabolic syndrome, followed by whites and blacks.

Other groups at increased risk for metabolic syndrome include:

- people who have a personal history of diabetes
- people who have a sibling or parent who has diabetes
- women when compared with men
- women who have a personal history of PCOS

Heart Disease Risk

Metabolic syndrome increases your risk for coronary heart disease. Other risk factors, besides metabolic syndrome, also increase your risk for heart disease. For example, a high low-density lipoprotein (LDL) ("bad") cholesterol level and smoking are major risk factors for heart disease.

Even if you don't have metabolic syndrome, you should find out your short-term risk for heart disease. The National Cholesterol Education Program (NCEP) divides short-term heart disease risk into four categories. Your risk category depends on which risk factors you have and how many you have.

Your risk factors are used to calculate your 10-year risk of developing heart disease.

- **High risk:** You're in this category if you already have heart disease or diabetes, or if your 10-year risk score is more than 20 percent.

- **Moderately high risk:** You're in this category if you have two or more risk factors and your 10-year risk score is 10 percent to 20 percent.

- **Moderate risk:** You're in this category if you have two or more risk factors and your 10-year risk score is less than 10 percent.

- **Lower risk:** You're in this category if you have zero or one risk factor.

Even if your 10-year risk score isn't high, metabolic syndrome will increase your risk for coronary heart disease over time.

What Are the Signs and Symptoms of Metabolic Syndrome?

Most of the metabolic risk factors have no signs or symptoms, although a large waistline is a visible sign.

Some people may have symptoms of high blood sugar if diabetes—especially type 2 diabetes—is present. Symptoms of high blood sugar often include increased thirst; increased urination, especially at night; fatigue (tiredness); and blurred vision.

High blood pressure usually has no signs or symptoms. However, some people in the early stages of high blood pressure may have dull headaches, dizzy spells, or more nosebleeds than usual.

How Is Metabolic Syndrome Diagnosed?

Your doctor will diagnose metabolic syndrome based on the results of a physical exam and blood tests. You must have at least three of the five metabolic risk factors to be diagnosed with metabolic syndrome.

Metabolic Risk Factors

A Large Waistline

Having a large waistline means that you carry excess weight around your waist (abdominal obesity). This is also called having an "apple-shaped" figure. Your doctor will measure your waist to find out whether you have a large waistline.

A waist measurement of 35 inches or more for women or 40 inches or more for men is a metabolic risk factor. A large waistline means you're at increased risk for heart disease and other health problems.

A High Triglyceride Level

Triglycerides are a type of fat found in the blood. A triglyceride level of 150 mg/dL or higher (or being on medicine to treat high triglycerides) is a metabolic risk factor. (The mg/dL is milligrams per deciliter—the units used to measure triglycerides, cholesterol, and blood sugar.)

A Low HDL Cholesterol Level

HDL cholesterol sometimes is called "good" cholesterol. This is because it helps remove cholesterol from your arteries.

An HDL cholesterol level of less than 50 mg/dL for women and less than 40 mg/dL for men (or being on medicine to treat low HDL cholesterol) is a metabolic risk factor.

High Blood Pressure

A blood pressure of 130/85 mmHg or higher (or being on medicine to treat high blood pressure) is a metabolic risk factor. (The mmHg is millimeters of mercury—the units used to measure blood pressure.)

If only one of your two blood pressure numbers is high, you're still at risk for metabolic syndrome.

High Fasting Blood Sugar

A normal fasting blood sugar level is less than 100 mg/dL. A fasting blood sugar level between 100–125 mg/dL is considered prediabetes. A fasting blood sugar level of 126 mg/dL or higher is considered diabetes.

A fasting blood sugar level of 100 mg/dL or higher (or being on medicine to treat high blood sugar) is a metabolic risk factor.

About 85 percent of people who have type 2 diabetes—the most common type of diabetes—also have metabolic syndrome. These people have a much higher risk for heart disease than the 15 percent of people who have type 2 diabetes without metabolic syndrome.

How Is Metabolic Syndrome Treated?

Heart-healthy lifestyle changes are the first line of treatment for metabolic syndrome. If heart-healthy lifestyle changes aren't enough, your doctor may prescribe medicines. Medicines are used to treat and control risk factors, such as high blood pressure, high triglycerides, low HDL ("good") cholesterol, and high blood sugar.

Goals of Treatment

The major goal of treating metabolic syndrome is to reduce the risk of coronary heart disease. Treatment is directed first at lowering LDL cholesterol and high blood pressure and managing diabetes (if these conditions are present).

The second goal of treatment is to prevent the onset of type 2 diabetes, if it hasn't already developed. Long-term complications of diabetes often include heart and kidney disease, vision loss, and foot or leg amputation. If diabetes is present, the goal of treatment is to reduce your risk for heart disease by controlling all of your risk factors.

Heart-Healthy Lifestyle Changes

Heart-healthy lifestyle changes include heart-healthy eating, aiming for a healthy weight, managing stress, physical activity, and quitting smoking.

Medicines

Sometimes lifestyle changes aren't enough to control your risk factors for metabolic syndrome. For example, you may need statin medications to control or lower your cholesterol. By lowering your blood cholesterol level, you can decrease your chance of having a heart attack or stroke. Doctors usually prescribe statins for people who have:

- diabetes

- heart disease or had a prior stroke

- high LDL cholesterol levels

Doctors may discuss beginning statin treatment with those who have an elevated risk for developing heart disease or having a stroke.

Your doctor also may prescribe other medications to:

- decrease your chance of having a heart attack or dying suddenly

- lower your blood pressure

- prevent blood clots, which can lead to heart attack or stroke

- reduce your heart's workload and relieve symptoms of coronary heart disease

Take all medicines regularly, as your doctor prescribes. Don't change the amount of your medicine or skip a dose unless your doctor tells you to. You should still follow a heart-healthy lifestyle, even if you take medicines to treat your risk factors for metabolic syndrome.

How Can Metabolic Syndrome Be Prevented?

The best way to prevent metabolic syndrom is to adopt heart-healthy lifestyle changes. Make sure to schedule routine doctor visits to keep track of your cholesterol, blood pressure, and blood sugar levels. Speak with your doctor about a blood test called a lipoprotein panel, which shows your levels of total cholesterol, LDL cholesterol, HDL cholesterol, and triglycerides.

Living with Metabolic Syndrome

Metabolic syndrome is a lifelong condition. However, lifestyle changes can help you control your risk factors and reduce your risk for coronary heart disease and diabetes.

If you already have heart disease or diabetes, lifestyle changes can help you prevent or delay related problems. Examples of these problems include heart attack, stroke, and diabetes-related complications (for example, damage to your eyes, nerves, kidneys, feet, and legs).

Heart-healthy lifestyle changes may include:

- heart-healthy eating

- aiming for a healthy weight

- managing stress

- physical activity

- quitting smoking

If lifestyle changes aren't enough, your doctor may recommend medicines. Take all of your medicines as prescribed by your doctor. Make realistic short- and long-term goals for yourself when you begin to make healthy lifestyle changes. Work closely with your doctor, and seek regular medical care.

Chapter 60

Multiple Endocrine Neoplasia Type 1 (MEN1)

What Is Multiple Endocrine Neoplasia Type 1 (MEN1)?

MEN1 is an inherited disorder that causes tumors in the endocrine glands and the duodenum, the first part of the small intestine. MEN1 is sometimes called multiple endocrine adenomatosis or Wermer syndrome, after one of the first doctors to recognize it. MEN1 is rare, occurring in about one in 30,000 people. The disorder affects both sexes equally and shows no geographical, racial, or ethnic preferences. Endocrine glands release hormones into the bloodstream. Hormones are powerful chemicals that travel through the blood, controlling and instructing the functions of various organs. Normally, the hormones released by endocrine glands are carefully balanced to meet the body's needs. In people with MEN1, multiple endocrine glands form tumors and become hormonally overactive, often at the same time. The overactive glands may include the parathyroids, pancreas, or pituitary. Most people who develop overactivity of only one endocrine gland do not have MEN1.

This chapter includes text excerpted from "Multiple Endocrine Neoplasia Type 1," National Institute of Diabetes and Digestive and Kidney Diseases (NIDDK), November 2009. Reviewed October 2016.

How Does MEN1 Affect the Endocrine Glands and the Duodenum?

The Parathyroid Glands

The parathyroids are the endocrine glands earliest and most often affected by MEN1. The body normally has four parathyroid glands, which are located close to the thyroid gland in the front of the neck. The parathyroids release into the bloodstream a chemical called parathyroid hormone (PTH), which helps maintain a normal supply of calcium in the blood, bones, and urine.

Hyperparathyroidism

In MEN1, all four parathyroid glands tend to be overactive, causing hyperparathyroidism. The parathyroid glands form tumors that release too much PTH, leading to excess calcium in the blood. High blood calcium, known as hypercalcemia, can exist for many years before it is found by accident or through screening for MEN1. Unrecognized hypercalcemia can cause excess calcium to spill into the urine, leading to kidney stones or kidney damage. Also, the bones may lose calcium and weaken.

Nearly everyone who inherits a susceptibility to MEN1 will develop hyperparathyroidism by age 50, but the disorder can often be detected before age 20. Hyperparathyroidism may cause no problems for many years, or it may cause tiredness, weakness, muscle or bone pain, constipation, indigestion, kidney stones, or thinning of bones.

Doctors must decide whether hyperparathyroidism in MEN1 is severe enough to need treatment, especially in a person who has no symptoms. The usual treatment is an operation to remove most or all of the parathyroid glands. One option is to remove the three largest glands and all but a small part of the fourth. Another is to remove all four glands and at the same time transplant a small part of one gland into the forearm. By maintaining a portion of one gland, the parathyroid transplant continues to release PTH into the bloodstream to do its job. After parathyroid surgery, regular testing of blood calcium should continue because often the small piece of remaining parathyroid tissue grows larger and causes recurrent hyperparathyroidism. If the remaining piece is in the forearm and additional surgery is needed to remove more parathyroid tissue, the arm operation can be performed under local anesthesia. Sometimes all four glands are completely removed to prevent recurrence or may be unintentionally removed during parathyroid surgery. People whose parathyroid glands have been completely removed must take daily supplements of calcium and vitamin D or another related treatment to prevent hypocalcemia, or low blood calcium.

The Pancreas and Duodenum

Located behind the stomach, the pancreas has two major roles: to release digestive juices into the intestines and key hormones into the bloodstream. The duodenum is the first part of the small intestine next to the pancreas. The pancreatic hormones are normally produced by small clusters of specialized cells called pancreatic islets. Some of the major hormones produced by the pancreatic islets are

- insulin—lowers blood glucose, also called blood sugar

- glucagon—raises blood glucose

- somatostatin—inhibits secretion of certain other hormones

- vasoactive intestinal peptide (VIP)— causes intestinal cells to secrete water into the intestine

- gastrin—causes the stomach to produce acid for digestion

Gastrinomas

In MEN1, gastrin may be oversecreted by tumors called gastrinomas in the pancreas, duodenum, and lymph glands. If exposed to too much gastrin, the stomach releases excess acid, leading to the formation of severe ulcers in the stomach and small intestine. In addition, too much gastrin usually causes serious diarrhea. People with MEN1 have about a 20 to 60 percent chance of developing gastrinomas. The illness associated with these tumors is called Zollinger-Ellison syndrome. The ulcers caused by untreated gastrinomas are much more dangerous than typical stomach or intestinal ulcers. Left untreated, they can cause rupture of the stomach or intestine and even death.

The gastrinomas associated with MEN1 are not easily cured through tumor surgery because finding the many small gastrinomas in the pancreas, duodenum, and lymph glands is difficult. The mainstay of treatment is powerful medicines called acid pump inhibitors that block stomach acid release. Taken by mouth, these medicines have proven effective in controlling the complications of excess gastrin in most cases of Zollinger-Ellison syndrome.

Rare Pancreatic Complications

Occasionally, a person who has MEN1 develops an islet tumor of the pancreas that secretes high levels of hormones. Insulinomas, for example, produce too much insulin, causing hypoglycemia, or low blood glucose. About 10 percent of adults with MEN1 develop insulinomas. Rare pancreatic tumors may secrete too much glucagon, which can cause diabetes, or too much VIP, which can cause watery diarrhea. Tumors that secrete adrenocorticotropin (ACTH) may also arise in the pancreas. ACTH is normally secreted by the pituitary gland and stimulates the adrenal glands to produce cortisol, a hormone that helps the body respond to stress. Tumors in the pancreas may also infrequently secrete gonadotropin-releasing hormone (GnRH). GnRH is normally secreted by the hypothalamus and stimulates the pituitary gland to release follicle stimulating hormone (FSH), which regulates fertility in men through sperm production and in women through ovulation. In general, surgery is the mainstay of treatment for these uncommon types of tumors.

The Pituitary Gland

The pituitary, a small gland located at the base of the brain, produces many important hormones that regulate basic body functions. The normal major pituitary hormones are

- prolactin—controls the formation of breast milk and influences fertility and bone strength
- growth hormone—regulates body growth, especially during adolescence
- ACTH—stimulates the adrenal glands to produce cortisol
- thyrotropin—stimulates the thyroid gland to produce thyroid hormones, which regulate metabolism
- luteinizing hormone—stimulates the ovaries or testes to produce sex hormones
- FSH—regulates fertility

Prolactinomas

The pituitary gland becomes overactive in about one in four people with MEN1. This overactivity can usually be traced to a small tumor in the gland that releases too much prolactin, called a prolactinoma.

High prolactin levels can cause excessive production of breast milk or interfere with fertility in women or with sex drive and fertility in men.

Treatment may not be needed for prolactinomas. If treatment is needed, a medicine known as a dopamine agonist can effectively shrink the tumor and lower the production of prolactin. Occasionally, prolactinomas do not respond well to this medication. In such cases, surgery, radiation, or both may be needed.

Rare Pituitary Complications

Rarely, MEN1 creates pituitary tumors that release high amounts of ACTH, which in turn stimulates the adrenal glands to produce excess cortisol. Too much cortisol can lead to muscle weakness, weakened bones and fractures, and thinning skin, among other problems. Pituitary tumors that produce growth hormone cause excessive bone growth or disfigurement. In general, surgery is the mainstay of treatment for these uncommon types of tumors.

Are the Tumors Associated with MEN1 Cancerous?

The tumors associated with MEN1 are usually benign, meaning they are not cancerous. However, they can disrupt normal function by releasing hormones or by crowding nearby tissue. For example, a prolactinoma may become quite large in someone with MEN1. As it grows, the tumor can press against and damage the normal part of the pituitary gland or the nerves for vision. Sometimes impaired vision is the first sign of a pituitary tumor in a person with MEN1. Another type of benign tumor seen in about one-third of people with MEN1 is a plumsized, fatty tumor called a lipoma, which grows under the skin. Lipomas cause no health problems and can be removed by simple cosmetic surgery if desired. Benign tumors do not spread to or invade other parts of the body. Cancer cells, by contrast, break away from the primary tumor and spread, or metastasize, to other parts of the body through the bloodstream or lymphatic system. The pancreatic islet tumors associated with MEN1 tend to be numerous and small, but most are benign and do not release active hormones into the blood. Over time, gastrinomas may become cancerous but are usually slow-growing. Eventually, about half of people with MEN1 will develop a cancerous pancreatic or carcinoid tumor. A carcinoid is a slow-growing endocrine tumor inside the chest or stomach of a person with MEN1. Although carcinoids arise from endocrine cells, which are present in many parts of the body, they rarely secrete a hormone in a person with MEN1. Carcinoids of the stomach usually do not require treatment.

Treatment of Pancreatic Endocrine Cancer in MEN1

Because the type of pancreatic endocrine cancer associated with MEN1 can be difficult to recognize, difficult to treat, and slow to progress, doctors have different views about the value of surgery in managing these tumors. One approach is to "watch and wait," using medical, or nonsurgical, treatments. According to this school of thought, pancreatic surgery has serious complications, so it should not be attempted unless it will cure a tumor or cure a hormone excess state. Another school advocates early surgery, perhaps when a tumor grows to a certain size, to prevent or treat pancreatic endocrine cancer—even if the tumor does not over secrete a hormone—before the cancer spreads. No clear evidence exists, however, that surgery to prevent pancreatic endocrine cancer from spreading actually leads to longer survival for patients with MEN1.

Doctors agree that excessive release of certain hormones—mainly gastrin—from pancreatic endocrine cancer in MEN1 needs to be treated, and medications are often effective in blocking the effects of these hormones. Some tumors, such as insulinomas, are usually benign and single and are curable by pancreatic surgery. Such surgery needs to be considered carefully in each patient's case.

Is MEN1 the Same in Everyone?

Although MEN1 tends to follow certain patterns, it can affect a person's health in many different ways. Not only do the tumors of MEN1 vary among members of the same family, but some families with MEN1 tend to have a higher rate of prolactin-secreting pituitary tumors and a much lower frequency of gastrin-secreting tumors. The age at which MEN1 can begin to cause endocrine gland overactivity can differ strikingly from one family member to another. One person may have only mild hyperparathyroidism beginning at age 50, while a relative may develop complications from tumors of the parathyroid, pancreas, and pituitary by age 18.

How Is MEN1 Detected?

MEN1 is detected by gene testing or, when gene testing is unavailable or yields a negative result, by laboratory tests that measure hormone levels. Less often, MEN1 is diagnosed based on an individual's medical and family history.

Can MEN1 Be Cured?

MEN1 cannot be cured, but regular testing can detect many of the problems caused by MEN1 tumors many years before serious complications develop. Finding these tumors early enables doctors to begin preventive treatment, reducing the chances that MEN1 will cause problems later. Even after treatment, residual tissue can grow back or different glands may become affected. Periodic and careful monitoring enables doctors to adjust an individual's treatment as needed and to check for any new problems caused by MEN1. Most people with MEN1 have a long and productive life.

Should a Person Who Has MEN1 Avoid Having Children?

A person who has MEN1 or who has a MEN1 gene mutation may have a hard time deciding whether to have a child. Some facts to consider include the following:

- A man or a woman with MEN1 has a 50-50 risk with each pregnancy of having a child with MEN1.

- MEN1 tends to fit a broad pattern within a given family, but the severity of the disorder varies widely from one family member to another. In particular, a parent's experience with MEN1 cannot be used to predict the eventual severity of MEN1 in a child.

- The tumors that result from MEN1 do not usually develop until adulthood. Treatment may require regular monitoring and considerable expense, but the disease usually does not prevent an active, productive adulthood.

- Prolactin-releasing tumors in a man or woman with MEN1 may inhibit fertility and make it difficult to conceive.

- Hyperparathyroidism during pregnancy may raise the risks of complications for mother and child.

- Pregnancy is usually normal for the mother or child who is a carrier of MEN1.

Genetic counselors and other professionals can provide information to help with the decision-making process, but they will not tell individuals or couples what decision to make or how to make it.

Part Eight

Additional Help and Information

Chapter 61

Glossary of Terms Related to Endocrine and Metabolic Disorders

acute: A short-term, intense health effect.

adenoma: A noncancerous tumor.

adrenal gland: A small gland that makes steroid hormones, adrenaline, and noradrenaline. These hormones help control heart rate, blood pressure, and other important body functions.

adverse reaction: An untoward (unfavorable) effect caused by a vaccine that is extraneous to (not in keeping with) the vaccine's primary purpose of production of immunity.

AIDS: Acquired immunodeficiency syndrome (AIDS) is a medical condition in which the immune system cannot function properly and protect the body from disease; as a result, the body cannot defend itself against infectious diseases.

antibiotic: A drug used to fight infections caused by bacteria.

antibodies: Special proteins made by the body in response to antigens (foreign substances.

antigen: Foreign substances (e.g., bacteria or viruses) in the body that are capable of causing disease; the presence of antigens in

This glossary contains terms excerpted from documents produced by several sources deemed reliable.

the body triggers an immune response, usually the production of antibodies.

arthritis: Inflammation of the joints that causes swelling, stiffness, and pain.

aspiration: Sucking of fluid or a foreign body into the airway when drawing breath or swallowing.

asthma: A chronic respiratory disease characterized by constriction of the bronchial tubes to the lungs, which causes sudden and recurring breathing problems, coughing, and chest tightness and wheezing.

bacteria: Single-celled microorganisms, some of which can cause disease.

benign: Not cancerous. Benign tumors may grow larger but do not spread to other parts of the body.

bilateral: Affecting both sides, as in both the right and left hand side of the body.

blood chemistry study: A procedure in which a sample of blood is examined to measure the amounts of certain substances made in the body.

bloodstream: The blood that flows through the blood vessels of the circulatory system.

bone marrow: Soft tissue located within bones that produces all blood cells, including the ones that fight infection.

calcium: A mineral found in teeth, bones, and other body tissues.

cancer: A term for diseases in which abnormal cells divide without control. Cancer cells can invade nearby tissues and can spread through the bloodstream and lymphatic system to other parts of the body.

carcinogens: Substances which can cause cancer.

cardiovascular: Related to the heart and blood vessels.

cataracts: Clouding of the lens of the eye that reduces the ability to see clearly; can lead to blindness.

catheter: A flexible tube used to deliver fluids into or withdraw fluids from the body.

cell: The individual unit that makes up the tissues of the body. All living things are made up of one or more cells.

central nervous system (CNS): The brain and spinal cord.

chemotherapy: Treatment with drugs that kill cancer cells.

chronic: Lasting for a long time or marked by frequent recurrence.

chronological age: The age of a person as measured from his or her birth.

computed tomography (CT) scan: A series of detailed pictures of areas inside the body taken from different angles; the pictures are created by a computer linked to an X-ray machine.

constipation: Passage of small amounts of hard, dry bowel movements, usually fewer than three times a week. Persons who are constipated may find it difficult and painful to have a bowel movement.

corticosteroids: A steroid hormone; when given as a medication, it suppresses the body's normal inflammatory reactions to infection. This increases the risk for serious infection.

craniotomy: An operation in which an opening is made in the skull.

de novo: A chromosome abnormality that occurred in the individual and was not inherited from the parents.

dehydration: Inadequate amount of water in the body; can occur from illness or from decreased or lack of fluid intake.

diabetes: A chronic health condition in which the body is unable to produce insulin and properly break down sugar (glucose) in the blood.

diagnosis: The process of identifying a disease by the signs and symptoms.

diarrhea: Abnormally watery bowel movements.

drug: Any substance, other than food, that is used to prevent, diagnose, treat or relieve symptoms of a disease or abnormal condition.

encephalitis: Inflammation of the brain caused by a virus; encephalitis can result in permanent brain damage or death.

exocrine glands: Glands that release the substances into a duct or opening to the inside or outside of the body.

external radiation: Radiation therapy that uses a machine to aim high-energy rays at the cancer. Also called external-beam radiation.

fatigue: Extreme tiredness or weariness.

functioning tumor: A tumor that is found in endocrine tissue and makes hormones.

gland: An organ that makes one or more substances, such as hormones, digestive juices, sweat, tears, saliva, or milk.

glucocorticoid: A compound that belongs to the family of compounds called corticosteroids (steroids). Glucocorticoids affect metabolism and have anti-inflammatory and immunosuppressive effects.

hormone: A chemical made by glands in the body. Hormones circulate in the bloodstream and control the actions of certain cells or organs.

hypercalcemia: Abnormally high blood calcium.

hyperparathyroidism: A condition in which the parathyroid gland (one of four pea-sized organs found on the thyroid) makes too much parathyroid hormone.

imaging: Tests that produce pictures of areas inside the body.

impotence: In medicine, refers to the inability to have an erection of the penis adequate for sexual intercourse.

inherited: Transmitted through genes that have been passed from parents to their offspring (children).

laboratory test: A medical procedure that involves testing a sample of blood, urine, or other substance from the body. Tests can help determine a diagnosis, plan treatment, check to see if treatment is working, or monitor the disease over time.

lymph node: A rounded mass of lymphatic tissue that is surrounded by a capsule of connective tissue. Lymph nodes filter lymph (lymphatic fluid), and they store lymphocytes (white blood cells).

medication: A legal drug that is used to prevent, treat, or relieve symptoms of a disease or abnormal condition. Also called medicine.

meiosis: Cell division resulting in gametes (eggs and sperm cells), each containing one set of chromosomes—that is, 23 single chromosomes—rather than the 23 paired sets of chromosomes in nonreproductive cells.

menstrual cycle: The monthly cycle of hormonal changes from the beginning of one menstrual period to the beginning of the next one.

metabolic: Relates to metabolism or processes in an organism that make energy.

metastasectomy: Surgery to remove one or more metastases (tumors formed from cells that have spread from the primary tumor).

metastasize: To spread from one part of the body to another. When cancer cells metastasize and form secondary tumors, the cells in the metastatic tumor are like those in the original (primary) tumor.

mitosis: Cell division resulting in cells that have paired sets of chromosomes.

mosaicism: Abnormal chromosome division resulting in two or more kinds of cells, each containing different numbers of chromosomes.

multiple endocrine neoplasia type 1 syndrome (MEN1 syndrome): A rare, inherited disorder that affects the endocrine glands and can cause tumors in the parathyroid and pituitary glands and the pancreas.

ovary: One of a pair of female reproductive glands in which the ova, or eggs, are formed.

pancreas: A glandular organ located in the abdomen. It makes pancreatic juices, which contain enzymes that aid in digestion, and it produces several hormones, including insulin.

parathyroid cancer: A rare cancer that forms in tissues of one or more of the parathyroid glands.

parathyroid gland: One of four pea-sized glands found on the thyroid. The parathyroid hormone produced by these glands increases the calcium level in the blood.

parathyroid hormone (PTH): A substance made by the parathyroid gland that helps the body store and use calcium.

pituitary gland: The pituitary is a peasized organ in the center of the brain above the back of the nose. It produces hormones that control other glands and many body functions, especially growth.

pituitary tumor: A tumor that forms in the pituitary gland. Most pituitary tumors are benign (not cancer).

prognosis: The likely outcome or course of a disease; the chance of recovery or recurrence.

radiation therapy: The use of high-energy radiation from X-rays, gamma rays, neutrons, and other sources to kill cancer cells and shrink tumors.

reciprocal translocation: Segments from two different chromosomes have changed places.

regional chemotherapy: Treatment with anticancer drugs directed to a specific area of the body.

resection: A procedure that uses surgery to remove tissue or part or all of an organ.

sonogram: A computer picture of areas inside the body created by bouncing high-energy sound waves (ultrasound) off internal tissues or organs.

staging: Performing exams and tests to learn the extent of the cancer within the body, especially whether the disease has spread from the original site to other parts of the body.

standard therapy: In medicine, treatment that experts agree is appropriate, accepted, and widely used.

supportive care: Care given to improve the quality of life of patients who have a serious or life-threatening disease.

thyroid gland: A gland located beneath the voice box (larynx) that produces thyroid hormone. The thyroid helps regulate growth and metabolism.

thyroid hormone: A hormone that affects heart rate, blood pressure, body temperature, and weight.

tumor: An abnormal mass of tissue that results when cells divide more than they should or do not die when they should. Tumors may be benign (not cancerous), or malignant (cancerous).

tumor debulking: Surgically removing as much of the tumor as possible.

X-ray: A type of high-energy radiation. In low doses, X-rays are used to diagnose diseases by making pictures of the inside of the body. In high doses, X-rays are used to treat cancer.

Chapter 62

Additional Resources for Information about Endocrine and Metabolic Disorders

Government Agencies That Provide Information about Endocrine and Metabolic Disorders

Eunice Kennedy Shriver
National Institute of
Child Health and Human
Development (NICHD)
Information Resource Center
P.O. Box 3006
Rockville, MD 20847
Toll-Free: 800-370-2943
Toll-Free TTY: 888-320-6942
Fax: 866-760-5947
Website: www.nichd.nih.gov
E-mail:
NICHDInformationResource
Center@mail.nih.gov

Genetic and Rare Diseases
Information Center (GARD)
P.O. Box 8126
Gaithersburg, MD 20898-8126
Toll-Free: 888-205-2311
Toll-Free TTY: 888-205-3223
Fax: 240-632-9164
Website: rarediseases.info.nih.
gov

Resources in this chapter were compiled from several sources deemed reliable; all contact information was verified and updated in November 2016.

501

National Cancer Institute (NCI)
9609 Medical Center Dr.
BG 9609 MSC 9760
Bethesda, MD 20892-9760
Toll-Free: 800-4-CANCER
(800-422-6237)
Toll-Free TTY: 800-332-8615
Website: www.cancer.gov
E-mail: cancergovstaff@mail.nih.gov

National Heart, Lung, and Blood Institute (NHLBI)
Health Information Center
P.O. Box 30105
Bethesda, MD 20824-0105
Phone: 301-592-8573
Fax: 301-592-8563
Website: www.nhlbi.nih.gov
E-mail: nhlbiinfo@nhlbi.nih.gov

National Human Genome Research Institute (NHGRI)
31 Center Dr., MSC 2152
9000 Rockville Pike
Bldg. 31, Rm. 4B09
Bethesda, MD 20892-2152
Phone: 301-402-0911
Fax: 301-402-2218
Website: www.genome.gov

National Institute of Diabetes and Digestive and Kidney Diseases (NIDDK)
Information Clearinghouse
9000 Rockville Pike
Bethesda, MD 20892-3560
Toll-Free: 800-860-8747
Website: www.niddk.nih.gov

National Institute of Environmental Health Sciences (NIEHS)
P.O. Box 12233
Research Triangle Park, NC 27709-2233
Phone: 919-541-3345
TTY: 919-541-0731
Fax: 301-480-2978
Website: www.niehs.nih.gov
E-mail: webcenter@niehs.nih.gov

National Institute of Neurological Disorders and Stroke (NINDS)
P.O. Box 5801
Bethesda, MD 20824
Toll-Free: 800-352-9424
Phone: 301-496-5751
Website: www.ninds.nih.gov

National Kidney and Urologic Diseases Information Clearinghouse (NKUDIC)
3 Information Way
Bethesda, MD 20892-3580
Toll-Free: 800-891-5390
Phone: 301-654-4415
Website: www.ninds.nih.gov
E-mail: nkudic@info.niddk.nih.gov

National Library of Medicine (NLM)
8600 Rockville Pike
Bethesda, MD 20894
Toll-Free: 888-FIND-NLM
(888-346-3656)
Phone: 301-594-5983
Toll-Free TDD: 800-735-2258
Fax: 301-402-0872
Website: www.nlm.nih.gov
E-mail: custserv@nlm.nih.gov

NIH Clinical Center
10 Center Dr.
Bethesda, MD 20892
Toll-Free: 800-411-1222
Phone: 301-496-2563
TTY: 866-411-1010
Fax: 301-402-2984
Website: www.cc.nih.gov/contact.
html
E-mail: prpl@mail.cc.nih.gov

Private Agencies That Provide Information about Endocrine and Metabolic Disorders

American Academy of Otolaryngology—Head and Neck Surgery (AAO–HNS)
1650 Diagonal Rd.
Alexandria, VA 22314-2857
Phone: 703-836-4444
Website: www.entnet.org
E-mail: memberservices@entnet.
org

American Association of Clinical Endocrinologists (AACE)
245 Riverside Ave., Ste. 200
Jacksonville, FL 32202
Phone: 904-353-7878
Fax: 904-353-8185
Website: www.aace.com

American Autoimmune-Related Diseases Association, Inc. (AARDA)
22100 Gratiot Ave.
Eastpointe, MI 48021
Phone: 586-776-3900
Fax: 586-776-3903

Website: www.aarda.org

American Diabetes Association (ADA)
1701 N. Beauregard St.
Alexandria, VA 22311
Toll-Free: 800-DIABETES
(800-342-2383)
Website: www.diabetes.org
E-mail: askada@diabetes.org

American Gastroenterological Association (AGA)
4930 Del Ray Ave.
Bethesda, MD 20814
Phone: 301-654-2055
Fax: 301-654-5920
Website: www.gastro.org
E-mail: member@gastro.org

American Porphyria Foundation (APF)
4900 Woodway
Ste. 780
Houston, TX 77056-1837
Toll-Free: 866-APF-3635
(866-273-3635)
Phone: 713-266-9617
Fax: 713-840-9552
Website: www.
porphyriafoundation.com
E-mail: porphyrus@
porphyriafoundation.com

American Society for Bone and Mineral Research (ASBMR)
2025 M St. N.W.
Ste. 800
Washington, DC 20036-3309
Phone: 202-367-1161
Fax: 202-367-2161
Website: www.asbmr.org/
E-mail: asbmr@asbmr.org

American Society for Reproductive Medicine (ASRM)
1209 Montgomery Hwy
Birmingham, AL 35216-2809
Phone: 205-978-5000
Fax: 205-978-5005
Website: www.asrm.org
E-mail: asrm@asrm.org

American Society of Human Genetics (ASHG)
9650 Rockville Pike
Bethesda, MD 20814
Toll-Free: 866-HUM-GENE
(866-486-4363)
Phone: 301-634-7300
Website: www.ashg.org
E-mail: society@ashg.org

American Thyroid Association (ATA)
6066 Leesburg Pike
Ste. 550
Falls Church, VA 22041
Phone: 703-998-8890
Fax: 703-998-8893
Website: www.thyroid.org
E-mail: thyroid@thyroid.org

Association for Glycogen-Storage Disease (AGSD)
P.O. Box 896
Durant, IA 52747
Phone: 563-785-6038
Fax: 563-514-4022
Website: www.agsdus.org
E-mail: info@agsdus.org

Association for Neuro-Metabolic Disorders (ANMD)
5223 Brookfield Ln.
Sylvania, OH 43560-1809
Phone: 419-885-1809
Website: healthfinder.gov/
FindServices/Organizations/
Organization.aspx?code=HR2289

Association of Occupational and Environmental Clinics (AOEC)
1010 Vermont Ave. N.W.
Ste. 513
Washington, DC 20005
Toll-Free: 888-347-AOEC
(888-347-2632)
Phone: 202-347-4976
Fax: 202-347-4950
Website: www.aoec.org
E-mail: aoec@aoec.org

CARES Foundation
2414 Morris Ave.
Ste. 110
Union, NJ 07083
Toll-Free: 866-CARES-37
(866-227-3737)
Phone: 908-364-0272
Fax: 908-686-2019
Website: www.caresfoundation.
org
E-mail: contact@
caresfoundation.org

Children's Gaucher Research Fund (CGRF)
8110 Warren Ct.
Granite Bay, CA 95746
Phone: 916-797-3700
Fax: 916-797-3707
Website: www.childrensgaucher.
org
E-mail: research@
childrensgaucher.org

Children's PKU Network (CPN)
3306 Bumann Rd.
Encinitas, CA 92024
Toll-Free: 800-377-6677
Phone: 858-756-0079
Fax: 858-756-1059
Website: www.pkunetwork.org
E-mail: pkunetwork@aol.com

Creutzfeldt-Jakob Disease Foundation Inc. (CJDF)
P.O. Box 5312
Akron, OH 44334
Toll-Free: 800-659-1991
Fax: 234-466-7077
Website: www.cjdfoundation.org
E-mail: help@cjdfoundation.org

Cushing's Support and Research Foundation, Inc. (CSRF)
60 Robbins Rd.
Ste. 12
Plymouth, MA 02360
Phone: 617-723-3674
Fax: 617-723-3674
Website: csrf.net
E-mail: cushinfo@csrf.net

Cystic Fibrosis Foundation (CFF)
6931 Arlington Rd., 2nd fl.
Bethesda, MD 20814
Toll-Free: 800-FIGHT-CF
(800-344-4823)
Phone: 301-951-4422
Website: www.cff.org
E-mail: info@cff.org

Endocrine Society
2055 L St. N.W.
Ste. 600
Washington, DC 20036
Toll-Free: 888-363-6274
Phone: 202-971-3636
Fax: 202-736-9705
Website: www.endocrine.org
E-mail: hormone@endocrine.org

**Fatty Oxidation Disorders
(FOD) Family Support
Group**
P.O. Box 54
Okemos, MI 48805-0054
Phone: 517-381-1940
Fax: 866-290-5206
Website: www.fodsupport.org
E-mail: deb@fodsupport.org

Genetic Alliance, Inc.
4301 Connecticut Ave. N.W.
Ste. 404
Washington, DC 20008-2369
Phone: 202-966-5557
Fax: 202-966-8553
Website: www.geneticalliance.
org
E-mail: info@geneticalliance.org

**Graves' Disease and Thyroid
Foundation (GDATF)**
P.O. Box 2793
Rancho Santa Fe, CA 92067
Toll-Free: 877-643-3123
Fax: 877-643-3123
Website: www.gdatf.org
E-mail: info@gdatf.org

**Human Growth Foundation
(HGF)**
997 Glencove Ave.
Ste. 5
Glenhead, NY 11545
Toll-Free: 800-451-6434
Fax: 516-671-4055
Website: hgfound.org
E-mail: hgf1@hgfound.org

**Hypoglycemia Support
Foundation, Inc. (HSF)**
P.O. Box 451778
Sunrise, FL 33345
Website: hypoglycemia.org
E-mail: rruggiero@hypoglycemia.
org

Iron Disorders Institute (IDI)
P.O. Box 675
Taylors, SC 29687
Website: www.irondisorders.org
E-mail: info@irondisorders.org

**Juvenile Diabetes Research
Foundation (JDRF)**
26 Broadway
14th fl.
New York, NY 10004
Toll-Free: 800-533-CURE
(800-533-2873)
Phone: 212-785-9595
Website: www.jdrf.org
Email: info@jdrf.org

The MAGIC Foundation
4200 Cantera Dr.
Ste. 106
Warrenville, IL 60555
Toll-Free: 800-362-4423
Phone: 630-836-8200
Fax: 630-836-8181
Website: www.magicfoundation.
org
E-mail: contactus@
magicfoundation.org

**March of Dimes National
Office**
1275 Mamaroneck Ave.
White Plains, NY 10605
Toll-Free: 888-MODIMES
(888-663-4637)
Phone: 914-997-4488
Fax: 914-428-8203
Website: www.marchofdimes.org
E-mail: askus@marchofdimes.
com

**Muscular Dystrophy
Association (MDA)**
222 S. Riverside Pl.
Ste. 1500
Chicago, IL 60606
Toll-Free: 800-572-1717
Website: www.mdausa.org
E-mail: mda@mdausa.org

**National Adrenal Diseases
Foundation (NADF)**
505 Northern Blvd.
Great Neck, NY 11021
Phone: 516-487-4992
Website: www.nadf.us
E-mail: nadfsupport@nadf.us

**National Gaucher
Foundation (NGF)**
5410 Edson Ln.
Ste. 220
Rockville, MD 20852
Toll-Free: 800-504-3189
Phone: 301-593-1452
Website: www.gaucherdisease.
org

National MPS Society
P.O. Box 14686
Durham, NC 27709-4686
Toll-Free: 877-MPS-1001
(877-677-1001)
Phone: 919-806-0101
Website: mpssociety.org
E-mail: info@mpssociety.org

**National Organization for
Rare Disorders (NORD)**
55 Kenosia Ave.
Danbury, CT 06810
Toll-Free: 800-999-6673
Phone: 203-744-0100
Fax: 203-263-9938
Website: www.rarediseases.org
E-mail: orphan@rarediseases.org

**National Osteoporosis
Foundation (NOF)**
251 18th St. S.
Ste. 630
Arlington, VA 22202
Toll-Free: 800-231-4222
Phone: 202-223-2226
Fax: 202-223-2237
Website: www.nof.org
E-mail: info@nof.org

National Urea Cycle Disorders Foundation (NUCDF)
75 S. Grand Ave.
Pasadena, CA 91105
Toll-Free: 800-38-NUCDF
(800-386-8233)
Phone: 626-578-0833
Fax: 626-578-0823
Website: www.nucdf.org
E-mail: info@nucdf.org

The Nemours Foundation / KidsHealth®
Website: kidshealth.org
E-mail: info@KidsHealth.org

Organic Acidemia Association, Inc. (OAA)
9040 Duluth St.
Golden Valley, MN 55427
Phone: 763-559-1797
Toll-Free Fax: 866-539-4060
Website: www.oaanews.org
E-mail: mkstagni@gmail.com

The Oxalosis and Hyperoxaluria Foundation (OHF)
201 E. 19th St.
Ste. 12E
New York, NY 10003
Toll-Free: 800-OHF-8699
(800-643-8699)
Website: ohf.org
E-mail:info@ohf.org

Pediatric Endocrine Society (PES)
6728 Old McLean Village Dr.
McLean, VA 22101
Phone: 703-556-9222
Fax: 703-556-8729
Website: www.pedsendo.org/
contact/index.cfm
E-mail: info@pedsendo.org

Pituitary Network Association (PNA)
P.O. Box 1958
Thousand Oaks, CA 91358
Phone: 805-499-9973
Fax: 805-480-0633
Website: pituitary.org
E-mail: info@pituitary.org

The Pituitary Society
423 E. 23rd St.
Rm. 16048aW
New York, NY 10010
Phone: 212-951-7035
Fax: 212-951-7050
Website: pituitarysociety.org/
content/contact-us

Pituitary Tumor Network Association (PTNA)
16350 Ventura Blvd.
Encino, CA 91436
Toll-Free: 800-642-9211
Phone: 805-499-9973
Fax: 805-499-1523
Website: neurosurgery.mgh.
harvard.edu/PTNA/default.htm
E-mail: ptna@triax.com

Society for Inherited Metabolic Disorders (SIMD)
18265 Lower Midhill Dr.
West Linn, OR 97068
Phone: 503-636-9228
Fax: 503-210-1511
Website: www.simd.org/Contact. asp
E-mail: lublinkl@ohsu.edu

United Leukodystrophy Foundation (ULF)
224 N. Second St., Ste. 2
DeKalb, IL 60115
Toll-Free: 800-728-5483
Phone: 815-748-3211
Fax: 815-748-0844
Website: ulf.org
E-mail: bobbi@ulf.org

Wilson Disease Association (WDA)
5572 N. Diversey Blvd.
Milwaukee, WI. 53217
Toll-Free: 866-961-0533
Phone: 414-961-0533
Website: wilsonsdisease.ca/ about-wda/contact-us
E-mail: info@wilsonsdisease.org

Index

Index